James R. Lehman
Kristine Diaz • Henry Ng
Elizabeth M. Petty
Meena Thatikunta • Kristen Eckstrand
Editors

The Equal Curriculum

The Student and Educator Guide to LGBTQ Health

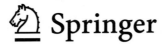

Springer

Editors
James R. Lehman
Department of Psychiatry
University of Wisconsin–Madison
Madison, WI
USA

Henry Ng
MetroHealth Medical Center
The MetroHealth System
Cleveland, OH
USA

Meena Thatikunta
University of Louisville
Louisville, KY
USA

Kristine Diaz
Medical Directorate
Defense Health Agency-National Capital
Bethesda, MD
USA

Elizabeth M. Petty
UW School of Medicine
and Public Health
University of Wisconsin–Madison
Madison, WI
USA

Kristen Eckstrand
Department of Psychiatry
University of Pittsburgh
Pittsburgh, PA
USA

ISBN 978-3-030-24024-0   ISBN 978-3-030-24025-7   (eBook)
https://doi.org/10.1007/978-3-030-24025-7

This Springer imprint is published by the registered company Springer Nature Switzerland AG
The registered company address is: Gewerbestrasse 11, 6330 Cham, Switzerland

Foreword

Ignorance as a Public Health Threat

There are an estimated 8.8 million LGBT-identifying individuals in the United States. (The use of *LGBT* versus *LGBTQ* – adding the Q for *queer* or *questioning* – in this text depends on the specific context of their use.) For our health care system to systematically ignore and at times abuse millions because of their identity and health needs is unjust. Through silence, ignorance, and hate we have created a second-class citizenry whose members suffer emotionally, physically, and mentally because they cannot obtain adequate health care.

According to the Center for American Progress, the LGBT population experiences significant health disparities that are attributable to a lack of quality health education and subsequent professional unpreparedness. A *JAMA* study found that 33.3% of medical schools dedicated zero hours of their curriculum to LGBT health. On average, medical schools dedicated just five hours to LGBT health education. The quality of this education varied widely; most is focused on HIV/AIDS, which represents just a sliver of the LGBTQ health spectrum. Ninety-two percent of medical students reported at least one clinical encounter with an (openly) LGBT-identifying patient. Despite predictable contact with LGBTQ patient(s), 46% of heterosexual medical students displayed explicit bias, defined as consciously expressed attitudes or beliefs, against gay men and lesbian women. Eighty-one percent of students displayed implicit bias, defined as subconscious attitudes or beliefs, against gay men and lesbian women. Furthermore, in a study of 1,335 medical students, a mere 12.9% passed a test assessing medical knowledge relevant to LGBT patient care. These statistics are alarming: the respondents represent the brightest students of our nation and future health care workforce. Medical education has so far left its students unprepared and the prognosis of the LGBTQ population's health rather grim.

Learning the Hard Way

Students often lament that the first time they realize how truly unprepared they were to care for LGBTQ patients is, not surprisingly, the first time they care for an LGBTQ patient. That experience came early for my own class in our second year of medical school.

Northeast Ohio Medical University (NEOMED), my alma mater, is unique in that it provides a lecture-based curriculum and experiential opportunities to interact with LGBTQ-identifying patients before clinical rotations. In one saturday session, we had four hours in which we organized into groups of four students and collectively interviewed a series of LGBTQ-identifying patients. There was no chief complaint, just a conversation about anything the students are curious. We were ill-prepared for such a situation. Why? First, there was no chief complaint, leaving us wondering what to explore. Second, the preparatory lecture meant to teach us about sexual orientation and gender identity lacked substantive recommendations. Therefore, we didn't know what was medically relevant to ask. Most students were flummoxed. Embarrassed. Quiet. I wouldn't have expected much more since we were so ill-equipped for the situation. We were unprepared to care for an LGBTQ-identifying patient, and we learned that lesson the hard way. (The curriculum has since been revised to better prepare students.)

Medical education is in clear need of reform.

A More Equal Curriculum

When reading a book, pay attention to what is said. Pay equal attention to what is not said.

This pearl from my high school English teacher, Ms. Connie Smith, has always stuck with me – it's part of being a critical learner, physician, and citizen. Analyze everything for what it is and for what it is not. That wisdom stayed with me even in medical school. Early on at Northeast Ohio Medical University (NEOMED), I realized that my education left me unprepared to care for an LGBTQ-identifying patient, leaving potential for patient discrimination, morbidity, and mortality. This is something that was, as Ms. Smith would say, "not said." An unspoken injustice.

"But, why? Why?" The question ran through my mind often. There was no good answer for me. I had grown up with a good number of friends and colleagues who identified with varying sexual orientations and gender identities. To me, it was normal and healthy to have this kind of diversity in one's life. It bothered me that medical education did not have the same expectations, especially for the LGBTQ population. So again, I asked, "Why is medical education ignoring this population?" No system is free of bias or injustice, even a system as altruistic as medical education. As it stood, the curriculum was *unequal* – teaching about some diseases and some populations and not others, simply because of ignorance. It was a medical education I could not swallow. I had discovered an inconvenient truth, and it gnawed at my conscience.

We needed a more equal curriculum.

I started looking at the data and ongoing efforts across the country. This "unequal curriculum" was actually a national problem. I saw a few people making effective headway at their own institutions, but no one effort was national in scope. The problem seemed unsolved to me. In order to gather more insight, I called leaders in LGBTQ health medical education. Essentially, I asked the same questions on every call, "What are we doing about this nationally? Why isn't there a widespread curriculum?" Most said, "Sure it makes sense to do something, but no one has. We are all at our own institutions fighting battles here to teach LGBTQ health effectively." It was true; I was doing the same at NEOMED. I consulted the incredible leaders I had met across the country on how to do this the right way at NEOMED.

Introducing Educational Reform

The first step was trying to understand the barriers to introducing LGBTQ health curriculum at any institution. I've briefly summarized those conversations into a list of considerations I had to make before I began the reform process:

- *New territory.* Only within the last decade have major organizations pushed for LGBTQ health competency as an educational standard. Additionally, we are still in the infancy stages of defining what those competencies even are.
- *Few qualified, institutional advocates.* Think of your own faculty. If they have never been taught LGBTQ health, it's unlikely that they will be able to teach it themselves. It is a cycle of ignorance and silence.
- *Insufficient comprehensive, introductory teaching resources.* Imagine again your faculty trying to teach themselves this topic so they can in turn teach you. Without introductory and summative learning resources, this is a challenging task indeed.
- *Limited curricular time.* Medical education is already saturated with material. How can we add on yet another competency area?
- *Stigma.* Medical education still has discriminatory practices related to race, gender, religion, age, socioeconomic class, sexual orientation, etc. Worse yet is medical education's "sweep under the rug" culture; medical education continues to be a risk-averse environment in which addressing controversial issues is not welcomed.

The educational leaders I consulted insisted that barriers should be acknowledged and addressed head on. We had a group of five truly passionate students who continued to push to reform and introduce new curriculum. In fact, the more we pushed, the more we received. The student feedback on the curriculum was incredible! We made a difference at NEOMED.

Still my wheels turned. The LGBTQ population is suffering because we haven't educated health care providers *en masse*. Widespread, national curriculum was *the answer*. Paul Farmer, MD writes in his book *Infections and*

Inequalities about a patient to whom he administers antibiotics for tuberculosis. Were it not for his volunteer service, she would have likely died of the disease. Those observing thought her recovery was a miracle. Dr. Farmer bluntly writes, "When she received⋯[the antibiotics], she soon began to respond – *almost as if she had a treatable infectious disease.*" Dr. Farmer means this is not rocket science; this is a problem with a concrete solution. Here the solution is a widely accessible, comprehensive educational resource⋯which is a tangible goal⋯Doable. Then, what were we waiting for? We know the LGBTQ population is suffering within the health care system. LGBTQ-identifying individuals need and deserve quality care from well-taught health professionals. It is our duty to help patients thrive despite injustice, invisibility, stigma, and abuse.

Committed Citizens

> *Never doubt that a small group of thoughtful, committed citizens can change the world; indeed it is the only thing that ever has.* – Margaret Mead

I was ready to start, and I called on leaders in LGBTQ health medical education to join me. Some thought I might be crazy. Most were intrigued. A few thought I might actually be on to something. It was those few who grew into our current team – initially over seventy some folks from all across the world. We all believed in this singular idea. That it *was* doable. Ah, how incredible.

Henry Ng, MD, MPH was one of my earliest teammates. I drove to his office in Cleveland to glean some insights and hopefully win him over. His career exemplifies such integrity, bravery, and justice; he is a real-life hero. Eventually, Dr. Ng joined as a Senior Editor. At that time, I still had no concrete strategy, just Dr. Ng's support. I kept going.

I had heard much about Kristen Eckstrand, PhD – now MD, PhD – a fellow medical student. She had her finger on what seemed like every LGBTQ health medical education initiative in the country. Kristen joined as a Senior Editor. I met her in-person a few months later at a conference. I offered to shake her hand; she refused and leaned in for a hug. It is one of the most meaningful hugs I have ever received.

Kristen connected me with Kristine Diaz, PsyD, and insisted that Kristine needed to be a Senior Editor as well. Kristine adds a much-needed perspective on the psychosocial aspects of LGBTQ health, as well as innovative approaches to medical education. She is a rare and powerful combination.

James R Lehman, MPH – now MD, MPH – a fellow medical student and advocate, came out of the blue. James found my online Prezi (a pitch for the project) and immediately understood the potential impact of *The Equal Curriculum*. Since then, James has been something of a secret weapon, making progress against all odds. He was an Associate Editor, then became the Managing Editor, then a Senior Editor.

James connected me with Elizabeth M. Petty, MD and insisted that she needed to be a Senior Editor. Dr. Petty knows medical education and knows medical students. It's an effective combination for leadership, especially on this project.

Next we gathered our most instrumental players, our many Associate Editors and primary authors. Many of them were students, which was by design. One of the barriers to LGBTQ health medical education reform is lack of faculty to teach such curricula. That faculty will come – they are today's students. *The Equal Curriculum* is an opportunity for students to lead and teach others. Moreover, *The Equal Curriculum* is a revolutionary effort to reform medical education nationally, and was humbly made possible by "thoughtful, committed citizens" who joined together.

Renewed Duty

I hope that you will read this text with a sense of duty. There are patients who need your help. Be knowledgeable. Be compassionate. Teach others, too. It is within your power to open minds and change systems. May you heal patients and our ailing health care system.

This text addresses only one barrier to LGBTQ health medical education reform: lack of comprehensive educational resources. It is a novel substrate but you are the catalyst. With your help we can galvanize LGBTQ medical education reform across the country, one institution at a time. Share this book with your peers, your faculty, and institutional leadership. Encourage them to read it and reform curricula. Together, we can come to expect an equal curriculum.

Thank you for all that you do.

Meena Thatikunta, MD
Founding Executive Director, Senior Editor

Acknowledgments

Thank you to the many physicians (Keisa Bennett, Mitchell Lunn, Greg Blaschke, Abbas Hyderi, William O'Byrne, Baligh Yehia, and others) who listened to my pitch for this project, offered advice, and connected me with other movers and shakers. Thank you to the entire *The Equal Curriculum* team for inspiring me with your sense of duty and daily work. I am so glad to have met all of you and to have created this work together. May you go on to do even greater things. Lastly, but certainly not the least, we are also grateful to NEOMED and its then College of Medicine Dean, Jeffrey Susman, MD, for their institutional and financial support of this project in its early stages.

References

Burke S, Dovidio J, Przedworski J et al. Do contact and empathy mitigate bias against gay and lesbian people among heterosexual first-year medical students? A report from the Medical Student CHANGE Study. Acad Med. 2015;90(5):645–51.

Center for American Progress. How to close the LGBT health disparities gap: 2009.

Lapinski J, Sexton P, Barker L. Acceptance of lesbian, gay, bisexual, and transgender patients, attitudes about their treatment, and related medical knowledge among osteopathic medical students. JAOA. 2014;114(10):788–96.

Obedin-Maliver J, Goldsmith E, Stewart L et al. Lesbian, gay, bisexual, and transgender related content in undergraduate medical education. JAMA. 2011;306(9).

Sanchez N, Rabatin J, Sanchez J, Hubbard S, Kalet A. Medical students' ability to care for lesbian, gay, bisexual, and transgendered patients. J Fam Med. 2006;38(1):22.

The Williams Institute. How many people are lesbian, gay, bisexual and transgender?: 2011.

Preface

It has been 50 years since the Stonewall Riots, regarded by many as the most significant event in LGBTQ history during the previous century. Since then, the story of LGBTQ Americans has had many twists and turns, from the HIV/AIDS epidemic, to policies like "Don't Ask, Don't Tell," and most recently, universal civil marriage equality. While organizations devoted to the health of sexual and gender minorities have labored for decades through these changes, it is only in the last several years that many government offices and mainstream health care organizations have openly acknowledged LGBTQ health as a priority.

Health care has had a parallel story. There is no shortage of examples of hostility and abuse – both interpersonal and structural – toward LGBTQ people. Though instances of severe abuse in the health system grow rarer, treatment and education practices have been sluggish in the realm of LGBTQ health. Where medicine previously grappled with tolerance, it now must evolve to provide treatment that is fully *inclusive* and *equitable*.

Many organizations, instructors, and trainees have started to develop and implement teaching about LGBTQ health. While these efforts have been excellent, they tend to address the needs of a specific time, place, and audience. The Association of American Medical Colleges has developed core competencies for LGBTQ medical education, giving educators – including us – a common concept of appropriate training outcomes.

In writing *The Equal Curriculum*, we have tried to create a comprehensive, high-quality resource that can serve as a foundation for LGBTQ health education across multiple disciplines. The subject matter has been organized for integration into preclinical work and clinical rotations, with careful attention to breadth and depth. Our hope is that a new generation of health professionals will have the tools that they need to deliver thoughtful and informed care to persons of all sexual orientations and gender identities.

Dozens of hardworking people contributed to this text. We would particularly like to thank our early phase copy-editor Kerry Bailey and our graphic designer Trent Waterman (https://www.trentwaterman.com), who were instrumental in making this work accessible and digestible for time-strapped trainees.

Washington, DC, USA   Kristine Diaz
Pittsburgh, PA, USA   Kristen Eckstrand
Madison, WI, USA   James R. Lehman
Berea, OH, USA   Henry Ng
Madison, WI, USA   Elizabeth M. Petty
Louisville, KY, USA   Meena Thatikunta

Contents

Contributors

Melanie Adams, MD Cape Breton Regional Hospital, Sydney, NS, Canada

Nadejda Bespalova, MD NYU Langone Medical Center, New York, NY, USA

Chris Beyrer, MD, MPH Johns Hopkins Bloomberg School of Public Health, Baltimore, MD, USA

Smitty Buckler-Amabilis Rad Care, Seattle, WA, USA

Stephan Carlson, MD Brookdale Hospital Medical Center, Brooklyn, NY, USA

Maria Carolina Casares, MD, MPH Georgia State University, Atlanta, GA, USA

Jeremy Connors, MD Rutgers New Jersey Medical School, Department of Medicine, Newark, NJ, USA

C. Nicholas Cuneo, MD Brigham and Women's Hospital, Boston Children's Hospital, Boston Medical Center, Boston, MA, USA

John A. Davis, PhD, MD University of California, San Francisco, San Francisco, CA, USA

Kristine Diaz, PsyD Defense Health Agency-National Capital, Bethesda, MD, USA

Jason D. Domogauer, MD, PhD Rutgers New Jersey Medical School, Newark, NJ, USA

Florence Doo, MD Mount Sinai West, New York, NY, USA

Kristen Eckstrand, MD, PhD Department of Psychiatry, University of Pittsburgh, Pittsburgh, PA, USA

Michele J. Eliason, PhD San Francisco State University, San Francisco, CA, USA

Christopher Estes, MD University of Miami, Miami, FL, USA

Lydia A. Fein, MD, MPH University of Miami Miller School of Medicine, Miami, FL, USA

Vanessa Ferrel, MD, MPH Montefiore Medical Center, The Bronx, NY, USA

Eric Fifield, MD University of Toronto, Toronto, ON, Canada

Ivy H. Gardner, MD Oregon Health & Science University, Portland, OR, USA

Jennifer L. Glick, PhD, MPH Johns Hopkins Bloomberg School of Public Health, Baltimore, MD, USA

Philipp Hannan, MD University of Arizona, Tucson, AZ, USA

Michael Haymer, MSW David Geffen School of Medicine, Los Angeles, CA, USA

Ronni Hayon, MD University of Wisconsin School of Medicine and Public Health, Madison, WI, USA

Michael C. Honigberg, MD, MPP Massachusetts General Hospital, Boston, MA, USA

Harvard Medical School, Boston, MA, USA

Elan L. Horesh, MD, MPH Mount Sinai Hospital, New York, NY, USA

Laura Irastorza, MD Arnold Palmer Children's Hospital, Orlando, FL, USA

Aron Janssen, MD New York University, New York, NY, USA

Laura Jennings, MHS, PA-C University of Pennsylvania Health System, Philadelphia, PA, USA

Kevin Johnson, MD Yale University, New Haven, CT, USA

Bobby Kelly, MD, MPH Geisel School of Medicine at Dartmouth, Hanover, NH, USA

Julie Kinzel, MEd, PA-C Drexel University Physician Assistant Program, Philadelphia, PA, USA

Brandyn D. Lau, MPH, CPH Johns Hopkins School of Medicine, Baltimore, MD, USA

Katherine Lawrence, MD, MPH New York University School of Medicine, New York, NY, USA

Rita S. Lee, MD University of Colorado School of Medicine, Aurora, CO, USA

James R. Lehman, MD, MPH Department of Psychiatry, University of Wisconsin–Madison, Madison, WI, USA

Kara Malone, MD The Ohio State University College of Medicine, Columbus, OH, USA

Ashley Rae Martinez, MD University of California, San Diego, La Jolla, CA, USA

W. Christopher Mathews, MD, MSPH Department of Medicine, University of California San Diego, La Jolla, CA, USA

Brent C. Monseur, MD, ScM Thomas Jefferson University Hospital, Philadelphia, PA, USA

Brian A. Nuyen, MD Stanford University School of Medicine, Stanford, CA, USA

Robert Obara, MB BCh BAO, MIPH Health Plus Medical Centre, Winnipeg, MB, USA

Poornima Oruganti, MD, MPH Loyola University Medical Center, Maywood, IL, USA

Shilpen Patel, MD University of Washington Department of Global Health, Redwood City, CA, USA

Andrew Petroll, MS, MD Medical College of Wisconsin, Wauwatosa, WI, USA

Marina Petsalis, BS University of Texas Health Science Center at Houston, Houston, TX, USA

Elizabeth M. Petty, MD UW School of Medicine and Public Health, University of Wisconsin–Madison, Madison, WI, USA

John R. Power, MD Vanderbilt University Medical Center, Nashville, TN, USA

Joyce Rosenfeld, MD Harrington Memorial Hospital, Southbridge, MA, USA

Christopher J. Salgado, MD University of Miami, Miami, FL, USA

Elizabeth A. Samuels, MD, MPH, MHS Alpert Medical School, Brown University, Providence, RI, USA

Ryan Smith, MD Yale New Haven Hospital, New Haven, CT, USA

Carl G. Streed Jr., MD, MPH Boston University School of Medicine, Center for Transgender Medicine & Surgery, Boston Medical Center, Boston, MA, USA

Erryn E. Tappy, MD, MPH George Washington University Hospital, Washington, DC, USA

Christopher Terndrup, MD Oregon Health & Science University, Portland, OR, USA

Meena Thatikunta, MD University of Louisville, Louisville, KY, USA

Marcus Tye, PhD College of Staten Island, City University of New York (CUNY), Staten Island, NY, USA

A. Ning Zhou, MD New York-Presbyterian, Columbia and Cornell, New York, NY, USA

Introduction

Education is the most powerful weapon, which you can use to change the world.

–Nelson Mandela

Over 100 years ago, Abraham Flexner released his 1910 report calling for necessary change in the foundations of medical education. Higher professional entry standards and rigorous, evidence-based curricula formed the core of the Flexner report, resulting in an academic system taking pride in research, evidence, analytic reasoning, and the overwhelming dissemination of this content to physicians in training. The resultant *structure and process education*, where students trained for a fixed time in a fixed curriculum, became the standard for medical education for nearly a century. Flexner's structure and process approach standardized medical education; however, it became clear that a fixed time curriculum led to variable outcomes. At the turn of the twenty-first century, accountability, responsibility, and quality of care for patients became equally recognized as core tenets of education. Indeed, it is not the structure and process of the education that needs to be fixed; rather it is the outcome of what defines a physician. This outcome should drive training, and it is this paradigm shift that leads us to *competency-based medical education* (CBME).

The Association of American Medical Colleges (AAMC) broadly defines CBME as an educational framework utilizing curricula and assessments that support the achievement of competence in clinical practice. *Competence* is "measurable or observable behaviors that combine knowledge, skills, and attitudes related to specific professional activities." Competencies are arranged across eight *competency domains*, each of which describes a particular theme in medicine. Competencies for graduating medical students are defined by Dr. Robert Englander's 2013 *Reference List of General Physician Competencies*. Finally, different competencies work in concert to describe *Entrustable Professional Activities* (EPAs), the essential professional tasks or responsibilities in which a trainee should demonstrate competence before being allowed to practice unsupervised. Figure I.1 demonstrates these key pieces of CBME. Importantly, this framework has already been adopted by the AAMC Advisory Committee on Sexual Orientation, Gender Identity, and Sex Development to describe the key features of competence in caring for individuals who are lesbian, gay, bisexual, and transgender (LGBT), gender nonconforming, and/or born with a difference of sex development (DSD).

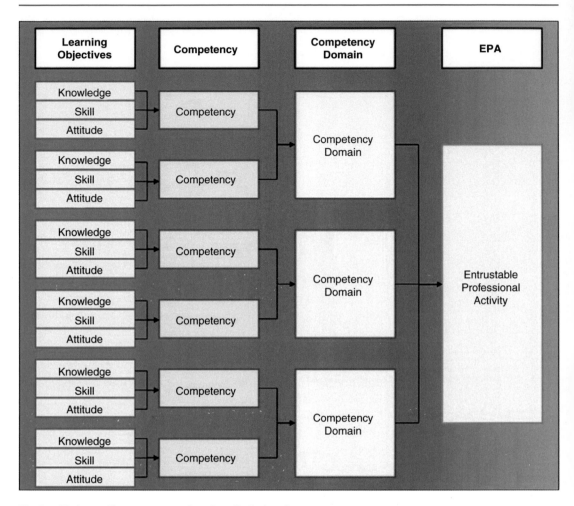

Fig. I.1 Understanding competency-based medical education

The Equal Curriculum strives to advance the work of the AAMC by creating the content necessary to support the acquisition of competence in caring for people who identify as LGBT. (In this section, we are using *LGBT* rather than *LGBTQ* or *sexual and gender minorities*, because that is the term used in the AAMC competencies.)

This textbook is designed to stimulate health educators' and students' interest and knowledge about issues that are relevant to the optimization of the health and well-being of LGBT individuals throughout their lifespan. Most importantly, it seeks to create an educational resource to address current unmet needs of learners across diverse health professional education and training programs. The textbook was developed with consideration of varying curriculum delivery formats – from problem-based learning to required didactic courses – that focus on LGBT health. We will highlight how this textbook may be integrated into the curriculum at your institution as well as strategies to evaluate the integration of LGBT health topics (Fig. I.2).

First, we will provide a brief overview of the chapters in the textbook. Chapters 1, 2, 3, and 4 cover general content that is highly relevant to all health professionals working with individuals who are LGBT; Chaps. 5, 6, 7,

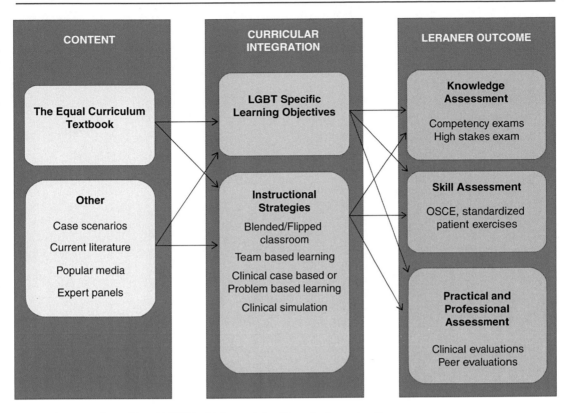

Fig. I.2 Framework to address LGBT health issues in health professions education

8, 9, 10, 11, and 12 focus on specific patient populations and areas of clinical delivery; and Chaps. 13 and 14 focus on special topics. Content was developed to highlight key points in each chapter to aid in the comprehension of each topic. Cases provided throughout the textbook will allow learners to apply the content to clinical scenarios in order to analyze how the application of relevant knowledge may impact health outcomes. Questions at the end of each chapter, which are usually written in National Board of Medical Examiners (NBME) style, assist in the application of content material.

The spirit of this textbook from its inception has been a learner-centered, collaborative approach to LGBT health education. While we acknowledge the limitations of time, necessary resources, and volume of material allotted for courses, we passionately advocate for the integration of LGBT health into all aspects of curricula. The *Equal Curriculum* serves as a guide to support curriculum development and integration. Without proper introduction, some LGBT topics may feel disingenuous (topic included just to meet an accreditation standard) or displaced in the context of the larger course. Knowledge-based activities (tables, charts, figures, guest speaker) in a traditional didactic, lecture format should be given in short time frames (<10 minute periods), alternating with active learning activities. Knowledge-based activities allow for cognitive dissonance in the learner about the differences in health issues and patient outcomes. Skill-based activities (clinical simulation, audio or video clips, case-based learning, clinical precepting of learners) allow learners to develop skills with clinical interviewing, assessment, medical decision-making, and treat-

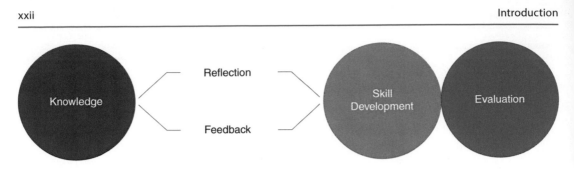

Fig. I.3 Maximizing intellectual capability, emotional intelligence, and clinical performance in learners

Fig. I.4 Evaluation of cultural competency in curriculum

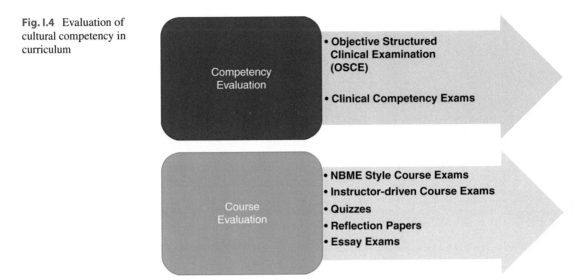

ment within a cultural framework. Ideally, the integration of LGBT health includes both educational and clinical training using multiple strategies to academically prepare health students to treat the LGBT patient population.

Next, we will identify several instructional strategies for potential in-classroom use in the integration of LGBT health topics into the curriculum. Instructional strategies will serve as an opportunity for the learner to use reflection and critical analysis of course material in the application of LGBT health topics to improve skill development in the treatment of the LGBT patient population (Fig. I.3). In-class instruction provides the learner with immediate feedback from the educator and peers in the comprehension and mastery of higher-order concepts. A process-oriented approach to the mastery of knowledge, attitude, and skill development of the learner may lead to a culturally competent health care provider.

Students early in their preclinical years may benefit from using the textbook as a primary resource in a course that addresses public health and/or behavioral science topics. Selected chapters may be used to present clinical scenarios in basic science courses for a full integration of LGBT health topics throughout the curriculum. Selected chapters may also be prerequisite reading as part of class preparation in a blended learning activity such as flipped classroom format (where content is presented outside of the classroom setting and then applied or discussed in a classroom or small group setting) or team-based learning activity (where peers work together to master the material

Table I.1 Competency-based approach to curriculum integration

Competency domain	Chapters
Interpersonal and communication skills	Chap. 3
Medical knowledge	Chaps. 5, 6, 7, 8, 9, 10, 11, 12
Patient care	Chaps. 3, 4
Practice-based learning and improvement	Chaps. 4, 14
Professionalism	Chap. 3
Systems-based practice	Chaps. 1, 2, 13
Personal and professional development	Chaps. 1, 2, 3
Interprofessional collaboration	Chap. 4

through consensus-based learning). Cases provided in the textbook can be used to facilitate in-class discussion, either in a large or small group format, as part of a problem-based or team-based learning activity. Students immersed in specialty-focused clinical rotations may benefit from reviewing chapters most relevant to those specialties in an easily accessible learning format. Student-driven selection of chapters may increase student engagement and learning of course material.

The impact and success of the integration of LGBT health education and instructional strategies is determined by the learners' outcomes on various evaluation measures. Patient simulation, standardized patients, clinical training, and high-risk exams provide quantitative data to evaluate the outcomes of a course or specific clinical training (Fig. I.4). Educators may want to assess learners' knowledge in LGBT health topics to obtain baseline data for quality improvement in curriculum integration. Using competency and course outcomes of LGBT health topics may be beneficial to promote and evaluate learning and retention of material.

The textbook has been divided according to competency domains for easy integration of this material into your curriculum. Table I.1 will assist in connecting course and lectures' objectives to competency domains for professional development to create a culturally competent health care provider.

References

Cox M, Irby DM, Cooke M, Irby DM, Sullivan W, Ludmerer KM. American medical education 100 years after the flexner report. New Engl J Med. 2006;355(13):1339–44.

Eckstrand KL, Leibowitz SL, Potter J, Dreger AD. Professional competencies to improve health care for people who are or may be LGBT, gender nonconforming, and/or born with DSD. In: Hollenbach A, Eckstrand KL, Dreger AD, eds. Implementing curricular and institutional climate changes to improve health care for individuals who are LGBT, gender nonconforming, or born with DSD: a resource for medical educators. Washington DC: Association of American Medical Colleges; 2014.

Englander R, Aschenbrener CA, Call SA, et al. Core entrustable professional activities for entering residency. MedEdPORTAL. 2014.

Englander R, Cameron T, Ballard AJ, Dodge J, Bull J, Aschenbrener CA. Toward a common taxonomy of competency domains for the health professions and competencies for physicians. Academic Medicine. 2013;88(8):1088–94.

Flexner A. Medical education in the United States and Canada: a report to the Carnegie Foundation for the Advancement of Teaching. New York: Carnegie Foundation for the Advancement of Teaching;1910.

Language and History of the LGBTQ Community

Michael Haymer, Smitty Buckler-Amabilis,
Katherine Lawrence, and Marcus Tye

Introduction

This chapter will provide guidance for the use of appropriate terms in the treatment of LGBTQ persons and will familiarize the reader with terminology used in subsequent chapters to ensure active engagement with the learning material. Simply mastering the terminology, however, is insufficient to ensure patient-centered care. The key concept of this chapter is that **patients should always feel comfortable and encouraged to use terminology representative of their authentic identities**. Examples in this chapter will highlight how terminology affects diverse LGBTQ people and their perception of health and health care and will show ways in which providers can best serve members of these populations. While the term *patient* and *provider* are used throughout this chapter, many concepts are applicable to workers and clients in non-health care fields.

The first listed author is the chapter's associate editor from The Equal Curriculum Project. The chapter authors are otherwise ordered according to their preference.

M. Haymer (✉)
David Geffen School of Medicine,
Los Angeles, CA, USA
e-mail: mhaymer@mednet.ucla.edu

S. Buckler-Amabilis
Rad Care, Seattle, WA, USA

K. Lawrence
New York University School of Medicine,
New York, NY, USA

M. Tye
College of Staten Island, City University
of New York (CUNY), Staten Island, NY, USA
e-mail: marcus.tye@csi.cuny.edu

Overview of LGBTQ Patient-Centered Terminology

Language and communication are foundational for high-quality patient-centered health care. The establishment of meaningful relationships with patients hinges on a health professional's ability to communicate in a culturally appropriate, nonjudgmental way. Health professionals must both understand and effectively use terminology that aligns with the perspectives and preferences of diverse patient populations. This is easier said than done. The terminology used to describe these populations is complex, and the terms used by their members represent the diversity that exists both between and within specific patient populations. This is even true of people encompassed by the familiar abbreviation *LGBT*.

LGBT is an umbrella term used to describe people who self-identify their sexual orientation as lesbian, gay, or bisexual and/or who self-identify their gender identity as transgender. The acronym became popular in the late twentieth century as a more inclusive way of describing the sexual and gender minorities. Although the terms *LGBT* and *LGBTQ* are used in this book, the reader must understand that sexual orientation and gender identity are different attributes, each existing along a continuum that may change over a person's lifespan. Health professionals should be encouraged to respect and celebrate patient's self-identifications and to use terms that patients and clients prefer.

Many iterations of the abbreviation *LGBT* have been developed to capture the range of identities one may encounter. The modern development of LGBT-related language reflects evolving sociopolitical attitudes and a broader understanding of diversity, equity, and inclusion. As individuals and communities begin to express themselves authentically, and as sociopolitical conversations regarding diversity evolve, the language used to describe distinct patient populations has become more complex. *LGBT* is frequently appended with additional letters to represent broader and more inclusive population. Letters may be subtracted when specific populations are being discussed (e.g., LG, LGB). The broadest contemporary term is ***sexual and gender minorities*** (SGM). Because *SGM* is a newer term, *LGBT* is often sloppily substituted – even in this book!

In care environments, it is ultimately the care provider's responsibility to ensure that each patient receives high-quality patient-centered care regardless of identity and/or expression. This does require the care provider to learn additional terms and their relevance to the patient, even amid competing demands on the professional's time and attention. However, the most basic understanding of LGBT-related vocabulary can go a long way toward building a therapeutic relationship. Health professionals who are not care providers, such as workers in public health departments or community health workers, likewise benefit from advancing their understanding of the language and identifiers used by populations they serve.

You may find yourself thinking, "What do all of these words *mean* in my life? Which of these terms applies to *me*? How do *I* self-identify?" This is a good thing! Curiosity and self-reflection encourage a critical understanding of the components of one's identity. Moreover, exploring self-identity is often the first step in understanding the identities of others. The terminology presented in this chapter is intended to help health professionals elicit valuable information about their patients' identities and life histories to improve overall health. Inherent in building these communication skills is the ability to better understand fundamental aspects of personhood, including development, relationships, family, mental health, sexual health, and other influential psychosocial factors.

Key Points
- Patients should always feel comfortable and encouraged to use terminology expressing their authentic identities. Health care professionals should respect their patients' identities and use the terms preferred by patients.
- The establishment of meaningful relationships with patients and their families often hinges on a provider's ability to communicate in a culturally appropriate and nonjudgmental manner, which requires knowledge of LGBT health terminology, history, and culture.
- Terminology used to describe various populations is complex; the terms used by their members represent the diversity that exists both between and within patient populations

External Resource 1.1
"Transgender Terms: Breaking Down Definitions and Do's and Don'ts": This video, produced by ABC News, reviews basic terminology relevant to LGBTQ persons. Total time: 2:34. http://bit.ly/TECe1ch01_01

Basic Terminology—Sex, Gender Identity, and Gender Expression

Many people assume that *sex* and *gender* are interchangeable. Indeed, they often appear on applications, intake forms, and other information-gathering tools as equivalent descriptors. In fact, *sex* and *gender* are not synonymous! The differences between these terms provide much of the framework for understanding how individuals realize their identities.

Sex, or **natal sex**, usually refers to the biological traits, including genotype (e.g., XX, XY, XXY) and sex phenotype (e.g., external genitalia, gonads, internal sex organs), with which a person was born. Natal sex can be projected in utero with the use of medical imaging. The aggregate of sex characteristics is typically used as the basis to determine the newborn's **gender assigned at birth,** usually using the gender-binary framework of male or female. **Gender** refers to the cultural, behavioral, and psychosocial characteristics that are typically associated with maleness and femaleness.

Although gender may align with sex, this is not always the case. Furthermore, people express their gender in many ways. **Gender expression**, the outward manifestation of one's self-identified gender, serves to communicate a person's identity in relation to a particular societal role. Gender expression includes personal characteristics, mannerisms, choice of clothing, hairstyle, and specific behaviors. One's **gender role**, which can be considered along a masculine-feminine spectrum in many cases, refers to the role a person plays or is expected to play within a specific sociocultural framework. The sex an individual is assigned at birth by others may not be congruent with that person's **gender identity**. Gender identity is a person's subjective inner sense of belonging to a particular gender. Gender identity usually solidifies by the age of six but may continue evolve across the lifespan. Here is just a sampling of gender identity terms: boy/man, girl/woman, transgender, transfeminine spectrum, transmasculine spectrum, gender-nonconforming, gender nonbinary.

Gender identity is often discussed in relation to people who identify as **transgender**—the T in LGBT. Another umbrella term, *transgender* captures the identities of a diverse group of people whose current gender identities or gender expressions do not align with the genders they were assigned at birth. This is also known as *gender incongruence* or *gender discordance*. For example, an individual might be born with male biological traits and assigned a male sex at birth but now self-identifies as a woman. ***Transsexual*** is an older term, popularized in the early 1900s, that refers to an individual who has undergone gender-affirming interventions such as hormone therapy or body-modifying surgery. This term is falling out of favor. Both the terms *transgender* and *transsexual* are sometimes shortened to *trans*.

Gender-nonconforming (or **gender-variant**) people do not conform to a specific society's established gender roles and/or gendered behaviors associated with the gender they were assigned at birth. Consider the example of a gender-nonconforming youth who was assigned female gender at birth yet prefers dressing in boys' clothes and wishes to play exclusively with boys at school. **Genderqueer** is a similar term that quite literally identifies people whose gender identity is queer—those who do not identify with the male/female binary. Some use the term **nonbinary**. This terminology has undergone significant evolution as pejorative terms are replaced by terminology that empowers individuals to accept and express gender identity in dynamic ways. Some terms intended to include all of the above are ***transgender/nonconforming*** (TGNC) and ***transgender/nonbinary*** (TGNB).

Nonbinary gender identities have been observed across different cultures for millennia. The reader is encouraged to pause and reflect on how gender identity and the categories the people identify with or use are a product of time, place, and culture. It can be challenging to think outside of available gender identity stereotypes in one's own culture and time. Chap. 14 discusses some gender identities found across the world.

For many, sex assigned at birth and gender identity are concordant. For example, a person born with female sex characteristics might be assigned a female sex at birth and now self-identifies as a woman. In this example, the person can be considered **cisgender**, meaning that her gender identity aligns with the sex assigned at birth. Simply speaking, *cisgender* refers to people who do not self-identify as transgender or gender-nonconforming. Those who use the term *cisgender* for themselves usually intend to convey sensitivity to transgender and gender-nonconforming people. When a health professional uses *cisgender* as a self-descriptor, it signals to others openness to diverse gender identities. However, the term *cisgender* is not without its complications. First, people who could be classified as *cisgender* may not choose that label for themselves. Secondly, some dislike the implication that anatomic sex and gender identity can be compared as binary variables that either match or mismatch, seeing it as reinforcing stereotypes of one or the other (recall the use of *genderqueer* to refer to nonbinary gender identities). For example, someone may prefer to philosophically challenge the concept of what womanhood is rather than ascribe some classically "unwomanly" traits to masculinity or gender nonconformity. As always, it is safe to use terms that a person uses for self-identification.

Key Points
- *Sex* and *gender* are not interchangeable words or concepts.
- Gender expression is the outward manifestation of one's self-identified gender and serves to communicate a person's identity in relation to a particular societal role.
- Gender identity is a person's subjective inner sense of self-belonging to a particular gender.
- *Transgender* is an umbrella term capturing the identities of a diverse group of people whose current gender identity or gender expression does not align with their gender assigned at birth.
- Gender nonconforming (or gender variant) people do not conform to a specific society's established gender roles and/or gendered behaviors associated with the gender assigned at birth.

Basic Terminology—Sexuality, Sexual Orientation, and Sexual Behavior

Whereas sex and gender pertain to a single person, **sexuality** is a relational term that broadly encompasses one's sexual self-expression, interest in others, and behaviors that one exhibits around others on the basis of sexual and emotional feelings. **Sexual orientation** is an individual's description of desire to feel sexual attraction and/or emotional connection to a particular identity or body type. Sexual orientation can be understood as consisting of three distinct dimensions: **sexual identity**, **sexual desire**, and **sexual behaviors** (Fig. 1.1).

These components, much like gender identity, are not always congruent in a person based on societal expectations. Indeed, aspects of one's identity and behaviors are influenced by many factors—culture and religion are notable examples—and combinations of these dimensions may not match and can shift over the lifespan. For instance, an individual may identify with a specific sexual orientation under the LGB umbrella yet engage in sexual behaviors that do not match this identity. **Of the three parts of sexual orientation, no inferences can be made about any one component from the others.**

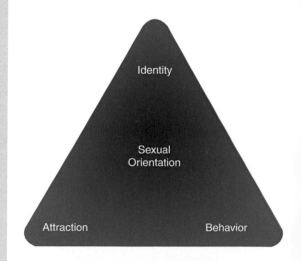

Fig. 1.1 Dimensions of sexual orientation

Heterosexual, when used as an adjective, describes opposite-sex or opposite-gender attraction. The term literally means "different sex." When used as a noun, *heterosexual* refers to someone who experiences romantic feelings, sexual attractions, and/or intimate interactions toward people of the opposite sex or gender. The term *straight* has also been used to describe this population. Of note, sexual orientation is a self-identity that is typically based on one's current gender identity and romantic attraction. Thus, an individual who identifies as male, whose sex assigned at birth was female, and who is attracted primarily to women may identify as straight.

Homosexual, literally meaning "same sex," is used as an adjective to describe same-sex or same-gender attraction. Despite sounding neutral, it has frequently referred to same-sex- or same-gender-loving people in a negative or dehumanizing way. The term introduces ambiguity because it is often applied as an identity label to a person or group based on their behaviors, not because of self-identified sexual orientation or sexual desires. In summary, in addition to having potentially negative connotation, *homosexual* is unclear as to what group of people it describes (a group classified by behaviors versus self-identification with the group), and, because of previous negative and dehumanizing connotations, should be used as an identifier for an individual or group cautiously.

Gay refers to a man who identifies his primary romantic feelings, sexual attractions, and/or intimate interactions toward people of the same sex or gender. *Lesbian* usually refers to a woman who identifies her primary romantic feelings, sexual attractions, and/or intimate interactions toward people of the same sex or gender, but some women prefer the term *gay*. *Bisexual* refers to people who are attracted to people of the opposite sex or gender in addition people of the same sex or gender. Bisexual people can also be thought of as having attractions to both men and women. These terms originated from a binary gender identity system and are popular labels for **sexual identity**. Other terms include

pansexual—individuals not limited in attraction with regard to biological sex, gender, or gender identity, and *asexual*—those without sexual feelings or associations.

It can be confusing that these terms are be used in multiple senses, sometimes referring to sexual desire and other times referring to self-identification. This text uses the term sexual orientation in the sense of sexual identity, essentially as synonyms. No person should assign a label of sexual identity to another. If someone reports a particular sexual attraction, that attraction is all that can be described about them. Ditto sexual behavior.

Queer may refer to individuals who identify with any, all, or none of the LGB part of the abbreviation, or who feel that their sexual orientation is not properly captured by any of these terms. Historically, *queer* has been used as a derogatory term to refer to a gay person. However, it is increasingly being reclaimed as an expression of self-empowerment by LGB-identifying individuals as well. It is important to note that *queer* is not necessarily an umbrella term for all those who do not identify as LGB; there are other identities on the LGBT spectrum. *Questioning*, distinct from *queer*, is a self-labeling term applied to individuals who may not have a fully developed sense of gender identity and/or sexual orientation. A questioning person may also be in the process of reconsidering and/or reconstructing their current gender identity and/or sexual orientation.

Henceforth, this text, when speaking broadly of sexual and gender minorities, will refer to LGBTQ people or to sexual and gender minorities (SGM). When referring to more specific populations, those populations will be named.

For certain epidemiologic and research purposes, a separate set of terms is used to classify people in terms of their sexual behavior rather than their identities:

- Men who have sex with men (MSM)
- Men who have sex with men and women (MSMW)

- Women who have sex with women (WSW)
- Women who have sex with men and women (WSMW)

These terms are crude and have sometimes been based on the natal sex of an individual and the natal sex of that individual's sexual partners (e.g., a transgender woman with a male partner could be classified as MSM). Unless stated otherwise, the MSM category fully includes all MSMW, and WSW fully includes all WSMW. **These terms should not generally be regarded as identity terms**. Journalists and researchers often mistakenly or simplistically translate *MSM* directly to "gay" or "gay and bisexual men" and neglect to conceptualize that the term also includes some straight-identifying natal males and transgender women. That is, they conflate sexual identity and behavior. The use of *MSM*, *MSMW*, *WSW*, and *WSMW* for classification purposes occurs most often in the context where health risks are related to one's own anatomy and the anatomy of one's sexual partners.

Key Points
- *Sexual orientation* is an individual's description of desire to feel sexual attraction and/or emotional connection to a particular identity or body type. It can be conceived as capturing three dimensions: sexual identity, sexual desire, and sexual behaviors.
- Sexual orientation is a self-identification selected by an individual, not another person.
- Some common sexual orientations are straight, gay, lesbian, and bisexual.
- The term *homosexual* is ambiguous and has negative or dehumanizing connotations based on historical use. It should be used cautiously.
- *Queer* may refer to individuals who identify with any, all, or none of the *LGB* abbreviation, or who feel their sex-

ual orientation is not properly captured by any of these terms.
- *Men who have sex with men (MSM), men who have sex with men and women (MSMW), women who have sex with women (WSW)*, and *women who have sex with men and women (WSMW)* are terms used for epidemiologic purposes, usually when an individual's sexual anatomy and the sexual anatomy of that person's partners are significant to health risks.

Language of Discrimination, Bias, and Shame

Sexual orientation and gender identity – and language – provide individuals with opportunities to describe, explore, and develop themselves. However, based on these identities, people may also become the objects of discriminatory cultural practices and beliefs. *Homophobia* refers to negative reactions to homosexuality, homosexual behavior, and people with same-gender attraction or behavior. *Transphobia* is the term for negative reactions towards transgender and/or gender-nonconforming people or behaviors. Homophobia and transphobia may even be directed at oneself. Anyone whose sexual orientation or gender identity is different from the major may experience the negative consequences of disempowerment, oppression, and underrepresentation because of that identity. Even people who do not identify with a minority sexual orientation or gender identity may face these kinds of discrimination based on others' perceptions that they belong to these groups.

Although discrimination is not always as overt as homophobia or transphobia, prevailing cultural norms that idealize **heterosexuality** imply that non-heterosexuals are anomalous. *Heterosexism* is a term used to describe a system of attitudes, bias, and discrimination favoring opposite-sex sexuality and relationships. Furthermore, it refers to stigmatization of same-sex sexuality and relationships. It is a result of **heteronormativity**, a prevalent cultural and sociopolitical ideology that normalizes heterosexuality and male/female and masculine/feminine binaries, consequently implying that other sex or gender constructs are deviant and inferior. Heteronormativity in professional fields, including health care, may result in **heterosexual bias**, or thoughts, beliefs, or behaviors that explicitly or implicitly show preference for heterosexuals and which may constitute discrimination against or neglect of those who do not identify with the predominant sexual and gender paradigms. It is sometimes called *heterocentric bias*. **Heterosexual bias includes the heterosexual assumption, the concept that everyone is—and should by default be treated as—heterosexual until there is an indication otherwise.** The heterosexual assumption is frequently used by health care providers when working with patients.

The process of discovering and developing one's sexual orientation and gender identity is complex, and an increasingly diverse terminology has flourished as people attempt to better capture their experiences. Many of these terms reflect the social and political evolution of communities that have struggled with self-identity or have been forcedly and discriminatorily identified as something they were not.

Key Points

- *Homophobia* refers to negative reactions to homosexuality, homosexual behavior, and people with same-gender attraction or behavior.
- *Transphobia* refers to negative reactions to persons identifying as transgender or gender nonconforming.
- Heterosexual bias and heterosexism may result from heteronormativity.

Identity Construction and Intersectionality

Identity and its significance to the health of individuals and populations can be examined through many different frameworks. Four frameworks are considered here: the life course theory, the social ecological model, the minority stress model, and intersectionality. These frameworks are useful for determining risk factors and protective factors for the health of individuals and populations. They are significant because health care has a relatively small impact on overall health status compared with the **social determinants of health**. These models are of importance for sociological, epidemiological and health outcomes researchers, as well as social workers, advocates, and public health officials.

Certain events in a person's life can be predictive of future events or health outcomes. The **life course theory** posits that people move through certain preprogrammed courses called *scripts*. Life course approaches tend to emphasize socioeconomic context and generational issues. In one common script, a person graduates from high school and pursues college. In another, a young adult gets married and starts a family, usually through reproduction with the spouse. Although LGBTQ people also have scripts, theirs tend to diverge from typical life course scripts, sometimes harmfully. For example, a person who faces high levels of familial rejection may be more likely to become homeless and not complete high school. **Coming out** is an example of a life script that is particular to LGBTQ people. *Coming out* is the process of disclosing one's sexual orientation and/or gender identity to others.

The **social ecological model** analyzes how multiple layers of influence, from the interpersonal and intrapersonal to physical environment and culture, affect health. Factors—both risk factors and protective factors—are classified as individual (intrapersonal), interpersonal, institutional, community, and societal. There are many variations of this model using different names and numbers of layers. This model is useful for those conceptualizing and implementing multi-level health interventions. For example, the risk for violence against transgender people may be understood within the social ecological framework. Individual risks include age, occupation, income, substance use, and history of abuse. Interpersonal risks include family dysfunction or familial rejection. Community risks include lack of access to safe housing, normalization of violence, and a weak or discriminatory local criminal justice system. Societal risks include transphobia and public policies, such as laws forcing transgender people to use identity-incongruent restrooms. The social ecological model is like the **biopsychosocial model**, which also incorporates biological (e.g., genetics, nutrition), psychological, and social factors, typically in the care of an individual. It is used most extensively in discussions of mental health. See Chap. 12 for a complete discussion.

The **minority stress model** considers how interpersonal prejudice, discrimination, and protective factors affect health outcomes. For example, constant bullying, harassment, and violence (distal stressors) in a gay man's high school years may result in hypervigilance (proximate stressor) and ultimately lead to depression or anxiety. This model is discussed extensively in Chap. 12.

Intersectionality is how social categorizations such as race, class, and gender overlap. Intersectionality is most often used to discuss how disadvantaged identities compound. That is, risk factors increase as the number of identities increases. For example, young black MSM were 55% of all incident HIV cases in 2010. In addition, people may place more importance or predominance on an identity or identities (e.g., a black transgender woman might identify most strongly as black or as a woman, with her transgender status not as important in her identity; a white gay transgender male immigrant might only identify as a gay man). Intersectionality may include—but is in no way limited to—categories of sexual orientation, gender identity, gender expression, race, ethnicity, socioeconomic status, age and generation, ability or disability, language, and immigration status.

Key Points
- Life course theory is a model for analyzing people's lives in structural, social, and cultural contexts in which people are described as following *scripts* as they move through life. Significant scripts may be disrupted in LGBTQ people. This theory posits that certain life events are predictive of future disease or health outcomes.
- The social ecological model analyzes how multiple layers of influence, from the interpersonal and intrapersonal to physical environment and culture, affect health. This model is useful in developing multi-level health interventions.
- The biopsychosocial model, typically used to consider factors that affect mental wellness and illness, classifies factors into three broad categories: biological, psychological, and social.
- The minority stress model considers how interpersonal prejudice, discrimination, and protective factors affect health outcomes.
- Intersectionality is how social categorizations such as race, class, and gender overlap.

History of LGBTQ Health Disparities and Discrimination in Health Care

An understanding of the history of LGBTQ culture and identity concepts is directly relevant to clinical practice for several reasons. First, it aids understanding the historical discrimination that has led to current health disparities. It also gives context to challenges in developing treatment relationships with LGBTQ patients, including older individuals who experienced the most pervasive discrimination firsthand. Indeed, younger patients may not have experienced the impact of medicine's **pathologization of homosexuality** as a psychiatric condition or the devastating effects of the HIV/AIDS epidemic. Prejudices have been embodied by medical professionals and maintained by the profession itself. Even now, health care providers' attitudes may be affected more by their biases or limited personal experiences than by their training, knowledge, or responsibility to the welfare of patients. For example, medical student and nursing students' knowledge and beliefs about LGBTQ parents seeking health care for their children are influenced in part by the students' racial community, political stance, religious beliefs, and the experience of having (or not having) friends who are LGBTQ.

Western culture has had a tradition of pathologizing variations in sexual behavior, sexual orientation, and gender identity based on moral beliefs and cultural attitudes. The perpetuation of prejudiced beliefs as science dates as far back as the 1700s. These pathologizing trends continued into the nineteenth century. The first physician to argue clearly for acceptance of sexual orientation and variations in gender expression was Magnus Hirschfeld, an early sexologist. During the "free love" movement of the late 1800s, Hirschfeld challenged the pervasive belief that same-sex sexual behavior was immoral. He founded what is considered the world's first LGBTQ rights organization, the Scientific Humanitarian Committee, in 1897 (In this section, the term *LGBTQ* is used as anachronism intentionally.).

With some notable exceptions, the medical establishment took many years to incorporate evidence and begin advocating strongly for equality. It took significant effort and time to overcome deeply entrenched cultural traditions and discriminatory laws. The first American LGBTQ rights organization, the Society for Human Rights, was founded in 1924. It was dismantled less than a year later. Despite its brief existence, the group's establishment sparked the modern LGBTQ rights movement, includ-

ing the work of Frank Kameny, the Mattachine Society, the Daughters of Bilitis into the 1960s. The LGBTQ rights movement reached a critical threshold with the 1969 police raid on the Stonewall Inn and subsequent riots in New York City. Deemed the **Stonewall Riots**, these events led to the formation of several advocacy organizations that sought the decriminalization of male same-sex sexual behaviors. Simultaneously, feminists, many of whom were lesbian and bisexual, began to demand greater protections for women and improved access to health care.

Propelled by these movements, psychologists and mental health professionals began to support depathologization of homosexuality. The American Psychiatric Association (APA) declassified homosexuality as a mental illness in 1973, though the category of ego-dystonic homosexuality remained in the *DSM-III* until the 1987 revision was released. Despite these strides, however, many individuals remained closeted because of the perceived stigma until the HIV/AIDS epidemic of the 1980s, when personal illness, loss of loved ones, and the fight for research funding led to significant changes in the visibility of lesbian, gay, and transgender people in the USA. Unfortunately, this increased visibility came at a cost. Fear of the "gay plague," compounded by existing homophobia in health care settings, led to increased interpersonal and institutional discrimination against gay men and unethical practices by health care providers. Patients seeking treatment were offered inappropriate care or refused care and often condemned for their sexual behaviors by their providers. Before the development of antiretroviral medications for HIV, the lack of effective treatment resulted in thousands of deaths. This tragedy inspired patients and their allies to demand equal treatment by the health care system, increased government support for research, and direct involvement in policy-making efforts.

Transgender rights and visibility have progressed more slowly until very recently. The aforementioned Magnus Hirschfeld, an early pioneer in transgender health, coined the term *transsexual* in 1923 to describe differences from transvestites. Harry Benjamin established *transsexual* as the term of choice in 1966 when he published his landmark book *The Transsexual Phenomenon*. It was the first major work to acknowledge a spectrum of gender variance, and it described the affirmative treatment path that Benjamin pioneered. One of Benjamin's patients, Christine Jorgenson, became the first American to undergo gender-affirming surgery in 1952. The surgery established her as an international sensation and brought publicity to gender nonconformity. Although significant advances in medical transitioning and gender-affirming procedures have been made since, transgender rights and social acceptance have lagged those afforded members of the lesbian, gay, and bisexual populations. From a medical perspective, transgender individuals face similar challenges in terms of having their identities pathologized. In fact, shortly after homosexuality was removed from the *Diagnostic and Statistical Manual of Mental Disorders, edition 2 (DSM-II)*, **gender identity disorder (GID)** was added to the *DSM-III* in 1980. GID is an older term that has been replaced in the *DSM-5* by **gender dysphoria** because of criticism that GID was stigmatizing. Some argue that the continued presence of gender dysphoria in *DSM-5* is also stigmatizing.

> **Key Points**
> - Historical prejudices in Western countries have often been mirrored by medical professionals and maintained by the profession of medicine itself.
> - Health care providers' attitudes may be affected more by their firsthand experiences and explicit and implicit biases than by their training or knowledge.
> - Two significant historical milestones for LGBTQ rights and health were the removal of homosexuality from the *DSM* and the HIV/AIDs epidemic.
> - The acceptance of transgender rights and visibility have moved more slowly but with tensions similar to those experienced by LGB people. Like homosexuality, **gender identity disorder** was removed from the *DSM* in part because it was stigmatizing.

Inclusive Language and the Patient-Provider Relationship

To establish a patient-provider relationship, it is vital for the provider to be sensitive to both personal and social contexts around sexuality. An understanding of historical and cultural influences regarding LGBTQ populations is helpful, particularly a patient's own cultural background, religious beliefs, age, and personal experiences. At the same time, one's lived experiences may vary according with geography, socioeconomic status, and demographic features such as culture, age, religion, and—of course—individuality. A preconceived idea of a patient's range of experiences is not necessarily accurate. This applies to the straight cisgender patient as well; *every* patient is unique. In many medical settings, time limitations reduce patient-provider interactions, and providers may find it difficult to become familiar with a patient's unique history.

Health professionals who self-identify as LGBTQ are not necessarily the best equipped to work with LGBTQ patients and clients. Simply identifying as LGBTQ does not qualify a provider to navigate an individual's problems simply because provider and patient may be more likely share some experiences. Similar backgrounds do not guarantee a strong patient-provider relationship. Some patients specifically prefer providers who are not like them in terms of identity.

On the other hand, many patients prefer congruence between their personal identity and that of their providers. The findings of patient satisfaction studies and health service research suggest that successful marketing to minority populations leads to improved enrollment in health clinics and education programs in urban settings. Specifically, investigators focused resources on establishments with considerable community influence, resulting in improved recruitment of low-income uninsured for routine health services. These establishments included barber shops and places of worship.

Encouraging patients to embrace their LGBTQ identity—by using inclusive language—is helpful during encounters. The use of inclusive language carries a risk of creating distance from a patient if he or she is uneducated about your use of gender-neutral, sexual orientation-inclusive, or sexual behavior-inclusive terminology. If a patient-provider relationship is hampered by inclusive language, it is likely an indication that the patient harbors homophobic or transphobic beliefs. However, a skilled interviewer is almost always able to use inclusive and non-presumptive language in a manner that maximizes feelings of safety, improves willingness to make sensitive disclosures, and minimizes the potential for personal offense.

The failure to use inclusive language can put a patient who has not disclosed an LGBTQ identity in a situation in which he or she may choose not to come out to the provider. For details on the components of creating a welcoming environment and conducting an inclusive history, refer to Chap. 3. **The failure to consider that a patient may be LGBTQ and assumptions about a patient's sexual orientation and gender identity constitute low-quality care.**

For elderly LGBTQ-identifying people, such disclosure may be new and uncomfortable, despite its relevance to their overall health. For the patient, failure to disclose information about one's identity may lead to poor health outcomes and diminished quality of life. The use of inclusive language and creation of a welcoming facility (e.g., magazines and LGBTQ-affirming symbols such as the rainbow flag and transgender flag) by health professionals may encourage disclosure without causing the individual to feel

forced to share such intimate information if not yet ready.

Above all, care providers must remember that although LGBTQ patients are unique, diverse individuals who benefit from a provider's vast knowledge, it is often the opportunity to be seen and respected as their authentic selves that they will consider the most valuable care.

Key Points

- Health professionals should be aware of cultural, historical, and social influences on LGBTQ people and how these may affect individuals.
- The failure to use inclusive language can put a patient who has not disclosed an LGBTQ identity in a situation in which he or she may not choose to come out to the provider.
- Patients should be encouraged to develop and express their identity within the health care setting. Providers can facilitate this with inclusive language. Failure to understand a patient's identity may result in a weak patient-provider relationship, poorer health outcomes, and diminished quality of life for the patient.
- Allowing patients to be seen and respected as their authentic selves is an important form of care.

Sources

A word about words. Gender spectrum. https://www.genderspectrum.org/images/stories/Resources/Family/A_Word_About_Words.pdf. Accessed 05 Apr 2017.

American Psychological Association Council of Representatives. Definition of terms: sex, gender identity, sexual orientation: the guidelines for psychological practice with lesbian, gay, and bisexual clients. American Psychological Association. http://www.apa.org/pi/lgbt/resources/guidelines.aspx. Accessed 16 June 2015.

Blanchard R. The concept of autogynephilia and the typology of male gender dysphoria. J Nerv Ment Dis. 1989;177:616–23. https://doi.org/10.1097/00005053-198910000-00004. ChPMID 2794988.

Chapman R, Watkins R, Zappia T, Nicol P, Shields L. Nursing and medical students' attitude, knowledge and beliefs regarding lesbian, gay, bisexual and transgender parents seeking health care for their children. J Clin Nurs. 2012;21(7–8):938–45. https://doi.org/10.1111/j.1365-2702.2011.03892.x.

Darby RJL. A surgical temptation: the demonization of the foreskin and the rise of circumcision in Britain. Chicago, IL: University of Chicago Press; 2005.

Definition of terms. Gender Equity Resource Center. http://ejce.berkeley.edu/geneq/resources/lgbtq-resources/definition-terms. Updated July 2013. Accessed 05 Apr 2017.

Gijs L, Carroll RA. Should transvestic fetishism be classified in DSM5? Recommendations from the WPATH consensus process for revision of the diagnosis of transvestic fetishism. Int J Transgend. 2011;12(4):189–97. https://doi.org/10.1080/15532739.2010.550766.

Knudson G, De Cuypere G, Bockting W. Second response of the World Professional Association for Transgender Health to the proposed revision of the diagnosis of transvestic disorder for DSM5. Int J Transgend. 2011;13:9–12. https://doi.org/10.1080/15532739.2011.606195.

Lautmann R. Categorization in concentration camps as a collective fate: a comparison of homosexuals, Jehovah's Witnesses, and political prisoners. J Homosex. 1990;19(1):67–88. https://doi.org/10.1300/J082v19n01_04.

Najmabadi A. Professing selves: transsexuality and same-sex desire in contemporary Iran. Durham, NC: Duke University Press; 2013.

Pharmacist conscience clauses: laws and information. National Conference of State Legislatures. May 2012. http://www.ncsl.org/research/health/pharmacist-conscience-clauses-laws-and-information.aspx. Accessed 26 Sept 2014.

Savin-Williams RC. The new gay teenager. Cambridge, MA: Harvard University Press; 2006.

Serano JM. The case against autogynephilia. Int J Transgend. 2010;12(3):176–87. http://www.informaworld.com/10.1080/15532739.2010.514223. Accessed 16 June 2015.

Sexual orientation and gender identity definitions. Human Rights Campaign. http://www.hrc.org/resources/entry/sexual-orientation-and-gender-identity-terminology-and-definitions. Accessed 16 June 2015.

Snyder JE. Trend analysis of medical publications about LGBT persons: 1950-2007. J Homosex. 2011;58(2):164–88. https://doi.org/10.1080/00918369.2011.540171.

Stulberg DB, Dude AM, Dahlquist I, Curlin FA. Obstetrician–gynecologists, religious institutions, and conflicts regarding patient care policies. Am J Obstet Gynecol. 2012;207(1):73.e1–5. https://doi.org/10.1016/j.ajog.2012.04.023.

Stulberg DB, Lawrence RE, Shattuck J, Curlin FA. Religious hospitals and primary care physicians: conflict over policies for patient care. J Gen Intern Med. 2010;25(7):725–30. https://doi.org/10.1007/s11606-010-1329-6.

Sweden to stop sex change sterilization. The Local: Sweden's News in English. January 11, 2013. http://www.thelocal.se/20130111/45550. Accessed 25 Sept 2014.

Tye MC. Sexuality and our diversity: integrating culture with the biopsychosocial. Washington, DC: Flat World Knowledge; 2013.

LGBTQIA Resource Center glossary. UC Davis LGBTQIA Resource Center. http://lgbtqia.ucdavis.edu/lgbt-education/lgbtqia-glossary. Accessed 16 June 2015.

von Krafft-Ebing R. Psychopathia sexualis. New York, NY: Medical Art Agency. 1906 translation, 1920 reprint. https://archive.org/stream/psychopathiasex01krafgoog#page/n590/mode/2up. Accessed 27 Sept 2014.

World Health Organization Human Reproduction Programme. Sexual and reproductive health. Geneva: World Health Organization. http://www.who.int/reproductivehealth/topics/sexual_health/sh_definitions/en/. Accessed 16 June 2015.

LGBTQ Health Disparities

2

Jeremy Connors, Maria Carolina Casares,
Michael C. Honigberg, and John A. Davis

The Historical Context of LGBTQ Populations in the US and Their Health Care

The history of societal and medical attitudes toward sexual orientation and gender identity have contributed to the current health and health care disparities experienced by LGBTQ people. Societal views of the early US immigrants from Europe regarding same-sex sexual activity were intolerant. Many early settlers immigrated for more freedom of religious practices, but these practices generally included intolerance and persecution of LGBTQ people. As mores and morals were written into law, the legal system became a tool of persecution. Societal pressure led most

---

The first listed author is the chapter's associate editor from The Equal Curriculum Project. The chapter authors are otherwise ordered according to their preference.

J. Connors (✉)
Rutgers New Jersey Medical School,
Department of Medicine, Newark, NJ, USA

M. C. Casares
Georgia State University, Atlanta, GA, USA
e-mail: casaresmc@comcast.net

M. C. Honigberg
Massachusetts General Hospital, Boston, MA, USA

Harvard Medical School, Boston, MA, USA

J. A. Davis
University of California, San Francisco,
San Francisco, CA, USA
e-mail: john.davis2@ucsf.edu

LGBTQ persons to conform or suffer dire consequences, including death.

The major shift of the common US view of sexual orientation and gender identity came with increasing interest of the medical/health care professions, often referred to as the **pathologization of homosexuality** and **pathologization of LGBTQ persons**. The major question was etiology: "What causes sexual orientation and gender identity?" Unfortunately, this question was usually motivated by the desire to prevent or alter LGBTQ identities.

Most of the research carried out from the late 1800s to early 1900s was conducted by mental health professionals, usually Europeans. Theories by Freud and others abounded regarding possible treatments. Medical literature in the US on topics of "sexual perversion" began in earnest near the end of the nineteenth century. Research of the time was focused on the "sexual invert," a concept that conflated sex, gender, and sexuality. Even in the 1930s and 1940s, when the concepts of male and female or masculine and feminine were increasingly viewed on a continuum rather than as a binary variable, underlying assumptions conflated the concepts. There was little concrete research on populations with **differences of sex development** or those with differences in gender expression or identity, though such populations were encountered in research. Medical culture in the US—most prominently psychiatrists and psychologists—advocated techniques aimed at treating patients with same-sex sexual attraction or gender-nonconforming behaviors. Treatments

© Springer Nature Switzerland AG 2020
J. R. Lehman et al. (eds.), *The Equal Curriculum*, https://doi.org/10.1007/978-3-030-24025-7_2

Table 2.1 Examples of historical anti-homosexual "therapies"

Psychotherapy
Depth psychotherapy (e.g., hypnosis)
Narcoanalysis/narcosynthesis
Reeducation
Changing the environment
Directive/nondirective therapies
Behavioral therapy
Conditioning (respondent, operant)
Desensitization
Chemotherapy and surgery
Chemical castration
Surgical castration

Modified from du Mas

of the time included psychotherapeutic, medical, and surgical approaches (Table 2.1). Most notable of these is **conversion therapy**, also known as *reparative therapy*, which claims to cure patients of homosexual desires and/or behaviors.

Around the mid-twentieth century, research on sexuality became less invested in labeling difference as pathology. Minority sexual orientation began to be viewed as variation rather than pathology. This marked a transition toward normalizing different sexual orientations. In 1973, the American Psychiatric Association removed homosexuality from the list of psychological disorders in the *Diagnostic and Statistical Manual of Mental Disorders (DSM)*. This change is discussed in Chaps. 1 and 12. Transgender and gender-nonconforming people have likewise—but more gradually—benefited from the move away from pathologizing variance. Even today, the presence of gender dysphoria in the *DSM-5* is debated as pathologizing and stigma-perpetuating. It has been suggested that sexual and gender minorities have benefited from a general shift toward biological rather than behavioral paradigms to explain the diversity of sexual identity and sexual behavior. Despite the overall trend away from pathologizing sexual orientation, some health care providers still maintain the belief that such people are aberrant, supporting efforts to prevent and treat their difference as disordered.

The HIV epidemic energized discourse around sexual orientation minorities. Many reactionaries called for reinstatement of previous laws and pas-

sage of new ones that would limit the liberties of gay men (or those "engaging in homosexual behavior"). HIV/AIDS brought about increased awareness to LGBTQ issues and discrimination. However, it has also at times overshadowed other LGBTQ issues, including some LGBTQ health issues.

The long history of LGBTQ persecution and the decades of civil rights advances led to a paradoxical situation in the late 1990s. On one hand, record-setting numbers of people attended gay pride parades and marches on Washington, and many prominent US figures came out as LGBTQ. On the other hand, notable anti-LGBTQ legislation and policies were put into place (the Defense of Marriage Act [DOMA], "Don't Ask, Don't Tell") as well as record rulings in courts against LGBTQ plaintiffs and passage of state referenda in the 1980s and '90s (*Bowers v Hardwick*, Colorado Initiative 2).

Now is an era of unprecedented advancement in LGBTQ rights, with the recent overturn of DOMA, the executive order requiring equal visitation rights for all in hospitals receiving federal funding, civil marriage equality, and the overturn of DOMA-like state laws. On the other hand, a major Institute of Medicine (IOM; now the National Academy of Medicine) report has drawn attention to the ongoing health and research disparities and inequities experienced by LGBT populations. Recognition and equality for LGBTQ persons continues to be subject to counteractive politicization and litigation at local, state, and federal levels.

Key Points
- Societal and medical attitudes toward sexual orientation and gender identity have contributed to LGBTQ health disparities that continue today.
- Inherited from the religious beliefs of European settlers, intolerance of same-sex sexual activity has been extensively enshrined in US laws.

- Medical interpretations of same-sex sexual orientation in the nineteenth century pathologized difference; by the mid–twentieth century, a shift toward understanding same-sex sexual orientation as a normal variant was under way.
- There still exists a minority of practitioners who believe that it is possible and desirable to change sexual orientation with reparative therapy.
- As the rights of LGBTQ advanced in the late twentieth century, counterreactions also intensified, culminating in such discriminatory policies as "Don't Ask, Don't Tell," and the Defense of Marriage Act.

Defining Disparity and Barriers to Care

By recent estimates, as much as 4% of the US population identifies as lesbian, gay, bisexual, or transgender. Though this is a sizable minority, even more people exhibit some aspect of same-sex sexual behavior in their lifetimes. LGBTQ persons are increasingly recognized as deserving of equal access to basic rights and opportunities, but the health status of LGBTQ populations is generally typically worse than that of the general population.

Defining Health and Health Care Disparities, Equity, and the Social Determinants of Health

The current legal definition of **health disparities**, as set forth in the Minority Health and Health Disparities Research and Education Act, can be interpreted as recognizing LGBTQ people as a health disparity population: "A population is a health disparity population if there is a significant disparity in the overall rate of disease incidence, prevalence, morbidity, mortality or survival rates in the population as compared to the health status of the general population." The term *health*

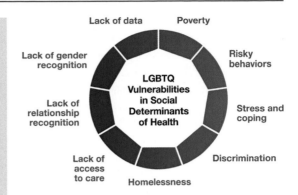

Fig. 2.1 LGBTQ vulnerabilities in social determinants of health

disparity is also applied to health determinants that differ among populations, such as income, smoking, and obesity. The term may also be applied to differences in access to health care and differences in quality of care received. The term *health inequity* is like *health disparities*: it refers to differences in health status or the health determinants in a population when the uneven distribution is unnecessary and unjust.

The **social determinants of health** are economic, environmental, and social conditions that determine health. Disparities in health and health care reflect ongoing injustices in our society or historical discriminatory practices, such as those related to race, ethnicity, socioeconomic status, and sexual or gender identity. Figure 2.1 illustrates social determinants of health that disproportionately affect LGBTQ populations. Health disparities of LGBTQ populations are largely effects of social disadvantage and systematic discrimination, including but not limited to legal discrimination in accessing health care, housing, and benefits; lack of laws protecting LGBTQ people; unavailability of social programs; and a shortage of culturally competent health care workers.

Health Disparities Affecting LGBTQ Populations

The health needs of LGBTQ populations can be examined with the use of models previously discussed in Chap. 1.

The IOM, in its 2011 report on LGBT health, applied the **life course framework** to discuss the health disparities faced by LGBT populations. The report highlights several health disparities across the life course that require special attention from health care professionals. Some of these disparities are listed in Table 2.2.

These disparities are linked to discrimination, social and sexual stigma, stereotyping, and denial of basic human and civil rights. Consequently, they are also health inequities. Discrimination is associated with higher incidences of suicide, substance use, and mental health problems. Additionally, stigma and stereotyping are related to abuse and violence, which decrease health-seeking behavior. These disparities can be assessed with the use of the **minority stress model**. LGBTQ persons may also belong to other minority communities and therefore face additional or exacerbated disparities, such as those based on minority race/ethnicity, limited English proficiency, disability, or low

Table 2.2 Some health and health care disparities of LGBT populations

LGBT people are less likely to have access to adequate and quality health care.
LGBT people are targets of stigma, discrimination, and violence because of their sexual and gender minority status.
LGBT youth and adults are at increased risk for depression, suicidal ideation, suicide attempts, and depression.
LGBT youth and adults are more likely to smoke, use alcohol, and abuse illicit substances than their heterosexual and cisgender counterparts.
LGBT youth are far more likely than their heterosexual peers to be homeless.
LGBT youth report increased levels of violence, victimization, and harassment.
HIV falls disproportionately affects men who have sex with men (MSM), particularly young black and Latino men.
Lesbians and bisexual women are less likely to use preventive health services than other women.
Lesbians and bisexual women are more likely to be overweight or obese than other women.
Lesbians and bisexual women have higher rates of breast cancer than other women.
Elderly LGBT people face the additional barriers of social isolation and lack of appropriate medical and social services.

socioeconomic status, as discussed previously in terms of **intersectionality**.

Barriers to Health Care

LGBTQ populations face many barriers to adequate health care. In *Unequal Treatment*, Smedley et al. redefined health care disparities and designated two categories of barriers: personal and structural.

Personal barriers are the attitudes, behaviors, and beliefs adopted by both care providers and patients in the health care system. These barriers encourage the persistence of stigma, biases, prejudices, stereotyping, and uncertainty in clinical communication and decision-making. Stigma can be differentiated into three types: enacted stigma (explicit behaviors that express stigma, such as verbal or physical abuse), felt stigma (perceived shame or embarrassment), and internalized stigma (acceptance of society's negative views). Whether deliberate or not, health care providers may harbor prejudices and be enactors of stigma and homophobia. For example, a 2018 study on physicians' attitudes toward homosexuality and HIV found that regarding discomfort treating patients, 7% reported discomfort treating homosexual patients, 22% transgender patients, and 13% HIV-positive patients. Regarding admission to medical school, 1% opposed admitting a homosexual applicant, 2% a transgender applicant, and 5% an HIV-positive applicant. However, compared with the results from previous surveys, these data suggest decreasing stigma associated with homosexuality and HIV.

In a 2010 study by Kitts, residents and attending physicians reported not engaging in best-practice techniques when working with LGBT adolescents. For instance, just 29% of surveyed physicians reported regularly discussing sexual orientation with adolescent patients, and 8.5% reported regularly discussing gender identity. Yet only 22% of surveyed physicians reported that they did not know of the link between LGBT status and depression in adolescents, and 33% reported that they did not know of the link between LGBT status and suicide in adolescents. In addition, 51% of surveyed physicians admitted that they did not believe that they had the skills to work effectively within the adolescent LGBT population. Little has been published recently to suggest that these numbers have changed significantly.

Patients may also be the source of personal barriers. Many LGBTQ people choose not to "**out**" themselves—including to their health care providers—as LGBTQ. Some are concerned about family and marital consequences; some simply do not self-identify as LGBTQ but engage in same-sex sexual activity; some are concerned that they will lose their jobs or face adverse employment consequences if their identity is disclosed; and some are worried about social stigma and moral condemnation. Some people may identify as LGBTQ but choose not to share particularly sensitive information about their sexual behavior with their health care providers, including information about fetishes, unprotected sex, number of sexual partners, and other high-risk behaviors such as recreational drug use.

Structural barriers are those that result from the stigma present in the health care system at the institutional level, such as limited or nonexistent employer coverage for LGBTQ individuals and same-sex couples and inadequate training for health care providers. Mayer discussed the barriers to accessing care and grouped them into four main issues:

1. The built environment may foster reluctance of some LGBTQ patients to disclose sexual or gender identity when seeking medical care (e.g., through inadequate privacy and other interferences with patient-provider communication, the absence of single-person or all-gender restrooms for transgender people).
2. Insufficient numbers of care providers are competent in dealing with LGBTQ issues as part of medical care.
3. Structural barriers impede access to health insurance and limit (or appear to limit) visitation and medical decision-making rights for LGBTQ persons and their families.
4. Culturally and anatomically appropriate prevention services are lacking.

Lack of health insurance has been a major barrier to quality health care for LGBTQ adults. It is partially a consequence of a lack of access to employer-sponsored insurance through civil marriage. However, the proportion of LGBTQ adults without insurance decreased with the implementation of the Patient Protection and Affordable Care Act. It is anticipated that the finding in favor of civil marriage equality by the Supreme Court in *Obergefell v. Hodges* will result in even greater access to insurance for LGBT adults and their children.

A recent Kaiser Family Foundation study found that rates of un-insurance decreased significantly among LGB adults (dropping from 19% in 2013 to 10% in 2016). In addition, Medicaid coverage increased from 7% to 15% during the same period, representing an estimated 511,000 more LGB individuals with Medicaid coverage. These coverage changes were similar to those seen in the heterosexual population.

Transition-related care for transgender people is usually not covered by insurance. For those with insurance, incongruence between recorded gender and certain sex-associated medical care can result in the denial of claims (e.g., a transgender man who has a uterus and cervix but is denied insurance payment for a Pap smear or cervical biopsy). In some cases, transgender people's claims have been denied merely based on being transgender—even for care that is related neither to transition nor to sexual/genitourinary anatomy.

The lack of robust research on LGBTQ people and culturally competent training for care providers are two of the biggest challenges to quality medical care for LGBTQ people. Optimal care of LGBTQ patients requires clinical and program environments that promote communication and that allow individuals to feel comfortable discussing their sexual orientation, behavior, attractions, and any conflicts they may be experiencing. Research suggests that an absence of cultural competency affects the quality of provider-patient communication. Poor communication is associated with poor health outcomes stemming from issues such as treatment nonadherence. Unfortunately, health care providers usually lack essential training on the needs of LGBTQ persons and populations and are ill equipped to provide these patients with culturally competent care in safe environments.

Key Points
- A population is a health disparity population if there is a significant disparity in the disease incidence, prevalence, morbidity, mortality, or survival rates in the population compared with the health status of the general population.
- Health disparities experienced by members of LGBTQ populations stem largely from the downstream effects of social disadvantage and systematic discrimination.
- Personal barriers and structural barriers to health care are reflections of the stigma experienced by many LGBTQ persons.
- Lack of health insurance has been a major barrier to quality health care for LGBTQ adults.

Eliminating LGBTQ Health Disparities

Correcting LGBTQ health inequities is crucial for a more just society. However, in the face of so much injustice, what should be expected from the expenditure of resources to address LGBTQ health disparities? Some of the benefits and anticipated obstacles are summarized in Table 2.3.

Strategies to reduce LGBTQ health disparities range in scope from the individual clinical encounter to federal legislation. Figure 2.2 provides a simplified schematic of potential areas of

Table 2.3 Societal benefits and barriers of addressing LGBT health disparities

Benefits
Decrease in transmission and progression of disease (e.g., HIV, other STIs)
Improved mental and physical wellbeing (supportive policies, culturally competent care)
Decreased health care costs (expansion of preventive and screening services)
Increased longevity (decreased preventable disease mortality rates)
Barriers
Shortage of data/data-collection methods for LGBT population
Lack of clarity regarding definitions (e.g., sexual orientation, gender identity)
Mistrust of health professions by LGBT populations
Limitations inherent in studying a population that is relatively small compared with the rest of the population

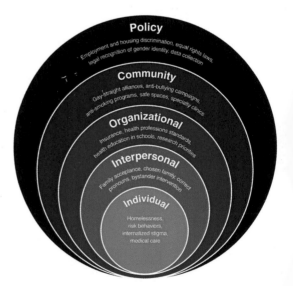

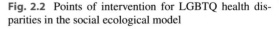

Fig. 2.2 Points of intervention for LGBTQ health disparities in the social ecological model

intervention. To meaningfully influence LGBTQ health disparities, clinicians, researchers, public health officials, and policymakers must employ a collaborative approach.

The Clinical Encounter

Clinicians must deliver patient-centered, evidence-based, individualized, and appropriate care to all LGBTQ patients. Broadly speaking, clinicians should be aware of the major health disparities affecting LGBTQ populations. Because of the relative paucity of rigorous data and evidence-based guidelines for many facets of LGBTQ health, clinical decision-making must be guided by a frank and detailed discussion of a patient's health-related behaviors and risk factors. Eliciting the patient's relevant history, particularly as it pertains to sexual health, must be done in a sensitive and nonjudgmental fashion. Ideally providers should employ shared decision-making in their counseling and treatment recommendations, asking about and incorporating patients' values and preferences.

LGBTQ health disparities are reviewed in general terms below. More extensive discussion of screening and risk reduction is provided in Chap. 5, except for a discussion of STIs, which can be found in Chaps. 8 and 11.

Mental Health

A 2008 systematic review reported increased suicidal ideation, self-harm, depression, and anxiety among LGB individuals compared with their heterosexual peers. Considering the especially pronounced and persistent stigma attached to transgender patients, the mental health disparities are greater for transgender people than LGB people.

Substance Use

LGBT populations appear to have higher prevalence of high-risk alcohol consumption, tobacco use, and illicit drug use. Lesbian and bisexual women appear to be at particularly elevated risk for alcohol abuse compared with heterosexual people. Recent US data show that sexual and gender minorities are at increased risk of tobacco use compared with heterosexuals, with bisexuals of both genders at highest risk. Among MSM, use of various illicit substances and heavy alcohol intake are associated with higher risk of unprotected oral and anal sex. This finding implies that taking a substance use history is an integral part of risk assessment and counseling for STIs and HIV prevention among MSM.

Cancer

Studies consistently show that women who have sex with women (WSW) are less likely than heterosexual women to undergo recommended Papanicolaou testing, even though WSW are still at risk for HPV infection and cervical cancer. A high proportion of WSW report prior sex with men, and female-female sexual contact also spreads HPV. Recent data suggest that female-to-male transgender individuals are less likely than non-transgender women, including WSW, to undergo Pap testing. Cervical cancer screening is indicated for any individual with a cervix, regardless of sexual orientation or gender identity. However, transgender men with a cervix appear to be much less likely than non-transgender women to be up to date on Pap tests.

HPV vaccination is likewise indicated regardless of natal sex, gender identity, or sexual orientation (and prevents genital warts and other cancers). WSW are also less likely than heterosexual women to undergo recommended mammography, even though WSW are more likely to have breast cancer risk factors (e.g., higher rates of obesity, alcohol use, and nulliparity). Among HIV-positive men who have sex with men (MSM), there is high prevalence of anal dysplasia, prompting recommendations for routine anal cytology (anal Paps) for this population.

Violence and Bullying

LGBTQ people, especially transgender people, are frequently the targets of violent victimization.

LGBTQ youth are at high risk for bullying, and not just physical bullying.

The findings of studies of intimate partner violence in LGBT populations are—partly for methodologic reasons—conflicting, with some indicating similar frequencies in same-sex and opposite-sex relationships and others finding increased frequencies in some LGBT groups. Screening recommendations and resources for intimate partner violence are largely targeted at straight women. Health care professionals may hold the implicit belief that men are not victims or that intimate partner violence is a specifically heterosexual phenomenon, and it has been suggested that people in in same-sex relationships are less likely to receive domestic violence screening. Community resources can be very limited for men and for transgender victims of intimate partner violence.

Seeking and Accessing Care

Accessibility

Lack of insurance and underinsurance are key barriers that prevent individuals from seeking care in the first place or from receiving certain treatments or services. Within the health care setting, barriers to care include practice environments that are perceived as unwelcoming or judgmental, and, related to this, a lack of cultural competence on the part of health care professionals.

Insurance Disparities

LGBT individuals and their children are less likely than heterosexual people and their children to have health insurance and therefore less likely to receive medical care. Men and women in same-sex relationships are less likely to have insurance and more likely to report unmet medical needs than are heterosexuals. Uninsured LGBT individuals and households stand to benefit from several provisions of federal health reform (e.g., [ACA] of 2010). However, the ACA did not require employers to offer equal insurance options to employees' same-sex partners in states where same-sex marriage had not been legalized.

Welcoming Health Care Settings

LGBTQ individuals often experience discrimination, whether explicit or implicit, active or passive. The same is true within health care. A nationally representative survey conducted in 2017 found that LGBTQ people experience discrimination in health care settings, deterring them from seeking care. The results revealed that for 8% of LGBQ and 29% of transgender respondents, a health care provider had refused to see them because of their actual or perceived sexual orientation or gender identity within the previous year.

A perception that a health care setting is unwelcoming to LGBTQ individuals may prevent patients from disclosing sexual orientation and relevant sexual health–related information and may deter them from seeking care at all. **Patients consciously and unconsciously assess health care settings for signs of safety and inclusiveness.** Front desk staff, for example, should use nonjudgmental language, avoid making assumptions about orientation or gender identity, and use patients' correct pronouns. Signs of inclusiveness (or lack thereof) are often nonverbal. Intake surveys should avoid assumptions about sexual orientation and gender identity and allow patients to indicate identification on the full continuum of identities and behaviors. Gender-neutral bathroom facilities should be available to promote the comfort of transgender patients. Informational materials (e.g., brochures) addressing LGBTQ health topics, as well as LGBTQ-oriented magazines in the waiting room, help foster a welcoming environment for LGBTQ patients.

External stakeholders have begun putting pressure on health organizations to provide welcoming and nondiscriminatory care to LGBTQ patients. In 2007, the Human Rights Campaign began publishing its Health Care Equality Index, which recognizes hospitals with policies of patient and employee nondiscrimination, equal visitation rights for same-sex partners, and staff training in LGBT care. In 2010, President Barack Obama ordered the Department of Health and Human Services to require equal visitation rights for same-sex partners in hospitals accepting money from Medicare and Medicaid. In 2011, the Department of Health and Human Services issued additional rules facilitating extension of health care proxy status to LGBTQ partners. Also in 2011, The Joint Commission introduced nondiscrimination and patient-centered communication standards, publishing an accompanying field guide to help organizations improve care for LGBT patients. These significant advances highlight the potential for payers, accreditation bodies, and watchdog organizations to improve health care for the LGBTQ community.

Cultural Competence of Care Providers

Sensitive and nonjudgmental treatment of LGBTQ individuals by clinicians is necessary both to establish a positive therapeutic relationship and to elicit clinically actionable information. Recent studies suggest that medical trainees receive inadequate exposure to LGBTQ health topics. A survey of allopathic and osteopathic medical schools in the United States and Canada in 2009 and 2010 found that medical students received a median five hours of instruction on LGBT health content across all of medical school. Seven percent of schools reported zero hours of LGBT-related instruction in the preclinical years, and one-third reported zero hours in the clinical years. Though nearly all schools reported that their students were instructed to ask patients, "Do you have sex with men, women, or both?" the coverage of other topics varied widely. Medical students received particularly little training in transgender health, potentially leaving them unequipped to understand distinctions among gender identity, gender expression, sexual orientation, attraction, and behavior that are important in caring for transgender individuals.

Data on LGBTQ content in other health professions training are lacking. The Association of American Medical Colleges has proposed a set of professional competencies related to LGBT health, spanning such areas as medical knowledge, patient care, communication skills, and professionalism.

The Accreditation Council for Graduate Medical Education (ACGME) defines sets of core competencies that residents are expected to meet by the end of training. Across specialties,

the ACGME states that residents are expected to demonstrate "sensitivity and responsiveness to a diverse patient population, including but not limited to diversity in gender…and sexual orientation." The limited available data suggest that this content is not being systematically taught. For example, in a survey of 229 US internal medicine residency programs, just 30% of programs reported having curricula on gay men's health, and only 11% reported curricula on lesbian health. In a survey of 427 LGBT physicians across specialties, most respondents reported zero curricular hours during residency devoted to gay (60%), lesbian (68%), bisexual (79%), or transgender (79%) health. Though many residents will experience some exposure to LGBTQ health through clinical care, a baseline amount of curricular content is essential, particularly for residents training in areas with smaller LGBTQ populations (e.g., rural settings), who may not knowingly care for a LGBTQ patient during residency.

A limited number of community health centers have established themselves as centers of excellence in LGBTQ care. The CDC has identified over a dozen such centers. Though these organizations provide outstanding patient-centered care, a significant proportion of the LGBTQ population lacks access to such centers. However, care providers everywhere may make use of excellent resources made available by these centers (see Appendices 1 and 2).

Public Policy and Cultural Climate

LGBTQ-Affirming Public Policies

Cultural views toward LGBTQ people remain highly variable across the United States, between urban and rural areas, and among different racial and ethnic groups. State-level laws and policies, such marriage recognition and employment protection for LGBTQ persons, have generally reflected the local climate. Evidence suggests that the cultural and policy climates both directly and indirectly affect the health of LGBTQ individuals.

Experiences of enacted, felt, and internalized stigma are believed to lead to worse

LGBTQ health outcomes. State bans on same-sex marriage, negative attitudes toward LGBTQ individuals, and lack of protection for sexual minorities against hate crimes and employment discrimination have been associated with higher rates of substance use and various psychiatric illnesses among LGBT people. The adoption of civil marriage equality in Massachusetts in 2003 led to reductions in medical and mental health visits among gay and bisexual men and to lower mental health spending. These studies suggest that public policies directly affect LGBTQ health, potentially through a reduction in stigma and the stress associated with minority status.

Myriad policies also indirectly affect the health of LGBTQ individuals—for instance, by influencing total and disposable income, one of the most significant social determinants of health. Access to employment—which depends, in part, on protection against employment discrimination based on sexual orientation and gender identity—provides many individuals with access to health insurance, in addition to subsistence. After the US Supreme Court's decision in *United States v. Windsor*, the Internal Revenue Service extended federal tax benefits to married same-sex couples. Before the Supreme Court's ruling in favor of civil marriage equality in *Obergefell v. Hodges,* these benefits only applied to those possessing a marriage certificate from a state with legalized civil marriage equality (not civil unions).

Schools are an obvious setting for interventions aimed at improving outcomes for LGBTQ youth. LGBTQ youth are at higher risk for depression, suicidal ideation, substance use, and homelessness than heterosexual youth. In a 2017 national survey of LGBT youth, more high school students self-identifying as lesbian, gay, or bisexual (LGB) reported having been bullied on school property (33%) and cyber-bullied (27%) in the past year, than their non-LGB peers (17% and 13%, respectively). More protective school climates are associated with fewer suicide attempts among LGBT youth. As of 2018, there are no federal laws addressing bullying based on sexual orientation or gender identity.

Research on LGBTQ Health and Disparities

Research priorities are an extension of public policy. More high-quality research on LGBTQ health and health disparities is critically needed. The ability of clinicians, public health officials, and policymakers to address LGBTQ health disparities is impaired by the paucity of high-quality research and, consequently, a limited understanding of disparities and their underlying causes. Between 1989 and 2011, only 0.1% of NIH-funded studies addressed LGBT health, excluding HIV/AIDS and sexual health. Of all LGBT-focused projects undertaken during this period, 86% were focused on gay and bisexual men, and just 7% addressed transgender health. Moreover, LGBTQ health research frequently relies on non-probability samples because of resource constraints, which may result in the overstatement of certain behaviors (e.g., alcohol use among individuals recruited at a nightclub), harming generalizability. Additionally, LGBTQ health research often lumps LGBTQ subpopulations together, limiting the possibility of elucidating these subpopulations' differences and unique disparities.

Consequently, the IOM report's first recommendation was for the NIH to formulate an LGBT research agenda. The IOM highlighted demographics, social influences in the lives of LGBT individuals, inequities, intervention research, and transgender health as key areas for future research. The integration of sexual orientation into the National Health Interview Survey started in 2013. It will facilitate further population-level LGB health research if data collection continues. As of 2018, it is unclear whether the National Health Interview Survey will incorporate gender identity, sexual attraction, or sexual behavior.

Key Points

- Strategies to eliminate LGBTQ health disparities range in scope from the individual clinical encounter to federal legislation.
- Significant areas of health disparity for LGBT populations include sexually transmitted infections, mental health, substance use, cancer, and violence.
- Significant points of intervention to improve LGBTQ experiences of health care include addressing insurance disparities, making health care settings more LGBTQ-friendly, and improving health professionals' cultural competence.
- High-quality research on LGBTQ health and health disparities is lacking; better research is critically needed.

Medicolegal Issues in Access and Treatment for LGBTQ Persons

Previous sections discussed the importance of civil marriage for insurance access, but there have been additional effects of civil marriage inequality. Same-sex couples without access to marriage have sometimes been prevented from seeing each other during hospital stays and could be prevented from providing consent for medical care or authorizing emergency treatment and health care decisions for non-biological children or children who are not jointly adopted. In fact, there are instances in which hospitals have denied these rights and privileges to family members even when legal relationships are in place.

Federal and state governments have imposed onerous requirements on transgender people who have transitioned and want updated legal and personal identification such as birth certificates and photo identification. For example, the US State Department and Social Security Administration had surgical requirements for change of gender on passports until 2010 and 2013, respectively. There are multiple reasons that a transgender person might not pursue surgery, including but not limited to satisfaction with nonsurgical transition modalities, medical contraindications to surgery, and inability to afford surgery. Many states still have requirements for surgeries or court orders to amend birth certificates.

For decades, every state in the country criminalized same-sex sexual conduct. As recently as 1986, the Supreme Court upheld the constitutionality of a Georgia law making it a crime to "perform or submit to any sexual act involving the sex organs of one person and the mouth or anus of another." Although the Georgia law could be applied to heterosexuals engaged in non-procreative sex, the law was applied to target homosexuals—a point that the Supreme Court emphasized in upholding the law against a constitutional challenge.

Discriminatory laws did not target only those who engaged in same-sex sexual conduct; they targeted people who merely *identified* as LGBTQ. For example, it was the policy of the US military for decades to discharge any member of the armed forces who merely *stated* that he or she was gay, lesbian, or bisexual. Known as "Don't Ask, Don't Tell," the law forced LGBTQ members of the armed forces to scrupulously hide traces of their sexual identity for fear of harassment and discharge.

The absence of legal protections for LGBTQ people leaves in place many of the existing societal barriers and discriminatory attitudes that set the community back. For example, although there are protections for women and racial minorities, there is still no federal law prohibiting employment discrimination on the basis of sexual orientation. In other words, an employer may fire someone for identifying as gay or transgender without fear of federal legal repercussions.

These laws and administrative policies are but a few examples, but they have each contributed materially to the stigmatization of LGBTQ people, affecting their ability and willingness to obtain medical care and undermining the ability of health care professionals to engage in frank discussions about the health of their LGBTQ patients.

But the landscape is changing. Recent polling suggests that the number of Americans who oppose same-sex marriage is decreasing and the number who approve of it is increasing—and that younger generations of Americans overwhelmingly support same-sex marriage. The Supreme Court reversed its prior decision upholding the constitutionality of Georgia's anti-sodomy law and struck down a Texas same-sex anti-sodomy law in 2003. The repeal of Don't Ask, Don't Tell has permitted LGBTQ service members to live openly without fear of legal repercussions or discharge. As mentioned several times before, the Supreme Court's 2015 decision in favor of nationwide civil marriage equality in *Obergefell v. Hodges* was monumental. Positive effects on the health and well-being of LGBTQ people are anticipated, but it is not expected that civil marriage equality will erase the effect of years of marginalization by the government.

Health policy barriers pose special obstacles for the transgender community in obtaining access to medically necessary health interventions. Discrimination based on gender identity has been commonplace in the insurance industry, and transgender-specific care is often excluded from private and public health insurance coverage. Fortunately, the trend is moving in the other direction. For example, the Department of Health and Human Services overturned its decades-old ban on Medicare coverage for gender-confirmation surgeries and other trans-sensitive care. State insurance commissioners have started issuing regulatory guidance indicating that transgender-specific exclusions violate state and federal nondiscrimination laws; as of this writing, 19 states and the District of Columbia prohibit transgender exclusion in health insurance.

The Affordable Care Act and the regulations promulgated under it prohibit insurance coverage plans sold on state and federal insurance exchanges from discriminating on the basis of gender identity. Additionally, insurers are prohibited from denying coverage or charging higher rates based on a patient's sexual orientation, and lifetime dollar limits on health insurance coverage are also prohibited—an important improvement for people with HIV/AIDS and other chronic diseases.

Key Points

- The LGBTQ community has faced decades of legal discrimination, including the criminalization of same-sex sexual activity, the prohibition of gay men and women from serving openly in the US military, and state constitutional amendments prohibiting state governments from recognizing same-sex marriages.

- Decades of legal discrimination have contributed to the stigmatization of the LGBTQ community. That stigma has kept LGBTQ people from being open and willing to seek out medical care.

- The history of legal discrimination against LGBTQ people and the closely related stigma of LGBTQ people is also the cause of their unwillingness to be open with their health care providers about sexual orientation and sexual activity.

- Conditions for the LGBTQ community are improving. The Patient Protection and Affordable Care Act authorized the integration of LGBTQ health data collection with national health data collection efforts. As civil marriage equality is enacted, employer-provided health insurance should provide health coverage for more LGBTQ people.

Case 2.1

A primary care provider meets a patient for the first time and takes the patient's basic health information. The patient is a man in his mid-30s. Although the primary care provider asks about the patient's sexual history, the man lies about his sexual history, failing to disclose that he has sex with men.

What are some of the reasons that the patient may have chosen to omit this information about his sexual history?

The patient might be concerned about negative consequences of disclosing his sexual history and possibly his sexual orientation (though we do not know whether he identifies as straight, gay, bisexual, or something else). In particular, he may be worried that disclosing his sexual history, even to his primary care provider, could result in his employer's learning about his sexual history, thereby jeopardizing his career because he perceives his employer as being unwelcoming to LGBTQ people. He may be concerned that his family will learn about his sexual history, leading to his being ostracized.

Case 2.2

Xander and Muhammad come to establish care in your clinic. Xander is a 37-year-old man and Muhammad is a 41-year old who recently retired from the Marines. Until this past year, Xander had been working two part-time jobs, neither of which offered health insurance. Though he and Muhammad have been together for 10 years. Muhammad hid their relationship until after he retired from the Marines. After they married, three months ago,

Xander was able to obtain health insurance through Muhammad's plan for retired members of the military.

What are the legal issues influencing Xander's and Muhmammad's access to health?

For Xander, the ability to obtain health insurance was affected by (1) the lack of domestic partnership benefits offered by the military, (2) the military's "Don't Ask, Don't Tell," policy, which forced Muhammad to hide their relationship, (3) the illegality of same-sex marriage in the state. With the change in DADT, Muhammad is now able to openly acknowledge their relationship. With the couple's new right to marry, Xander is able to obtain health insurance as a spousal benefit.

For Muhammad, years of hiding their relationship may have caused significant stress and resultant mental health issues. Even though Muhammad had health insurance, he may not have received optimal health care because he may not have disclosed certain behaviors under the DADT policy.

Conclusion

This chapter explored many of the health care disparities encountered by LGBTQ populations today and discussed examples and suggestions for how to make health care more inclusive of—and equitable for—LGBTQ populations. A listing of some of these ideas is provided in Table 2.4. Many of these suggestions come from published guidelines, policy papers, and best practices offered by leading and official groups. American society, including professional and health care organizations, is becoming more aware of health disparities and the need to

Table 2.4 How health professionals can improve LGBT health and reduce disparities

Ensure a welcoming climate
Understand specific needs and health disparities of LGBT patients
Inquire about and be supportive of sexual orientation and gender identity
Use gender-neutral language when discussing personal relationships
Create a welcoming environment to facilitate engagement in health care
Ensure that all forms are inclusive of sexual orientation, gender identity, and family unit identification
Incorporate LGBT topics into health professions education curricula and continuing education
Ensure that health care professions students can engage in an adequate number and variety of LGBT patient encounters
Develop/implement programs within LGBT communities to address health needs
Foster a supportive environment for LGBT youth
Effectively advocate for policy change at the state and federal levels
Assist government and community agencies in becoming LGBT-inclusive in all programs and in creating new LGBT-specific programs

address them for reasons including health promotion, cost, and social justice. All of society would benefit from a commitment to eliminating health disparities for LGBTQ persons and other historically marginalized groups.

Boards-Style Application Questions

Question 1. A 17-year-old boy comes to the physician for a precollege examination. He has no history of serious illness. He does not smoke cigarettes or drink alcohol, and he is not currently sexually active. Examination shows no abnormalities. During a discussion of sexual activity, the patient acknowledges that he is attracted to another boy and that they have been seeing each other. Though he has been abstinent, he reports that he is thinking about becoming sexually active with the other boy but wants to prevent sexually transmitted diseases. He asks for advice

about safer sex. What is the most appropriate recommendation for this patient?

A. Abstinence from sex
B. Avoiding oral sex
C. Avoiding symptomatic partners
D. Correct and consistent condom use
E. Limiting his number of sexual partners

Question 2. During a routine examination, a 25-year-old natal female who self-identifies as male and has not decided to alter his body hormonally or surgically expresses concern about his risk for ovarian cancer because his mother died of the disease. The patient uses he/him/his pronouns. Which of the following terms best describes this individual's gender identity?

A. Gay.
B. Lesbian.
C. Transgender.
D. Transvestite.
E. Transitioning.

What is the most appropriate course of action?

A. Annual CT scan of the patient's abdomen
B. Obtaining a more detailed family history of cancer
C. Reassuring him that ovarian cancer is not hereditary
D. Recommending a diet high in beta-carotene
E. Recommending prophylactic oophorectomy

Question 3. A previously healthy 32-year-old man comes to the emergency department with a three-day history of pain and swelling of his right knee. Two weeks ago he injured the knee during a touch football game and had more swelling and bruising than expected. One week ago, he underwent extraction of a molar for severe dental caries. He is sexually active with one male partner and uses condoms consistently. HIV antibody testing was negative three months ago. Temperature is 39.2 ° C (102.6 ° F), pulse is 106 beats/min, and blood pressure is 125/65 mm Hg. Examination of the right knee reveals warmth, erythema, and joint effusion. Flexion and extension of the right knee are severely limited. An x-ray of the knee confirms the joint effusion. What is the most appropriate next step in diagnosis?

A. Arthrocentesis
B. Arthroscopic exploration of the knee
C. Bone scan
D. MRI of the knee
E. Venous doppler ultrasonography

Question 4. An otherwise healthy 27-year-old man is referred to a cardiologist after three episodes of severe palpitations, dull chest discomfort, and a choking sensation. The episodes occur suddenly and are associated with nausea, faintness, trembling, sweating, and tingling of the extremities; he feels as if he is dying. Within a few hours of each episode, physical examination and laboratory tests show no abnormalities. The patient, who works as a welder, is afraid that the episodes will significantly affect his work. During a recent lunchtime conversation, he was outed by a co-worker who saw him leaving a popular gay bar. Since then he has felt that his co-workers have been treating him differently and keeping him at arm's length. He does not use drugs or alcohol and has no history of interpersonal problems. What is the most likely diagnosis?

A. Delusional disorder
B. Generalized anxiety disorder
C. Hypochondriasis (Illness Anxiety Disorder)
D. Panic attack
E. Somatization disorder

What is a good course of action?

A. Advising him to change jobs and to keep his sexual orientation a secret
B. Listening to and acknowledging his concerns, discussing possible courses of action, and continuing to monitor the patient

C. Prescribing anti-anxiety medication and telling him to ignore the situation
D. Referring him for psychiatric evaluation
E. Telling him he is just having panic attacks and that they will eventually pass without treatment

Question 5. Which of the following statements are true?

A. LGBTQ youth are less likely than heterosexual youth to be homeless.
B. The burden of HIV falls disproportionately on white men who have sex with men.
C. Elderly LGBTQ people no longer face social isolation and lack of appropriate services.
D. Lesbians and bisexual women have higher rates of breast cancer than heterosexual women.
E. LGBTQ youth and adults are at increased risk for suicidal ideation and attempts, as well as depression.
F. Lesbians and bisexual women are more likely than their heterosexual counterparts to use preventive health services.
G. In general, LGBTQ people are more likely than heterosexual ones to have access to adequate and quality health care
H. LGBTQ youth and adults have lower rates of smoking, alcohol consumption, and substance use than heterosexual ones.
I. LGBTQ people are frequently the targets of stigma, discrimination, and violence because of their sexual and gender minority status.

Boards-Style Application Questions Answer Key

Question 1. (D) A common mistake would be to identify this youth as "high risk" based on his sexual identification. The course of action for this youth is the same as for any youth with no risk factors and abstinent, which is correct and consistent condom use. All remaining answers are not supported in evidence-based STI prevention guidelines. Option A has been demonstrated ineffective, and the remaining options do not effectively mitigate risk.

Question 2. Part 1. (C). Part 2. (B) Transgender is an umbrella term for people whose gender identity and/or gender expression differs from what is typically associated with the sex they were assigned at birth. In part 1, options A, B, and C are sexual orientations, and E is not an identity term. While many transgender people are prescribed hormones, and some undergo surgery, not all transgender people can or will take those steps, and a transgender identity is not dependent upon physical appearance or medical procedures. As for part 2, the correct course of action for this patient is obtaining a more detailed family history of cancer to assess his level of risk for developing ovarian cancer. A, D, and E would not at this early juncture be indicated for a natal female with a family history of ovarian cancer without better history. Option C is a false statement.

Question 3. (A) This patient has the same exact risk factors as his heterosexual counterparts. Therefore, an arthrocentesis should be performed to establish a diagnosis and treatment. The patient's history of trauma two weeks prior with unusually pain and swelling suggest hemarthrosis. However, a significant tooth extraction without the mention of prescribed antibiotic prophylaxis raises the possibility of an infectious process requiring prompt treatment of a joint infection to preserve the joint integrity. Items B, C, D, and E do little to nothing to establish the presence or identity of an infectious agent. This question is a reminder to proceed rationally with differential diagnosis and not fixate on minority characteristics.

Question 4. Part 1. (D). Part 2. (B) Somewhere between 30 and 60 percent of LGBT people deal with anxiety and depression at some point in their lives. That rate is higher than that of their straight or gender-conforming counterparts. This otherwise healthy individual is clearly suffering from panic attacks brought on by being outed at work. The description of his physical and mental experience is classic for a panic attack. There are no data to support delusional thinking (A), longstanding anxiety symptoms across multiple domains of life (B), excessive attention to the possibility of illness (C), or a broader pattern of fixation on somatic symptoms (E). As for part 2, his perceived fear of being discriminated against by his co-workers and possibly losing his job are real in context with his profession as a welder. Panic attacks can be very frightening and can cause the individual severe anxiety. The sense of losing control, having a heart attack, or even dying are highly distressing. Initial treatment should focus on listening to and acknowledging specific concerns, discussing choices, and continuing to monitor his progress. Reassurance and encouraging insight may be sufficient for this patient given recent onset. Options A, C, and E are dismissive of the underlying cause, and due to his clear history, he does not need referral to a specialist level of care yet (option D).

Question 5. F, T, T, F, F, F, F, T, F

Sources

Accreditation Council for Graduate Medical Education. ACGME Program Requirements for Graduate Medical Education in Internal Medicine. September 16, 2008. http://www.acgme.org/portals/0/pfassets/programrequirements/140_internal_medicine_2016.pdf. Accessed 05 Apr 2017.

Adler NE, Rehkopf DH. US disparities in health: descriptions, causes, and mechanisms. Annu Rev Public Health. 2008;29:35–252.

Advancing Effective Communication, Cultural Competence, and Patient- and Family-Centered Care for the Lesbian, Gay, Bisexual, and Transgender (LGBT) Community: A Field Guide. Oak Brook, IL: The Joint Commission; 2011. http://www.joint-commission.org/assets/1/18/LGBTFieldGuide.pdf. Accessed 05 Apr 2017.

American Association of Medical Colleges. Implementing curricular and institutional climate changes to improve health care for individuals who are LGBT, gender nonconforming, or born with DSD: a resource for medical educators. Washington DC: AAMC; 2014. https://www.aamc.org/download/414172/data/lgbt.pdf. Accessed 05 Apr 2017.

Ard KL, Makadon HJ. Addressing intimate partner violence in lesbian, gay, bisexual, and transgender patients. J Gen Intern Med. 2011;26:930–3.

Awosogba T, Betancourt JR, Conyers FG, Estapé ES, Francois F, Gard SJ, et al. Prioritizing health disparities in medical education to improve care. Ann N Y Acad Sci. 2013;1287:17–30.

Bayer R. Homosexuality and American psychiatry: the politics of diagnosis. Princeton, NJ: Princeton University Press; 1987.

Bockting WO, Miner MH, Swinburne Romine RE, Hamilton A, Coleman E. Stigma, mental health, and resilience in an online sample of the US transgender population. Am J Public Health. 2013;103:943–51.

Braveman P. Health disparities and health equity: concepts and measurement. Annu Rev Public Health. 2006;27:167–94.

Buchmueller T, Carpenter CS. Disparities in health insurance coverage, access, and outcomes for individuals in same-sex versus different-sex relationships, 2000-2007. Am J Public Health. 2010;100:489–95.

Case P, Austin SB, Hunter DJ, Manson JE, Malspeis S, Willett WC, et al. Sexual orientation, health risk factors, and physical functioning in the Nurses' Health Study II. J Womens Health (Larchmt). 2004;13:1033–47.

Center for American Progress. Discrimination prevents LGBTQ people from accessing health care. https://www.americanprogress.org/issues/lgbt/news/2018/01/18/445130/discrimination-prevents-lgbtq-people-accessing-health-care/. Posted January 18, 2018. Accessed 02 Dec 2018.

Centers for Disease Control and Prevention. Lesbian, gay, bisexual and transgender health: health services. Atlanta, GA: CDC; 2018. Published March 26, 2018. Accessed 02 Dec 2018. http://www.cdc.gov/lgbthealth/health-services.htm.

Centers for Disease Control and Prevention. Lesbian, gay, bisexual and transgender health: health services. Atlanta, GA: CDC; 2014. Published March 24, 2014. Accessed 12 Sept 2014. http://www.cdc.gov/lgbthealth/health-services.htm.

Coulter RW, Kenst KS, Bowen DJ, Scout. Research funded by the National Institutes of Health on the health of lesbian, gay, bisexual, and transgender populations. Am J Public Health. 2014;104:e105–12.

Diamant AL, Schuster MA, McGuigan K, Lever J. Lesbians' sexual history with men: implications for taking a sexual history. Arch Intern Med. 1999;159:2730–6.

du Mas FM. Gay is not good. Nashville, TN: Thomas Nelson Publishers; 1979.

Eliason MJ, Dibble SL, Robertson PA. Lesbian, gay, bisexual, and transgender (LGBT) physicians' experiences in the workplace. J Homosex. 2011;58:1355–71.

Fallin A, Goodin A, Lee YO, Bennett K. Smoking characteristics among lesbian, gay, and bisexual adults. Prev Med. 2015;74:123–30.

Gaisa M, Sigel K, Hand J, Goldstone S. High rates of anal dysplasia in HIV-infected men who have sex with men, women, and heterosexual men. AIDS. 2014;28:215–22.

Gates GJ. Demographics and LGBT health. J Health Soc Behavior. 2013;54:72–4.

Gates GJ. In U.S., LGBT more likely than non-LGBT to be uninsured. Washington, DC: Gallup; 2014. http://www.gallup.com/poll/175445/lgbt-likely-non-lgbt-uninsured.aspx. Accessed 05 Apr 2017.

Goldie SJ, Kuntz KM, Weinstein MC, Freedberg KA, Welton ML, Palefsky JM. The clinical effectiveness and cost-effectiveness of screening for anal squamous intraepithelial lesions in homosexual and bisexual HIV-positive men. JAMA. 1999;281:1822–9.

Grant JM, Koskovich G, Somjen Frazer M, Bjerk S, Services and Advocacy for GLBT Elders. Outing age 2010: public policy issues affecting lesbian, gay, bisexual, and transgender elders. Washington, DC: National Gay and Lesbian Task Force Policy Institute; 2010. http://www.thetaskforce.org/downloads/reports/reports/outingage_final.pdf. Accessed 05 Apr 2017.

Gruskin EP, Hart S, Gordon N, Ackerson L. Patterns of cigarette smoking and alcohol use among lesbians and bisexual women enrolled in a large health maintenance organization. Am J Public Health. 2001;91:976–9.

Hatzenbuehler ML, Birkett M, Van Wagenen A, Meyer IH. Protective school climates and reduced risk for suicide ideation in sexual minority youths. Am J Public Health. 2014;104:279–86.

Hatzenbuehler ML, Keyes KM, Hasin DS. State-level policies and psychiatric morbidity in lesbian, gay, and bisexual populations. Am J Public Health. 2009;99:2275–81.

Hatzenbuehler ML, Keyes KM. Inclusive anti-bullying policies and reduced risk of suicide attempts in lesbian and gay youth. J Adolesc Health. 2013;53:S21–6.

Hatzenbuehler ML, McLaughlin KA, Keyes KM, Hasin DS. The impact of institutional discrimination on psychiatric disorders in lesbian, gay, and bisexual populations: a prospective study. Am J Public Health. 2010;100:452–9.

Hatzenbuehler ML, O'Cleirigh C, Grasso C, Mayer K, Safren S, Bradford J. Effect of same-sex marriage laws on health care use and expenditures in sexual minority men: a quasi-natural experiment. Am J Public Health. 2012;102:285–91.

Healthy People 2020. Lesbian, gay, bisexual, and transgender health. Washington, DC: US Department of Health and Human Services; 2013. Accessed 17 Mar 2014. http://www.healthypeople.gov/2020/topicsobjectives2020/overview.aspx?topicid=25.

Healthy People 2020. Lesbian, gay, bisexual, and transgender. Washington, DC: Office of Disease Prevention and Health Promotion. Accessed 06 Mar 2014. http://www.healthypeople.gov/2020/topicsobjectives2020/overview.aspx?topicid=25#one.

Improving Data Collection for the LGBT Community. Washington, DC: US Department of Health and Human Services. http://minorityhealth.hhs.gov/assets/pdf/checked/1/Fact_Sheet_LGBT.pdf. Accessed 14 Sept 2014.

Institute of Medicine. The health of lesbian, gay, bisexual, and transgender people: building a Foundation for Better Understanding. Washington, DC: National Academies Press; 2011.

Kaiser Family Foundation. The affordable care act and insurance coverage changes by sexual orientation. https://www.kff.org/disparities-policy/issue-brief/the-affordable-care-act-and-insurance-coverage-changes-by-sexual-orientation/. Published May 2018. Accessed 20 Nov 2018.

Kann L, McManus T, Harris WA, et al. Youth risk behavior surveillance - United States, 2017. MMWR Surveill Summ. 2018;67:1–114. https://www.cdc.gov/mmwr/volumes/67/ss/pdfs/ss6708a1-h.pdf. Accessed 02 Dec 2018.

Kerker BD, Mostashari F, Thorpe L. Health care access and utilization among women who have sex with women: sexual behavior and identity. J Urban Health. 2006;83:970–9.

King M, Semlyen J, Tai SS, Killaspy H, Osborn D, Popelyuk D, et al. A systematic review of mental disorder, suicide, and deliberate self harm in lesbian, gay and bisexual people. BMC Psychiatr. 2008;8:70.

Kinsey A, Pomeroy W, Martin C. Sexual behavior in the human male. Philadelphia, PA: W.B. Saunders; 1948.

Kitts RL. Barriers to optimal care between physicians and lesbian, gay, bisexual, transgender, and questioning adolescent patients. J Homosex. 2010;57(6):730–47. https://doi.org/10.1080/00918369.2010.485872.

Koblin BA, Chesney MA, Husnik M, Bozeman S, Celum CL, et al. High-risk behaviors among men who have sex with men in 6 US cities: baseline data from the EXPLORE Study. Am J Public Health. 2003;93:926–32.

Kosciw JG, Diaz A, Greytak EA. 2007 National School Climate Survey: The Experiences of Lesbian, Gay, Bisexual and Transgender Youth in Our Nation's Schools. New York, NY: The Gay, Lesbian and Straight Education Network; 2008.

Makadon HJ, Mayer KH, Potter J, Goldhammer H. Fenway guide to lesbian, gay, bisexual, and transgender health. Philadelphia, PA: American College of Physicians; 2008.

Marlin R, Kadakia A, Ethridge B, Mathews WC. Physician attitudes toward homosexuality and HIV: the PATHH-III survey. LGBT Health. 2018;5(7):431–42.

Marrazzo JM, Koutsky LA, Kiviat NB, Kuypers JM, Stine K. Papanicolaou test screening and prevalence of genital human papillomavirus among women who have sex with women. Am J Public Health. 2001;91:947–52.

Mayer KH, Bradford JB, Makadon HJ, Stall R, Goldhammer H, Landers S. Sexual and gender minority health: what we know and what needs to be done. Am J Public Health. 2008;98:989–95.

McGarry KA, Clarke JG, Landau C, Cyr MG. Caring for vulnerable populations: curricula in U.S. internal medicine residencies. J Homosex. 2008;54:225–32.

Minority Health and Health Disparities Research and Education Act United States Public Law 106-525. 2000; 2498 Web site. http://www.gpo.gov/fdsys/pkg/PLAW-106publ525/pdf/PLAW-106publ525.pdf. Accessed 10 Mar 2014.

Mollon L. The forgotten minorities: health disparities of the lesbian, gay, bisexual, and transgendered communities. J Health Care Poor Underserved. 2012;23(1):1–6.

Obedin-Maliver J, Goldsmith ES, Stewart L, White W, Tran E, Brenman S, et al. Lesbian, gay, bisexual, and transgender-related content in undergraduate medical education. JAMA. 2011;306:971–7.

Olden K, White SL. Health-related disparities: influence of environmental factors. Med Clin North Am. 2005;89(4):721–38.

Pachankis JE, Hatzenbuehler ML, Starks TJ. The influence of structural stigma and rejection sensitivity on young sexual minority men's daily tobacco and alcohol use. Soc Sci Med. 2014;103:67–75.

Peitzmeier SM, Khullar K, Reisner SL, Potter J. Pap test use is lower among female-to-male patients than nontransgender women. Am J Prev Med. 2014;47:808–12.

Peterkin A, Risdon C. Caring for lesbian and gay people: a clinical guide. Toronto, ON: University of Toronto Press; 2003.

Presidential Memorandum – Hospital Visitation. The White House Office of the Press Secretary. http://www.whitehouse.gov/the-press-office/presidential-memorandum-hospital-visitation. Published April 15, 2010. Accessed 12 Sept 2014.

Report on the United States of America: Universal Periodic Review on Sexual Rights, Ninth Round. National Council for LGBT Health and Sexuality Information and Education Council of the United States; 2010. Accessed 22 Mar 2014. http://lib.ohchr.org/HRBodies/UPR/Documents/session9/US/JS10_JointSubmission10.pdf.

Smedley B, Stith A, Nelson A. Introduction and literature review. In: Unequal treatment: confronting racial and ethnic disparities in health care. Washington, DC: The National Academies Press; 2003. p. 29–77.

Smith DM. Mathews. Physicians' attitudes toward homosexuality and HIV: survey of a California Medical Society- revisited (PATHH-II). J Homosex. 2007;52(3–4):1–9.

Smyczek P, Singh AE, Romanowski B. Anal intraepithelial neoplasia: review and recommendations for screening and management. Int J STD AIDS. 2013;24:843–51.

Social determinants of health: the solid facts. 2nd ed. Geneva, Switzerland: World Health Organiation; 2003. Accessed 06 Mar 2014. http://www.euro.who.int/__data/assets/pdf_file/0005/98438/e81384.pdf

Soto-Salgado M, Colón-López V, Perez C, et al. Same-sex behavior and its relationship with sexual and health-related practices among a population-based sample of women in Puerto Rico: implications for cancer prevention and control. Int J Sex Health. 2016;28(4):296–305.

Terry J. An American obsession: science, medicine, and homosexuality in modern society. Chicago, IL: University of Chicago Press; 1999.

The Health care Equality Index Core Four Leader Criteria. Washington, DC: Human Rights Campaign.

http://www.hrc.org/hei/the-core-four-leader-criteria. Accessed 12 Sept 2014.

The Health of Lesbian, Gay, Bisexual, and Transgender People: Building a Foundation for Better Understanding. Washington, DC: Institute of Medicine; 2011.

Tripp CA. The Homosexual Matrix. 2nd ed. New York, NY: New American Library; 1987.

When Health Care Isn't Caring: Lambda Legal's Survey of Discrimination Against LGBT People and People with HIV. New York, NY: Lambda Legal; 2010. http:// www.lambdalegal.org/sites/default/files/publications/ downloads/whcic-report_when-health-care-isnt-caring.pdf. Accessed 05 Apr 2017.

The LGBTQ-Friendly Clinic Encounter

3

Brian A. Nuyen, Maria Carolina Casares,
Eric Fifield, Kevin Johnson, and Rita S. Lee

The Impact of Patient-Centered LGBTQ-Friendly Clinical Encounter on Patient Care and Health Outcomes

Core Issues for LGBTQ Patients

An important first step in becoming an LGBTQ-friendly clinician is learning about the historical conflicts between medical culture and the LGBTQ community that cause or perpetuate distrust of the healthcare system.

The first listed author is the chapter's associate editor from The Equal Curriculum Project. The chapter authors are otherwise ordered according to their preference.

B. A. Nuyen (✉)
Stanford University School of Medicine,
Stanford, CA, USA

M. C. Casares
Georgia State University, Atlanta, GA, USA
e-mail: casaresmc@comcast.net

E. Fifield
University of Toronto, Toronto, ON, Canada

K. Johnson
Yale University, New Haven, CT, USA
e-mail: kevin@transbodies.com

R. S. Lee
University of Colorado School of Medicine,
Aurora, CO, USA
e-mail: rita.lee@ucdenver.edu

Historical Pathologization of Homosexuality

Before 1973, the *Diagnostic and Statistical Manual of Mental Disorders* (*DSM*) defined same-sex attraction as a mental illness, justifying the existence of **conversion therapy** groups to "cure" individuals with same-sex attractions and/or behaviors. These therapies involved electroshock therapy, genital mutilation, and even castration. The stigmatization of same-sex attraction as a mental illness has led to lasting distrust between some LGB persons and healthcare professionals.

Clinicians as Gatekeepers of Health Care Access

Transgender and gender-nonconforming individuals may find themselves in conflict with clinicians because of the clinician's implied role of gatekeeper to such services as hormone therapy and gender-affirming surgeries.

Past and Present Discrimination by Health Care Providers

Care providers (not limited to physicians) have an unfortunate track record of discrimination against their LGBTQ patients, leading to these patients' delaying care or avoiding it altogether. At times these discriminatory attitudes have led to outright refusal of care. In the National Transgender Discrimination Survey (2015), nearly one in five respondents reported being refused health care because they identified as transgender or gender-nonconforming.

© Springer Nature Switzerland AG 2020
J. R. Lehman et al. (eds.), *The Equal Curriculum*, https://doi.org/10.1007/978-3-030-24025-7_3

Institutional Discrimination

Policies such as the United States military's "Don't Ask, Don't Tell" (DADT) policy, which barred LGB service members from publicly disclosing their sexual orientation or partners, led to a 30.8% underutilization of health care and a 14.9% circumvention of military health care for various LGBTQ health issues. The diagnosis and treatment of STIs and mental health care were negatively influenced by this policy.

Lack of Knowledgeable Health Care Providers

When deciding whether to disclose sexual orientation or gender identity to a healthcare provider, many LGBTQ people consider the provider's knowledge of LGBTQ health issues (or their perception thereof). A lack of knowledge of LGBTQ health care may lead providers to unknowingly ignore health concerns, leading in turn to poor health outcomes.

LGBTQ-Friendly Clinicians and Health Promotion

Because of the above historical context, many patients still fear that providers will refuse to treat them, will humiliate them, or will fail to understand them. In a 2011 survey of more than 1000 LGBT Coloradans, 55% feared that their healthcare providers would treat them differently if they were to learn that they were LGBT. Sixty-five percent felt there were not enough adequately trained or culturally competent health professionals.

Ensuring that clinicians are LGBTQ-friendly not only helps patients feel more at ease but also improves health promotion among LGBTQ individuals. LGBTQ patients with providers who were knowledgeable of LGBTQ health and who used inclusive gender-neutral language were more likely to report having seen their providers in the previous six months, having received a flu shot in the past year, and having gotten an HIV test. Gay and bisexual men who attended an LGBT-centered substance use treatment program reported higher levels of therapeutic support, were less likely to leave treatment before completion, and were better able to abstain from drug use.

After Massachusetts legalized same-sex marriage, health centers reported fewer medical care visits and mental health care visits, resulting in lower healthcare costs. Comparative studies also revealed that LGBT people living in states that allowed same-sex marriage had lower prevalence of depression, anxiety, and alcohol use disorder.

Key Points
- Historical pathologization of homosexuality, the role of physicians as gatekeepers to care, institutional and provider discrimination against LGBTQ patients, and a lack of knowledgeable providers all contribute to substandard care of LGBTQ persons.
- Many LGBTQ patients fear disclosing their orientation or gender identity to providers because of mistrust and anticipation of discrimination or harm based on the historical and continued poor treatment of LGBTQ persons.
- Care in an LGBTQ-friendly environment or from an LGBTQ-friendly provider can result in improved health outcomes.

Case 3.1
Edwin is an 86-year-old man who has come to your family practice office with his daughter. Edwin has lived in a long-term care home for several years and is well known to you and your practice. Because you have become quite close to Edwin and his family over the years, you ask whether anything exciting or new has happened. Edwin's daughter tells you that he recently became romantically involved with another male resident. Before she can finish her sentence, Edwin quickly cuts her off and changes the subject.

What are some reasons that Edwin might be reluctant to discuss his relationship?

How can the PCP delve further into Edwin's situation?

Is Edwin's new relationship a health-relevant concern?

What other topics should be discussed with Edwin?

Though Edwin may simply be shy about disclosing details of his romantic endeavors to people outside his family, it is important for you to be aware of the cultural and historical reasons that could explain this reluctance. Because Edwin is an older gentleman, he has lived through the time when homosexuality was listed in the DSM. He may also have experienced discrimination by past providers because of his same-sex attraction. Edwin is also a resident of a long-term care home, where same-sex romance may be frowned upon and he may be discriminated against by other residents. This could have caused Edwin to fear further discrimination and avoid revealing these details. It is especially important to take the historical context into consideration when dealing with LGBTQ patients. (See Chap. 7 for further discussion of LGBTQ elders.)

Edwin's new relationship is of importance to a PCP for two reasons: (1) Knowing more about it will better help you understand the patient and strengthen the provider-patient relationship; and (2) it will enable you to identify any relevant health concerns related to Edwin's identity and romantic relationship. Relevant health concerns are discussed extensively in other chapters.

The PCP may initiate the conversation by stating, "I understand that you may be reluctant to share details of your relationship with me. Please know that in my role as your provider, I'm here to understand and support you, and I'd love to discuss

your new relationship whenever you are ready." Edwin may not understand the relevance of this new relationship to his health, and this may likewise be addressed with him.

It's notable that Edwin is displaying male same-sex behaviors; he has not stated his sexual orientation. Providers should not assume or label a patient without first verifying how that person self-identifies.

Coming Out: Patient Disclosure and Provider Response

For the LGBTQ patient, coming out is a multi-step process that starts with becoming self-aware of one's orientation and gender identity and progresses to sharing this awareness with others. Coming out can generally be split into three main stages:

1. The personal phase: becoming self-aware of orientation and/or gender identity
2. The private phase: beginning to share orientation and/or identity with others
3. The public phase: living life openly in regard to sexual orientation and/or gender identity

Every patient is in one of these three stages of coming out, so disclosures will vary. Working through the process of coming out allows a person to integrate their identity into everyday life, thus improving their mental health and overall well-being. Individuals do not progress through these stages in a linear fashion. Instead, environments or circumstances can provoke a person to move forward or backward though the stages. For instance, a person who is typically open sexual orientation may feel uncomfortable in an unwelcoming medical environment and revert to the private phase.

Patients tend to consider three factors when deciding to come out to their healthcare providers: personal characteristics (e.g., relationship status, attitudes about health care, comfort with identity), context of health care (the setting of the medical interaction), and relevance of the information (i.e., some patients are more likely to disclose when the information is directly related to their primary concern).

By taking these factors into consideration, a patient may decide whether to disclose sexual orientation and/or gender identity and to choose the nature of that disclosure. In general, patients will use either an active or passive method of disclosure. **Active disclosure** involves directly telling a healthcare provider one's orientation or gender identity; **passive disclosure** consists of giving hints about one's orientation or identity (e.g., mentioning a "partner" without gender pronouns or changing one's clothing to be more like normative clothing for a particular gender identity). Active disclosure is more likely when a healthcare provider is rated highly on warmth, amount of eye contact, use of inclusive language, knowledge of LGBTQ health, and communication skills.

Discussing sexual orientation or gender identity can be a way to enhance care, build trust, and improve communication between provider and patient. Despite these benefits, many people are afraid to come out to their healthcare providers, fearing negative consequences or lack of confidentiality or viewing disclosure as unimportant. In one study, 15% of LGB youth perceived discrimination when they came out to their healthcare providers. Additionally, LGB youth may not feel safe disclosing, fear their parents will find out, or assume their health care provider is against sexual minorities. These fears are not limited to LGBTQ youth, as LGBTQ veterans have expressed concerns about disclosure and its potential negative consequences when engaging with the Veteran Affairs health care system. Due to these fears and negative perceptions, it is important to create a safe and welcoming environment that facilitates disclosure.

A patient-centered, LGBTQ-friendly approach requires specific knowledge, skills, attitudes, and behaviors. It is important that healthcare providers identify at the minimum the sexual orientation and gender identity of each patient as a routine part of the clinical encounter. Many studies have shown that this benefits patients and helps avoid alienating them. Among LGBTQ communities, acknowledgment of sexual orientation and/ or gender-identity facilitates essential screening for suicidal ideation, mental health issues, violence, tobacco and substance use disorders, infectious diseases, and certain cancers for which these populations are at higher risk.

Developing a nonjudgmental method for obtaining this information is essential. Clinical questions should be inclusive and avoid making assumptions about the patient's sexual behavior or relationships. Not every LGBTQ patient— even when asked—will disclose sexual orientation or gender identity. Therefore, care must be taken to avoid pressuring patients to discuss orientation or gender concerns. In addition, clinical questions should be restricted to those necessary to address the issue with explanations on why the information is needed to avoid the perception of intrusion. For example:

- "I'm going to ask you some questions about your sexual health that I ask of all my patients."
- "It's important for me to know the answers to these questions so I'll know how to keep you healthy. As with everything else I learn during this this visit, this information is confidential."
- "I routinely ask patients about sexual orientation to assess them for health risks."
- "What gender pronouns should I use to make you feel comfortable?"

Key Points
- A patient's willingness to come out to a provider depends on several factors, including the relevance of this information, personal and provider characteristics, and the context of the health care.
- Though there are many benefits to coming out to a health care provider, many LGBTQ people may have fears related

to coming out. It is up to the health care provider to create a welcoming environment to alleviate these fears.
- Developing a thoughtful patient-centered approach to interacting with patients is important for healthcare providers in training.

will disclose orientation and/or gender identity and how they will go about disclosing it.

Some patients may also fear a negative reaction from a provider or a lack of confidentiality. As providers, it is important for us to address these fears and provide a welcoming environment for disclosure. Patients should feel supported but not pressured to disclose.

Case 3.2

Smriti, a 57-year-old lesbian, visits your family practice. Because she is a new patient, you start a general assessment. Over the course of your conversation, she reveals that she emigrated from India five years ago and that she is now working in the service industry. After establishing a rapport with Smiriti, you begin to assess her sexual health by inquiring about her sexual orientation. At this point, you notice that her demeanor changes and she becomes uncomfortable.

What could be going through Smiriti's mind at this point?

Why might she be feeling uncomfortable?

How might her Indian heritage contribute to her discomfort?

Patients deciding whether to come out to their health care providers tend to consider three factors: (1) personal characteristics, (2) health care context, and (3) relevance of the information.

Based on these factors, the patient may feel uncomfortable disclosing her orientation. For instance, she may feel that you were not friendly enough during the interview, or she may not believe that revealing her sexual orientation is important. As an older Indian immigrant, Smriti may have experienced a more hostile and homophobic environment in India for the greater part of her life. Each patient will have a unique approach to deciding whether they

The Development of a Patient-Centered Approach to Appropriate Usage of LGBTQ-Friendly Language in a Clinical Setting

Asking About Sexual Orientation and Sexual Behavior

Some health care providers fail to address sexual orientation because they do not have time or they assume that their patients are heterosexual. In one study, 58% of LGB patients affected by cancer admitted bringing up their sexual orientation or gender identity as a way to correct a mistaken (often heterosexual) assumption; only 17% reported being asked directly. When they do address sexuality, they may ask whether their patients are sexually active with men, women, or both – and they typically stop there. This section is focused broadly on a patient-centered approach to discussing sexual orientation and sexual behavior. Chap. 8 discusses the sexual health history in depth.

Not all people who identify as LGB are sexually active or engage in exclusively same-sex sexual contact. Likewise, those who identify as heterosexual may also engage in same-sex sexual behavior. In one survey, 9.4% of straight-identified men reported having sex with at least one man (and no women) in the preceding 12 months. Still, those who identify as LGB are significantly more likely to report suicidal behavior than those who indicated same-sex attraction or behavior but identified as heterosexual. Simply asking whether a person has sex with men, women, or both will miss this significant difference between heterosexual and LGB patients. It will also yield incomplete or inaccurate information if the patient or patient's partner(s) is transgender or non-binary. Hence it is important to differentiate between sexual orientation and sexual behavior to appropriately screen patients for health concerns.

In all patient-centered encounters, starting with open-ended, inclusive questions is key. Providers should avoid presumptive questions or language implying that the patient is heterosexual or conforming to a set of stereotypes (e.g., "Are you in a married?" "What form of birth control do you use?" "When did you last have intercourse?"). Hence it is preferable to use gender-neutral terms and pronouns when referring to partners until behavior and orientation become clearer. Table 3.1 contains non-presumptive questions about sexual orientation and sexual behavior.

Asking About Gender Identity

Assuming gender identity in clinical practice is common, but these assumptions are stigmatizing for any patient who does not identify as cisgender. Some transgender patients will be immediately open about their identity, whereas others

may not disclose their identity. Providers may also encounter patients who are gender nonconforming, questioning their gender, or unsure how to express their gender concerns.

The first important step in rendering friendly transgender and gender-nonconforming care is establishing the patient's correct gender pronouns. They may be feminine (*she, her, hers*), masculine (*he, him, his*), or gender-neutral (*they, them, their; ze, hir, hirs*). A patient's pronouns may not match the gender that is listed in the chart, or even previously documented gender pronouns, if gender assumptions were made. An example of this inquiry: "Out of respect for my patients' right to self-identify, I ask all my patients what gender pronouns I should use for them. What pronouns would you like me to use for you?"

Some patients may request that that the provider avoid pronouns altogether; others may not care which pronouns providers use; and still others may move fluidly between identities over time and avoid labels altogether. Table 3.2 contains some sample questions related to gender identity.

Talking about bodies, sexuality, and sexual health may be stressful for transgender individuals. They may feel uncomfortable referring to their body parts with gendered terms and instead use more gender-neutral terminology, such as *chest* (instead of *breasts*); *man-hole, front-hole,* or *fun-hole* (instead of *vagina*); and *dicklet* or *little bit* (instead of *clitoris*). Instead of applying labels to gendered body parts, it is critical to allow patients

Table 3.1 Sample questions about self-identification, attraction, and behavior

Who lives with you?
Who do you consider to be your family?
What are your relationships with the people in your home?
Are you in a romantic relationship right now?
Do you have a significant other, partner, or spouse?
What are the genders of the individuals with whom you're sexually active?
When was the last time you had sexual contact? (Note the use of "contact" instead of "intercourse.")
What body parts do you make sexual contact with?
Do you have any plans to start a family?
Are you out to your family? Friends? Co-workers?
Do you have any concerns or questions about your sexuality, sexual identity, or sexual desires?
How can I support you through your coming out process?

Table 3.2 Sample questions about gender identity

"Because so many people are affected by gender issues, I've begun asking all of my patients whether they have concerns about their gender. Anything you do say about gender issues will be kept confidential. If this topic isn't relevant to you, tell me and I'll move on."
"Do you agree with the gender you were assigned at birth?"
"The medical record lists your legal name as X. How would you like me to address you?"
"Out of respect for my patients' right to self-identify, I ask all my patients what gender pronouns they'd prefer I use for them. What pronouns would you like me to use for you?"
"How would you describe your gender identity?"

to take the lead when it comes to determining how they want to describe themselves. Providers should never hesitate to nonjudgmentally ask for clarification: "Which body parts do you use to have sex?" "What words do you prefer that I use to describe your genital region?" Providers should ask patients about sexual orientation and gender identity as separate items, because they are independent of each other.

In addition to asking patients in a considerate manner that includes all possibilities, it is important to be aware of the basic language a patient may use when **coming out**, including terminology for sexual orientation, sexual behavior, and gender identity. **Each of these terms is independent of others, meaning that a person's sexual orientation, sexual behavior, and gender identity cannot be inferred from each other.** Sexuality is also fluid, so a woman who currently identifies as a lesbian may have identified as heterosexual in the past and may have a sexual history with men.

External Resource 3.1
This video by the Vlogbrothers called **"Human Sexuality is Complicated..."** illustrates the differences and relationships between terms. Total time 3:48. http://bit.ly/TECe1ch03_01

A patient's sexual orientation or gender identity does not exist as a discrete entity. It is affected by race, ethnicity, religion, socioeconomic status, and/or country of origin. For this reason, it is essential to acknowledge the intersections between different forms of oppression, stigma, and discrimination. Being a member of other stigmatized populations can add to a person's mistrust of health care providers or fear of stigma. Furthermore, patients may describe themselves in culturally bound terms that are not limited to descriptors such as *lesbian*, *gay*, *bisexual*, or *transgender*. For instance, patients may describe themselves as **genderqueer,** subscribing to neither gender, between genders, or a combination of genders. Likewise, a person may identify as **pangender**, a combination of several gender identities. **Two-spirited** is a term used by Native people to describe a person who has attributes of both genders and who typically plays a distinct role within a tribe. The definition of the term varies, depending on which tribe the person belongs to.

The terminology and slang that LGBTQ communities use vary with time and **intersectionality**. To help manage these challenges, clinicians should nonjudgmentally clarify unfamiliar words with the patient or align the patient's term with their own understanding to avoid miscommunication. For example:

> Patient: "I live at home with my lady friend; she's genderqueer, too."
>
> Following the patient's lead: "I noticed that you identified yourself and your lady friend as genderqueer. Could you tell me a little more about what that means for you?"

It is understandable for the clinician to feel uncomfortable at times, as long the discomfort is acknowledged and the clinician reflects upon where it arises. Some clinicians may feel that this discomfort stems from a religious or personal apprehension against being LGBTQ. However, in patient-centered care, the focus on the patient's well-being and health outcomes makes failure to establish rapport unsustainable. To avoid patient alienation, the first step is acknowledging one's own discomfort. Clinicians may alleviate their discomfort with further education about LGBTQ health, discussion with a colleague or supervisor, or—if truly necessary—referral of care of LGBTQ patients to other providers who are more qualified or comfortable. Either way, the health and wellness of the patient comes first.

Key Points
- When interviewing patients, it is important for providers to avoid presumptive language and any assumptions regarding a patient's sexual orientation, sexual behavior, or gender identity.

- Recognizing the difference between sexual orientation and sexual behavior allows providers to identity opportunities for health promotion and provide appropriate care.
- Providers should be familiar with the language that transgender and gender-nonconforming patients may use, including gender pronouns and alternate terms for their body parts.
- A patient's race, ethnicity, religion, socioeconomic status, and/or country of origin may play a role in how patients identify and can affect the words they use to describe themselves.
- Feeling uncomfortable as a provider is acceptable as long as steps are taken to address, understand, and overcome this discomfort.

Case 3.3

Tahlia is a 39-year-old woman referred to your obstetrics practice. Because she is new to your practice, you begin with a general assessment of the patient. As a seasoned clinician, you know that obtaining a sexual history is integral to elucidating Tahlia's chief complaint.

How would you broach this subject with your patient?

If Tahlia initially states that she is straight, will this change your approach? How can you assess the details of Tahlia's gender identity?

It is important that you avoid using presumptive language and avoid making any assumptions regarding her orientation, sexual behavior, or gender identity. Some questions you could use to initially address this topic:

- *With whom do you live?*
- *Who do you include in your family?*

- *Are you currently sexually active?*
- *Are you currently in a relationship?*
- *Do you have a partner or spouse?*
- *When was the last time you had sexual contact with someone?*

Sexual orientation and sexual behavior are not mutually dependent. A person who identifies as gay or lesbian may still have sexual contact with people of the opposite gender. Likewise, someone who identifies as straight/heterosexual may have sexual contact with people of the same gender. It is important to differentiate sexual behavior and sexual orientation when you interview patients. Some examples of how to differentiate these terms:

- *I understand that you identify as straight, but to allow me to screen you for all health risks, would you tell me whether you have sexual contact with men, women, or both?*
- *What are the genders of the people you're sexually active with?*

Understanding your patient's gender identity is important, because it can influence the language both you and your patient use and the way in which you care for the patient.

Examples of how to assess gender identity:

- *"Because so many people are affected by gender issues, I've started asking all of my patients whether they have concerns about their gender. Anything you do say about gender issues will be kept confidential. If this topic isn't relevant to you, just tell me, and I'll move on."*
- *"How would you describe your gender identity?"*
- *"Do you have any concerns about your gender identity?"*

> • *"Out of respect for my patients' right to self-identify, I ask all my patients what gender pronouns they prefer for me to use for them. What pronoun would you like for me to use for you?"*

Effect of Physical Environment, Support Staff, and Policies on LGBTQ Care

Though the tendency is to focus on the interaction between a healthcare provider and the patient, it is important to think about the entire context in which a patient receives care. If the healthcare context, which includes everything from support staff to office space layout, is not welcoming, it can negatively affect the patient's healthcare experience and, ultimately, well-being.

Some patients may look for signals that coming out is accepted and encouraged as part of a protective strategy, wherein they scan the environment and monitor staff and their healthcare provider's behavior before deciding to disclose. Patients are more likely to disclose if the context of care, such as the physical environment of the office, supports disclosure. Additionally, patient flow, or the series of interactions with individuals and environments that a patient encounters during an appointment, plays a large role in determining a patient's comfort. It is important to think about all interactions a patient will have during a visit, including security guards, administrative assistants, medical assistants, other patients and physicians, and nursing staff.

The various aspects of the healthcare environment can be classed into the following three categories.

Nursing Staff and Support Staff Interactions

Patients will first encounter nurses and support staff, such as administrative assistants, front desk staff, and security guards. Staff set the tone for the patient's experience. For instance, a friendly staff is one of the most important factors LGBTQ youth use to rank a healthcare facility. Culturally responsive care and a nondiscriminatory environment lead to ease of disclosure, so having all staff trained in LGBTQ matters is very important. Such staff training should include such topics as the use of appropriate language, important LGBTQ health issues, office nondiscrimination policies, and identifying and dealing with any internalized discriminatory beliefs. Providers may also consider having their staff sign or acknowledge a confidentiality policy, which has been discussed as a priority of many LGBTQ patients.

Of particular importance is training staff with a basic understanding of transgender health care, which involves providing appropriate and responsive care to trans-identifying patients. Because trans patients may present with unexpected gender expression, a staff member who is obviously uncomfortable or awkward with such expression may alienate the patient and deliver lower-quality care. Having staff trained to navigate relevant aspects of trans care (e.g., using patients' correct gender pronouns and preferred name) prevents negative experiences.

> **External Resource 3.2**
> This video by Medical Queeries called **"Medical Queeries: Transcare"** provides a comprehensive overview of the basics of transcare. Total time 7:35. http://bit.ly/TECe1ch03_02

The Physical Environment

Patients who use a protective strategy to come out actively scan the environment for cues supporting disclosure, including:

- Prominently displayed LGBTQ symbols such as the pink triangle or rainbow flag
- Brochures about LGBTQ health concerns displayed in the waiting room

- Relevant LGBTQ media such as magazines or newsletters
- Single-person gender-neutral bathrooms
- Presence of other media bearing LGBTQ-affirming images
- Posted patient nondiscrimination policies if they are inclusive of sexual orientation and gender identity/expression

Office and Hospital Policies

Office and hospital policies also affect a patient's healthcare experience. As previously mentioned, confidentiality may be a pressing concern for patients, so a well-publicized confidentiality policy that applies to all types of clinical interactions (online, in-person, over the phone, documentation, intake forms, etc.) is critical. A prominently displayed nondiscrimination policy protecting sexual and gender minorities both in the office and online may make patients feel more comfortable. A clear means of recourse should be available for patients when necessary.

As mentioned previously, community and government policies such as hospital visitation, insurance coverage for trans care, and access to civil marriage and its benefits have positive effects on LGBTQ health.

External Resource 3.3

The **Healthcare Equality Index (HEI)** is the national LGBTQ benchmarking tool that evaluates healthcare facilities' policies and practices related to the equity and inclusion of their LGBTQ patients, visitors, and employees. http://bit.ly/TECe1ch03_03

The **Human Rights Campaign** has released several maps summarizing the status of laws and policies affecting LGBTQ people on a state-by-state basis. http://bit.ly/TECe1ch03_04

Key Points

- Some patients will look for external indications that coming out is accepted and encouraged. It is important to recognize how the physical environment, ancillary staff, and office policies can affect LGBTQ patients.
- Because patients often first encounter ancillary and nursing staff, staff training and a clear nondiscrimination policy are important.
- Clues in the physical environment, such as LGBTQ-related magazines and posters, can put LGBTQ patients at ease.
- It is important to be up to date on health policies in your region and to understand how these policies can affect your LGBTQ patients.

Case 3.4

Vanessa, a 36-year-old woman whom you have recently hired to work at the front desk, confides that she gets nervous when talking with your transgender patients. She says that she never knows what pronouns to use and is afraid of offending patients by choosing the wrong words.

What can you do to help Vanessa?

In what other ways can you make your practice more LGBTQ-friendly?

The most important intervention for making your office more LGBTQ-friendly is staff training. Vanessa's concerns are not trivial; desk staff and other ancillary workers are often the first point of contact patients have with your practice. This interaction can influence whether the patient has an overall positive or negative experience.

Staff training should include teaching in the use of appropriate language, office nondiscrimination policy, LGBTQ health topics, and management of any internalized homophobia or transphobia. Role play is an effective way for staff to become more comfortable using appropriate language and to practice in a nonjudgmental setting. A better understanding of LGBTQ health topics can foster in staff members an appreciation for the concerns of LGBTQ people.

In addition to staff training, existing office or hospital policies can be modified to make them more LGBTQ-friendly. Simply having an awareness of these policies can help clinicians and other staff deliver more effective care to LGBTQ patients.

Documentation of Sexual Orientation and Gender Identity in Health Records

In 2011, The Joint Commission highlighted the critical importance of including and protecting the LGBT population in health care when it issued its *Field Guide* to providing culturally competent patient- and family-centered care for the LGBT community.

External Resource 3.4

The Joint Commission: Advancing Effective Communication, Cultural Competence, and Patient- and Family-Centered Care for the Lesbian, Gay, Bisexual, and Transgender (LGBT) Community: A Field Guide. http://bit.ly/TECe1ch03_05

The *Field Guide* lists recommended elements in appropriate care:

1. All forms should contain inclusive gender-neutral language that permits self-identification of LGBT individuals
2. Clinics and hospitals should identify opportunities to collect LGBT-relevant data and information during the healthcare encounter:
   (a) At registration or admission
   (b) By way of patient portals or health history questionnaires (e.g., self-reported sexual orientation and gender identity information)
   (c) During the clinical encounter
3. Healthcare providers and hospitals should provide information about sexual orientation and gender identity in patient surveys

The Joint Commission recommends that medical records provide ways to document sexual orientation and gender identity. Electronic medical records may include fill-in fields or drop-down menus to improve documentation and aid research. All such information should be kept under strong privacy protections. Documentation issues are discussed thoroughly in Chap. 13. Figure 3.1 is an example of a simple interface that could be used to record the personal and clinical data discussed in this section.

Though there is no single accepted method of documenting sexual orientation and gender identity in health research or EMRs, most literature and advocacy groups support the recording of certain variables: sexual orientation, sexual behavior, gender identity, preferred name, preferred pronoun, and relationship status. The specific wording depends on the audience, the format, and the intended use.

As discussed in greater detail in Chap. 1, sexual orientation is comprised of three main dimensions: self-identification (how one identifies one's sexual orientation), behavior (types of sexual contact), and attraction (the sex or gender someone feels attracted to). The best practice is to include questions that address all dimensions of sexual orientation.

Regarding sexual orientation, the following wording is suitable for many intake forms and surveys:

Do you think of yourself as

• *Heterosexual or straight (that is, sexually attracted only to women/men);*
• *Homosexual or gay/lesbian (that is, sexually attracted only to men/women);*

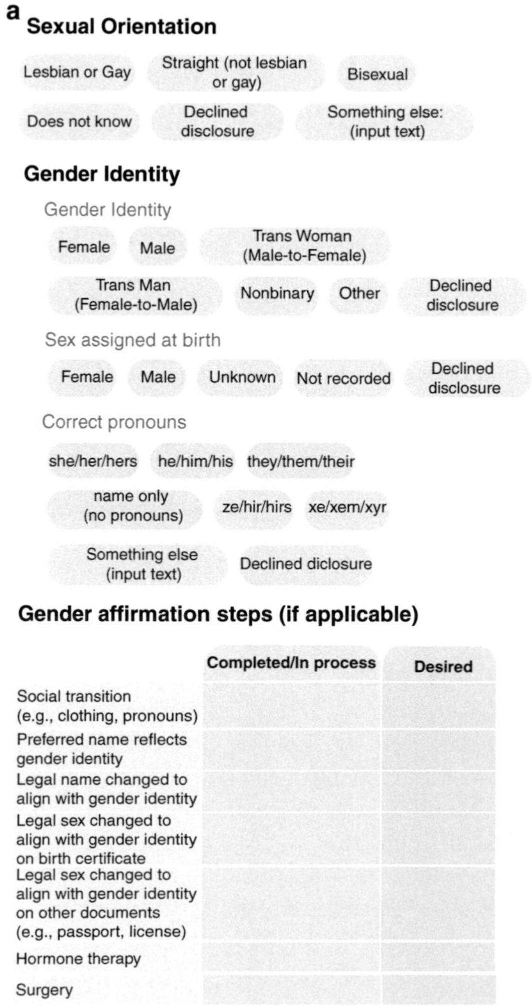

a **Sexual Orientation**

| Lesbian or Gay | Straight (not lesbian or gay) | Bisexual |
| Does not know | Declined disclosure | Something else: (input text) |

Gender Identity

Gender Identity

| Female | Male | Trans Woman (Male-to-Female) |
| Trans Man (Female-to-Male) | Nonbinary | Other | Declined disclosure |

Sex assigned at birth

| Female | Male | Unknown | Not recorded | Declined disclosure |

Correct pronouns

she/her/hers	he/him/his	they/them/their
name only (no pronouns)	ze/hir/hirs	xe/xem/xyr
Something else (input text)	Declined diclosure

Gender affirmation steps (if applicable)

	Completed/In process	Desired
Social transition (e.g., clothing, pronouns)		
Preferred name reflects gender identity		
Legal name changed to align with gender identity		
Legal sex changed to align with gender identity on birth certificate		
Legal sex changed to align with gender identity on other documents (e.g., passport, license)		
Hormone therapy		
Surgery		

Fig. 3.1 Example of an inclusive clinician interface for documenting sexual orientation and gender identity data

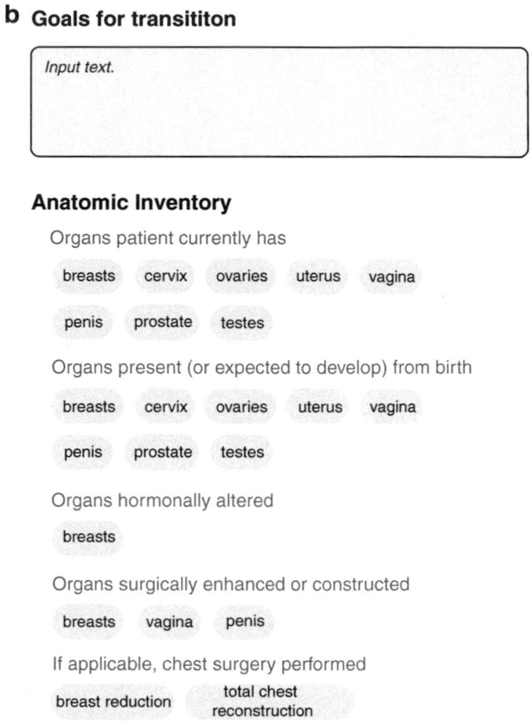

b Goals for transititon

| Input text. |

Anatomic Inventory

Organs patient currently has

| breasts | cervix | ovaries | uterus | vagina |
| penis | prostate | testes |

Organs present (or expected to develop) from birth

| breasts | cervix | ovaries | uterus | vagina |
| penis | prostate | testes |

Organs hormonally altered

| breasts |

Organs surgically enhanced or constructed

| breasts | vagina | penis |

If applicable, chest surgery performed

| breast reduction | total chest reconstruction |

Fig. 3.1 (continued)

• *Bisexual (that is, sexually attracted to men and women);*
• *Something else*
• *You're not sure?*

Regarding sexual attraction, this wording is suitable:

People are different in their sexual attraction to other people. Which best describes your feelings? Are you:

• *Only attracted to women?*
• *Mostly attracted to women?*
• *Equally attracted to women and men?*
• *Mostly attracted to men?*
• *Only attracted to men?*
• *Not sure?*

Gender Identity

Appropriate documentation of gender identity is a complex task. Inclusion of gender identity requires not only notation of gender identity status but also a way to include preferred pronoun and to inventory a patient's current anatomy and medical transition (if applicable). A two-step question is recommended to ask about gender identity:

1. *What is your current gender identity? Check all that apply.*
   - *Male*
   - *Female*
   - *Female-to-male (FtM)/transgender male/ trans man*
   - *Male-to-female (MtF)/transgender female/ trans woman*
   - *Genderqueer—neither exclusively male nor female*
   - *Additional gender category/(or other)— please specify*
   - *Decline to answer—please explain why*
2. *What sex were you assigned at birth on your original birth certificate? Check one.*
   - *Male*
   - *Female*
   - *Decline to answer—please explain why*

When studied in a variety of clinical settings, these questions were found to be acceptable to patients from a variety of sexual orientation and gender identity groups.

The increasing number of practices that are using electronic medical records yields additional challenges for documentation of gender identity. The World Professional Association for Transgender Health (WPATH) EMR working group recommended that EMRs have the following capabilities:

(a) Preferred name, gender identity, and pronoun preference, as identified by patients, should be included as demographic variables.
(b) A means of maintaining an inventory of a patient's medical transition history, current anatomy (also called **anatomic inventory**), and clinical care should be provided. This would include the capacity to document a physical exam, procedures, and surgeries that are uncoupled from a gender-coded

template (e.g., to document orchiectomy in a female patient or a pelvic exam and cervical cytology [Papanicolao smear] in a male one).
(c) The system should permit smooth transition from one listed name, anatomical inventory, and/or sex to another without affecting the integrity of the remainder of the patient's record.
(d) A system should exist by which to notify providers and clinic staff of a patient's correct name and correct pronoun (if either or both of these differ from the current legal documented name/sex).

Patients may request their own records and can see the language that is used to describe them. The use of the patient's non-preferred name and incorrect pronouns may be experienced as degrading and injure the patient's perception of providers and health care. Documentation is an opportunity to accurately describe the patient's circumstances and communicate preferred name and correct pronouns to other members of the care team, whether inpatient or outpatient. An example of a good identification line at the beginning of the note is as follows:

> *Dominic Johnson is a 32-year-old trans man (correct pronouns: he/him/his; EMR and legal documents currently list name as Kylie Johnson and gender as female) presents today for evaluation of a new rash...*

It is helpful to reinforce pronouns in the summary statement in the assessment:

> *Dominic Johnson is a 32-year-old trans man (correct pronouns: he/him/his) with a PMH significant for asthma presenting for evaluation of a morbilliform-appearing rash occurring in the context of starting erythromycin...*

Care providers can use EMR search functions to weed out incorrect pronouns before submitting. Providers struggling grammatically with pronouns such as the singular *they* always have the option to use the patient's preferred name or "the patient."

Key Points

- All hospitals and clinics should identify opportunities to collect LGBTQ-relevant data. These data should include sexual orientation, sexual behavior, gender identity, preferred name, preferred pronoun, and relationship status.
- All forms should contain inclusive, gender-neutral language that permits self-identification by LGBTQ individuals.
- A two-step question is recommended for the assessment of gender identity.
- Electronic health records should be capable of appropriately recording elements of sexual orientation, sexual behavior, gender identity, preferred name, preferred pronoun, relationship status, and transgender-related care (e.g., transition history, current anatomy, procedures and physical exam uncoupled from gender.).

Case 3.5

Maddux is a 25-year-old female-to-male transgender patient who presents to the clinic to establish care with you. He is undergoing testosterone therapy but has not had gender-reassignment surgery. Maddux self-identifies as a gay man and has had three sexual partners in his life-time—two male and one female. He wonders whether the clinic's new electronic medical record system will support his care.

What demographic data must the EMR capture to support Maddux's care adequately?

At what points in Maddux's care should the provider ask for these demographic data?

What features should an EMR have to ensure adequate documentation of Maddux's medical history?

Electronic medical records should support care for a diverse patient population by including the appropriate fields for demographic data collection. Key demographics include two-step gender identity, sexual orientation, preferred name, preferred pronouns, and relationship status. These fields should be easily accessible by the treating clinician.

Demographic data should be collected at multiple points—at patient registration, at time of scheduling, through electronic patient portals, and during clinical encounters—to increase the likelihood of data capture. While data should be asked of patients at multiple points, patients should always be allowed the option to not answer if they so desire.

In addition to being capable of documenting key demographics in the ways listed above, EMRs should also permit adequate documentation of transgender-related care. This includes a complete transition history, medication history, and physical exam, procedures, and surgeries that are uncoupled from the patient's gender. In Maddux's case, breast and gynecologic exam findings and Pap testing would be documented, even though his listed gender is male.

Mitigating LGBTQ-"Unfriendly" Clinical Encounters

Undoing the damage caused by LGBTQ-"unfriendly" encounters at the time of their occurrence is a challenging but critical part of promoting a safe environment. Much of the literature on this topic comes from anti-bullying efforts in schools but can be translated into the clinical setting. Key recommendations focus on intervening when bullying or unfriendly behavior is seen in the clinic, with the use of statements such as, "You may not have meant to hurt anyone, but saying 'That's gay' can hurt those around you…In the future I expect you to use that word respectfully and not in a hurtful way;" or "It is unacceptable to say that. All people are welcome here." The Teaching Tolerance project, part of the Southern Poverty Law Center, created a Speak Up Against Bias guide that can be used to combat everyday bias.

External Resource 3.5
Teaching Tolerance, a project of the Southern Poverty Law Center, has created a **Speak Up Against Bias pocket guide** that can be used to combat everyday bias. http://bit.ly/TECe1ch03_06
Additional resources can be found at the **Teaching Tolerance** website. https://www.tolerance.org/

The guide highlights four key steps:

- **Interrupt.** Speak up against biased remarks whenever they are heard. Consider what you might say ahead of time, such as "That statement is hurtful."
- **Question.** Ask simple questions in response to hateful or hurtful remarks to determine why the speaker made the offensive comment. This helps clarify how to best address the situation. Examples: "Why do you say that?" "What do you mean?"
- **Educate.** Explain why words or phrases are offensive and educate the speaker on other words or expressions he or she could choose instead.
- **Echo.** Express support and reiterate an anti-bias message whenever one is heard.

Another critical component of mitigating unfriendly encounters is creating an LGBTQ-inclusive environment. Best practices for improving the institutional climate include:

- Support from key administrators/personnel
- Specific training on LGBTQ inclusivity

- Inclusive policies and programs covering both employees and patients. Employee-level material should cover nondiscrimination and anti-bullying policies, same-sex partner benefits, and Family Medical Leave Act benefits. Patient-level material should cover nondiscrimination in the healthcare setting, decision-making (including health proxies and same-sex parent decision-making for minors), equal visitation, gender-neutral restrooms, and policies for bed assignments for trans patients.

There are no substantial data demonstrating the efficacy of speaker panels or diversity training in improving LGBTQ-friendliness. The most effective approaches rely on the following:

- **Framing LGBTQ-supportive measures** in ways that appeal to varying perspectives, such as improving productivity, appealing to a sense of fairness and equality, or supporting patient-centered care
- **Legitimizing policy proposals** by providing data or arguments to support the creation of new policies (including showing a need for the policy change, data from other organizations in which similar policies have been implemented [and their outcomes], and potential gains from policy implementation)
- **Creating inter-organizational networks** by connecting with other organizations that support proposed changes
- **Mobilizing people** by encouraging colleagues and supporters to play an active role or voice their concerns on an issue

Key Points
- Mitigating LGBTQ-unfriendly encounters begins with the creation of an LGBTQ-inclusive environment. This process should include support from key administrators and personnel, specific training on LGBTQ inclusion, and the creation of LGBTQ-inclusive policies.

- LGBTQ-inclusive policies should include those devoted to nondiscrimination, anti-bullying measures, same-sex partner benefits, Family Medical Leave Act benefits, decision-making (including health proxies and same-sex parent decision-making for minors), equal visitation, gender-neutral restrooms, and bed assignments for transgender patients.
- When bullying or discriminatory behavior is witnessed, the behavior should be addressed immediately through the use of peaceful responses.

Case 3.6

Lorna is a third-year medical student who is rotating on clerkships. While sitting in a hospital work area, she overhears two medical students talking about their weekend: "I can't believe the plot in that movie. It's so gay!"

What should Lorna do?

First, Lorna should assess her safety in this situation. If she deems her environment safe, she should:

Interrupt by making a statement such as "I know that you don't mean to be hurtful, but saying things like 'That's so gay' can hurt people around you."

Ask the speaker why he or she made the offensive comment—for instance, "What did you mean by that phrase?"

Educate the speaker on why words or phrases can be offensive and provide some other expressions that could be used instead: "The phrase 'That's so gay' is offensive because it equates being gay with being stupid, dumb, worthless, or hideous, which it is not. Next time, if you think the plot doesn't make sense, just say, "The plot doesn't make sense.'"

Boards-Style Application Questions

Question 1. A previously healthy 59-year-old woman reluctantly visits her physician almost one year after noticing a lump in her right axilla. She and her partner are concerned that the lump is cancer, because both her mother and aunt died of breast cancer. However, she has to this point avoided her physician since finding the lump and still refuses to get a mammogram. Which of these experiences could be the reason for the patient's reluctance to visit the physician?

A. Fear of the consequences of a cancer diagnosis
B. Fear of revealing her sexual orientation to her physician
C. Trouble obtaining coverage under her partner's insurance
D. A lack of material in the waiting room pertaining to lesbian and gay health
E. Assumption by a clinician on the patient's last visit that the patient had a male partner
F. Any of the above

Question 2. A 29-year-old man comes to the clinic with a one-week history of painful urination and a clear urethral discharge. Three months ago he had similar complaints and completed a course of ceftriaxone and doxycycline for a gonorrheal infection. A urine polymerase chain reaction test is positive for *Chlamydia trachomatis*. The patient cautiously reveals that in addition to being sexually active with his female spouse for nine years he has been sexually active with several anonymous male partners, of whom his wife is unaware. You inform the patient that chlamydia must be reported confidentially to the health department. Once you've tested the patient for all sexually transmitted diseases, including HIV, which of the following actions is the best next step?

A. Immediately documenting the patient's sexual orientation
B. Requiring the patient to inform his spouse of the other partners

C. Encouraging the patient to stop having sex with male sexual partners
D. Encouraging the patient to get his spouse and male partners tested for sexually transmitted infections
E. None of the above

Question 3. Miguel, a 43-year old divorced man, presents to your office complaining of burning with urination. While taking a sexual history, you learn that he was married to a woman previously but has, since his divorce, been sexually active with men. How do you describe his sexual orientation?

A. Bisexual
B. Formerly straight but now gay
C. Straight, despite currently being sexually active with men, because he was once married to a woman
D. Gay, despite having been married to a woman in the past, because he is now sexually active with men
E. Not enough information to answer this question

Question 4. Ryan is a 27-year old man who is new to your practice. During his first visit to your office, you take a general history as a means of getting to know him better. When you begin asking about his sexual history, Ryan becomes uncomfortable. Eventually he admits that he has recently begun sexually experimenting with men and is questioning his sexual orientation, and he asks you to keep this information private. What is the most appropriate next step?

A. Assuring Ryan that it's not a big deal and continuing with the interview
B. Allowing Ryan to control the course of the conversation because he was initially uncomfortable
C. Inquiring more about Ryan's recent experimenting, including condom use and number of sexual partners
D. Thanking Ryan for being comfortable enough to share this information with you and assuring him that it will be kept confidential

Question 5. You are an outpatient gynecologist who is scheduled to see a 31-year-old woman with a medical history of HPV and stable cervical dysplasia for her annual Pap examination. After taking the patient's weight and vital signs, the nurse brings the patient to your office. You immediately notice that the patient is wearing men's clothing and has a full beard. What's the most appropriate course of action?

A. Politely clarifying the patient's preferred gender pronouns by asking the patient directly
B. Confidently continuing to use the feminine pronouns used in the patient's earlier medical records
C. Strictly avoiding the use of pronouns during the clinical encounter and when writing notes on the encounter
D. Confidently using masculine pronouns when referring to the patient because of the patient's masculine appearance
E. Clarifying the patient's preferred gender pronouns by privately checking with the nurse ahead of time to avoid embarrassing the patient

Question 6. A 14-year-old boy is brought to the physician by his mother for a follow-up examination. He has been complaining of stomach pain since starting at a new school. After the mother is asked to leave the room, the boy confesses that he's been struggling with a sexual attraction to another boy in his class that has been making him feel "sick to his stomach." He asks, "Does this mean I'm gay?" What is the most appropriate response by the physician with which to begin a discussion centered on this patient's question?

A. "Are you sexually active?"
B. "Are you attracted to girls as well?"
C. "How do you feel about these attractions?"
D. "Do you think you're just going through a phase?"
E. "You may be gay, and there's nothing wrong with that."

Question 7. In recent months, several LGBTQ-identified patients have come separately to you, their family physician, and told you that they feel uncomfortable in your office. When you ask why, they tell you that your receptionist has made discriminatory comments, that there's a lack of LGBTQ-related material in the waiting room, that the bathrooms are gendered, and that the intake forms provide no way for them to identify their sexuality. What is the most appropriate first step in addressing these issues?

A. Staff training to address discrimination by staff members
B. Placing LGBTQ-focused magazines and brochures in the waiting room
C. Providing gender-neutral bathrooms instead of separately gendered ones
D. Reviewing and editing intake forms to ensure that they are LGBTQ-friendly

Question 8. Some young colleagues of yours have come to the realization that their practice is not LGBTQ-friendly. Because you're considered the local expert on LGBTQ health, they turn to you to help make their practice more culturally responsive. What is the most appropriate piece of advice for you to give your colleagues?

A. Use pink triangle stickers to show that your practice is LGBTQ-friendly
B. Read more about LGBTQ health to educate yourself about the specific healthcare needs of this population
C. Change intake forms and allow other changes to occur organically as the practice accumulates more LGBTQ patients
D. Begin by assessing the practice—both its physical environment and the staff's attitude toward and knowledge of LGBTQ health

Question 9. Janté is a 45-year old man who has been seen regularly for annual exams. After Janté complains several times of lower abdominal pain, stage III cervical cancer is diagnosed. Which problem with Janté's medical record may have contributed to the delayed diagnosis?

A. The record did not provide a place in which to document sexual behavior

B. The record did not have a place in which to document pronoun preference
C. The medical record did not have a place in which to document gender identity
D. The medical record did not have a place in which to document medical and surgical transition history

Question 10. All of the following features are recommended for sensitive, appropriate electronic medical record documentation **except**:

A. A way to document preferred name and pronoun preference
B. Uncoupling of procedures and surgeries from gender-coded templates
C. A way to document the patient's sex assigned at birth and current gender identity
D. Mandatory documentation of sexual orientation at the time of patient registration

Question 11. All of the following strategies have been shown to be effective in improving LGBTQ climate except:

A. Training
B. Gay-straight alliances
C. Anti-discrimination policies
D. Training in combination with gay-straight alliances

Question 12. Dionne, a medical student, overhears another student joking with a colleague and exclaiming, "That's so gay!" How should Dionne respond?

A. "You're right—it is *so* homosexual!"
B. "I'm going to report you to the school professionalism committee."
C. "We have a nondiscrimination policy that you really need to adhere to."
D. "You may not have meant to hurt anyone, but saying things like "That's gay" can hurt people around you. In the future I expect you to use that word respectfully, not in a hurtful way."
E. No response

Boards-Style Application Questions Answer Key

Question 1. The correct answer is F. Fear of obtaining a diagnosis is common (option A). Some of the most common cultural influences on clinical encounters with LGBTQ-identified patients include being stigmatized/discriminated against by physicians (option B), being less likely to be covered by insurance (option C), and the frequent (and often inappropriate) assumption of heterosexuality (option E). Hence some LGBTQ-identifying patients employ the protective strategy of seeking LGBTQ-friendly clinicians as a means of avoiding further discrimination. The patient looks for environmental cues that indicate whether a practice or hospital is LGBTQ-friendly—for instance, brochures about LGBTQ health concerns, relevant LGBTQ media such as magazines or newsletters, single-person or gender-neutral bathrooms, and media containing LGBTQ-affirming images (option D).

Question 2. The correct answer is D. In all newly diagnosed cases of STI, encouraging the patient to inform recent sexual partners and recommend that they get tested is the most appropriate option. Depending on the state, partner services may then ask for the patient's contacts and facilitate getting sexual partners tested. It is important to recognize that sexual behavior is separate from sexual orientation. Though this man is having sex with both male and female partners, it is not possible to discern, from the information provided, to know how he self-identifies his sexual orientation (option A). Though encouraging patients to reduce their risk by limiting their sexual partners and practicing safer sex is appropriate, forcing them to disclose sexual behavior to others (option B) or asking patients to stop having sex with certain sexual partners (option C) is not appropriate.

Question 3. The correct answer is E. There is not enough information in the scenario for you to answer this question accurately. It is not possible to determine someone's sexual identity on the basis of current or past sexual activity (options A, B, C, and D); sexual identity is a personally defined characteristic. To get an answer this question, you must ask Miguel how he identifies.

Question 4. The correct answer is D. When a patient comes out to you, it is important to respond in a positive manner, because coming out may have been a stressful experience for the patient. Failure to do so may cause the patient to feel the need to be vague when giving you information in the future. Because Ryan also has concerns about the confidentiality of the information, it is important to assure him that everything he tells you will remain confidential. Trivializing his coming out to you (option A) belittles the patient. Though it's important to eventually ask Ryan about his sexual behaviors and risks (option B), the first step is responding to his coming out. Finally, though it's a good idea to follow Ryan's lead through the rest of the conversation (option C), an empathetic response to his coming out and concerns about confidentiality first is the priority.

Question 5. The correct answer is option A. The choice of pronouns to be used to identify a patient always lies with the patient. Someone may prefer masculine pronouns (*he*, *him*), feminine pronouns (*she*, *her*), or gender-neutral pronouns (*they*, ze, *hir*, etc.), that person may want to avoid pronouns altogether. Whenever you are unsure of a patient's preferred gender pronouns, it is **always** appropriate to ask for clarification. Avoid assuming someone's pronouns on the basis of the medical record (option B), current gender presentation (option D), or others' accounts of the person (option E). Though avoiding pronouns altogether (option C) may be appropriate if you are unsure at the beginning of an encounter, you should ask for clarification as soon as possible to ensure that the patient's wishes are honored.

Question 6. The correct answer is option C. Healthcare providers are often the first professionals to whom young patients come out, so it is important for clinicians to avoid even the appearance of passing judgment. This patient reveals that he is struggling with same-sex attraction and expresses discomfort and uncertainty about it but does not mention that he identifies with a specific sexual orientation. Asking open-ended questions like the one in option C ("How do you feel about these attractions?") and avoiding conclusions (options D, "Do you think you're just going through a phase"? and E, "You may be gay, and there's nothing wrong with that") can start a discussion and help the patient from feeling that he or she is being judged or stigmatized. Though asking about sexual behavior (option A) and opposite-sex attraction (option B) may be appropriate in this context, these are not the best questions with which to start a discussion of sexual attraction.

Question 7. The best answer is option A. Although all of these areas should eventually be addressed, staff training is the most crucial intervention. Staff training will address any discriminatory beliefs and behaviors by staff members, who are often the first point of contact with a patient. A friendly staff has been shown to be one of the most important factors that LGB youth use to choose a physician. After staff training, adding LGBTQ brochures and reading materials (option B), gender-neutral bathrooms (option C), safe- zone stickers, and LGBTQ-inclusive forms (option D) can all improve the environment for LGBTQ patients.

Question 8. The best answer is option D. Before advertising your practice as LGBTQ-friendly, you must assess the physical environment, staff attitudes, and staff/provider knowledge of LGBTQ health to ensure that it actually is. This needs assessment will determine which strategies are most important for the practice to pursue. It would be inappropriate to advertise a practice as LGBTQ-friendly (the pink triangle stickers in option A) without first ensuring that it is. Once the needs assessment has been conducted, the practice may find it necessary to improve staff education on LGBTQ health (option B) or change intake forms (option C), but it would be naïve to assume that other changes will occur organically over time.

Question 9. The correct answer is option D. Because the medical record did not provide a place to document medical and surgical transition history, there was no place to note that Janté, a female-to-male transgender person, had not undergone hysterectomy as part of sex-reassignment surgery, and because Janté's sex was noted as male in the medical record, his providers did not realize that he required routine cervical cancer screening. Though medical records should provide a way to document sexual behavior (option A) and pronoun preference (option B), knowing this information alone would not have alerted the providers to Janté's current anatomy and gotten him the screening that he needed. Providing a way to document gender identity (option C) might have alerted to the healthcare providers to the need to ask Janté more information, but it would not guarantee that he got the care he needed.

Question 10. The correct answer is option D. Though every EMR should make it possible to document sexual orientation, disclosure should be voluntary and permitted at multiple points during the patient encounter. The World Professional Association for Transgender Health convened an EMR working group that recommended that EMRs have the following documentation capabilities: preferred name and pronouns (option A) and gender identity; a means of maintaining a patient's medical transition history and current anatomy, including a way to document a physical examination that is uncoupled from a gender-coded template (e.g., exam of cervix, uterus, and ovaries in a patient listed as male) (option B); a smooth transition from one listed name, anatomical inventory, and/or sex to another without affecting the integrity of the remainder of the patient's record; a way to notify providers and clinic staff of a patient's preferred name and/or pronoun (if either or both of these differ from the current legal documented name/sex). Several organizations recommend the use of a two-step question for gender identity that includes current gender identity and sex assigned at birth (option C).

Question 11. The correct answer is option A. Training alone has not been shown to be effective in improving the climate for LGBTQ people. Antidiscrimination policies (option B), gay-straight alliances (GSAs; option C), and training in combination with GSAs (option D) have all been shown to improve the climate for LGBTQ people.

Question 12. The best answer is option D. The best way to transform a culture is to intervene in a non-aggressive manner when bullying or bias-based behavior is witnessed. Often people will make remarks without recognizing their potential negative impact. Speaking up, understanding what the person meant to say, and educating the person on other words they could use instead would be a more productive way to combat bias. Mocking someone who engages in such behavior by making a joke about it, as in option A: ("You're right—it is *so* homosexual!") may trigger anger or embarrassment without understanding of the implications of the statement. If a person repeatedly bullies or makes biased remarks after confrontation regarding the impact of the behavior, it may be appropriate to report the person to a professionalism committee (option B), but this should not be the first response. Although the statement "That's so gay" implies bias, it does not on its own violate a nondiscrimination policy (option C). Refraining from responding (option E) implies agreement with the statement and will not change the institutional culture.

Sources

A Resource Guide to Coming Out. The Human Rights Campaign. http://www.hrc.org/resources/entry/resource-guide-to-coming-out. Updated April 2013. Accessed 10 Jun 2014.

American College of Obstetricians and Gynecologists. Healthcare for transgender individuals: committee opinion no. Obstet Gynecol. 2011;118(512):1454–8.

American Psychological Association. Sexual orientation and homosexuality. www.apa.org/topics/sorientation.pdf. Accessed 07 Jul 2014.

Anton B. Proceedings of the American Psychological Association for the legislative year 2009: minutes of the annual meeting of the Council of Representatives and minutes of the meetings of the Board of Directors. Am Psychol. 2010;65:385–475. https://doi.org/10.10377/a0019553.

APA Task Force on Appropriate Therapeutic Responses to Sexual Orientation. Report of the task force on appropriate therapeutic responses to sexual orientation. American Psychological Association. https://www.apa.org/pi/lgbt/resources/therapeutic-response.pdf. Published 2009. Accessed 21 Jan 2019.

Baker K. Gathering sexual orientation and gender identity data in health IT. Center for American Progress. www.americanprogress.org/issues/lgbt/news/2012/02/09/11146/gathering-sexual-orientation-and-gender-identity-data-in-health-it/. Published 2012. Accessed 13 Mar 2015.

Baker K. Top 10 things health reform does for gay and transgender Americans. Center for American Progress. http://www.americanprogress.org/issues/lgbt/news/2012/03/26/11246/top-10-things-health-reform-does-for-gay-and-transgender-americans/. Published 2012. Accessed 04 Sept 2014.

Baker KE, Durso LE, Cray A. Moving the needle: the impact of the affordable care act on LGBT communities. Center for American Progress. cdn.americanprogress.org/wp-content/uploads/2014/11/LGBTandACA-report.pdf. Published 2014. Accessed 13 Mar 2015.

Barbara AM, Quandt SA, Anderson RT. Experiences of lesbians in the health care environment. Women Health. 2001;34(1):45–62.

Barry J. Health disparities for LGBT military members serving under "Don't Ask, Don't Tell": quantifying health care utilization and circumvention. Lecture presented at: LGBTQ Health Workforce Conference, Center for Gay and Lesbian Studies, City University of New York. May 2, 2014. New York, NY.

Baskin v Bogan, 766 F.3d 648 (7th Cir 2014).

Bostic v Schaefer, 760 F.3d 352 (4th Cir 2014).

Bowers v Hardwick, 478 U.S. 187-88, n. 1 (1986).

Burke BP, White JC. Wellbeing of gay, lesbian, and bisexual doctors. BMJ. 2001;322:422–5.

Betancourt JR, Green AR, Carillo JE, Ananeh-Firempong O. Defining cultural competence: a practical framework for addressing racial/ethnic disparities in health and health care. Public Health Rep. 2003;118(4):293–302.

Bumiller E. Obama ends "don't ask, don't tell" policy. The New York Times. July 22, 2011. www.nytimes.com/2011/07/23/us/23military.html. Accessed 14 Sept 2014.

Context for LGBT health status in the United States. In: The health of lesbian, gay, bisexual, and transgender people. Washington, DC: National Academies Press; 2011. p. 36.

Coren JS, Coren CM, Pagliaro SN, Weiss LB. Assessing your office for care of lesbian, gay, bisexual, and transgender patients. Health Care Manag. 2011;30(1):66–70.

Creed WED. Seven conversations about the same thing: homophobia and heterosexism in the workplace. In:

Konrad AM, Prasad P, Pringle PK, editors. Handbook of workplace diversity. Thousand Oaks, CA: Sage; 2006. p. 371.

Degrees of Equality: A National Study Examining Workplace Climate for LGBT Employees. Human Rights Campaign. www.hrc.org/files/assets/resources/DegreesOfEquality_2009.pdf. Published 2009. Accessed 15 Mar 2015.

DeMaio TJ, Bates N. New relationship and marital status questions: a reflection of changes to the social and legal recognition of same-sex couples in the U.S.. https://www.census.gov/srd/papers/pdf/rsm2012-02.pdf. Published 2012. Accessed 22 Jan 2019.

Deutsch M, Green J, Keatley J, Mayer G, Hastings J, Hall AM. Electronic medical records and the transgender patient: recommendations from the World Professional Association for Transgender Health EMR Working Group. JAMIA. 2013;20(4):700–3. https://doi.org/10.1136/amiajnl-2012-001472.

Eliason MJ, Schope R. Does "Don't ask don't tell" apply to health care? Lesbian, gay, and bisexual people's disclosure to health care providers. J Gay Lesbian Med Assoc. 2001;5(4):125–34.

Equal Employment Opportunity Commission. 42 U.S.C. § 2000e.

Erickson-Schroth L. Trans bodies, trans selves: a resource for the transgender community. Oxford, UK: Oxford University Press; 2014.

Fact Sheet: Improving Data Collection for the LGBT Community. U.S. Department of Health and Human Services. http://minorityhealth.hhs.gov/lgbt/. Published 2011. Accessed 01 Jul 2014.

Feldman JL, Goldberg J. Transgender primary medical care: suggested guidelines for clinicians in British Columbia. Vancouver Coastal Health Transgender Health Program. http://lgbtqpn.ca/wp-content/uploads/woocommerce_uploads/2014/08/Guidelines-primarycare.pdf. Published 2006. Accessed 22 Jan 2019.

Gonzales G. Same-sex marriage: a prescription for better health. N Engl J Med. 2012;370:1373–6.

Grant JM, Mottlet LA, Tanis J, Harrison J, Herman JL, Keisling M. Injustice at every turn: a report of the National Transgender Discrimination Survey. National Gay and Lesbian Task Force. http://www.thetaskforce.org/static_html/downloads/reports/reports/ntds_full.pdf. Published 2011. Accessed 25 May 2014.

Griffin P, Ouellett ML. Going beyond gay-straight alliances to make schools safe for lesbian, gay, bisexual, and transgender students. Dent Angles. 2002;6(1):1–8.

Guidelines for Care of Lesbian, Gay, Bisexual, and Transgender Patients. Gay and Lesbian Medical Association. http://glma.org/_data/n_0001/resources/live/GLMA%20guidelines%202006%20FINAL.pdf. Published 2006. Accessed 21 Jan 2019.

Hitchcock JE. Personal risking: the decision-making process of lesbians regarding self-disclosure of sexual orientation to health providers [dissertation]. San Francisco: University of California; 1989.

Holyk G. Americans' ideology and age drive gay marriage views. ABC News website. http://abcnews.go.com/blogs/politics/2014/06/americans-ideology-and-age-drive-gay-marriage-views/. Published 2014. Accessed 21 Jan 2019.

Hatzenbuhler M, O'Cleirigh C, Grasso C, Mayer K, Safren S, Bradford J. Effect of same-sex marriage laws on health care use and expenditures in sexual minority men: a quasi-natural experiment. J Public Health. 2012;102:285–91.

Healthcare Equality Index. Human Rights Campaign website. www.hrc.org/hei. Accessed 24 Jun 2014.

Hoffman ND, Freeman K, Swann S. Healthcare preferences of lesbian, gay, bisexual, transgender and questioning youth. J Adolesc Health. 2009;45(3):222–9.

Institute of Medicine. Collecting sexual orientation and gender identity data in electronic health records: workshop summary. Washington, DC: The National Academies Press; 2013.

Istar Lev A. The mental health professional as gatekeeper. In: Transgender emergence: therapeutic guidelines for working with gender-variant people and their families. New York, NY: The Haworth Press. p. 2004.

Just the Facts About Sexual Orientation and Youth: A Primer for Principals, Educators, and School Personnel. American Psychological Association. www.apa.org/pi/lgbc/publications/justthefacts.html. Published 2008. Accessed 25 May 2014.

Kitchen v Herbert, 755 F.3d 1193 (10th Cir. 2014).

Kosenko K, Rintamaki L, Raney S, Maness K. Transgender patient perceptions of stigma in health care contexts. Med Care. 2013;51(9):819–22.

Lawrence v Texas, 539 US 558 (2003).

Low SM. The cultural basis of health, illness and disease. Soc Work Health Care. 1984;9:13–23.

Margolies L, Scout NFN. LGBT patient-centered outcomes: cancer survivors teach us how to improve care for all. National LGBT Cancer Network. www.cancernetwork.org/patient_centered_outcomes. Published 2013. Accessed 22 Jan 2019.

Marriage and family building equality for lesbian, gay, bisexual, transgender, queer, intersex, asexual, and gender nonconforming individuals. The American College of Obstetricians and Gynecologists. https://www.acog.org/-/media/Committee-Opinions/Committee-on-Health-Care-for-Underserved-Women/co749.pdf?dmc=1&ts=20180810T1021458170. Published 2018. Accessed 22 Jan 2019.

McBride B. Four cases that paved the way for marriage equality and a reminder of the work ahead. Human Rights Campaign. https://www.hrc.org/blog/four-cases-that-paved-the-way-for-marriage-equality-and-a-reminder-of-the-w. Published 2017. Accessed 22 Jan 2019.

RP MN, Hegarty K, Taft A. From silence to sensitivity: a new identity disclosure model to facilitate disclosure for same-sex attracted women in general practice consultations. Soc Sci Med. 2012;75(1):208–16.

National Defense Authorization Act for Fiscal Year 1994, P.L. 103-160 (codified at 10 U.S.C. §654).

National LGBT Health Education Center: Ending Invisibility: Better Care for LGBT Populations

(Module 1). Boston, MA: The Fenway Institute. 2009. http://www.lgbthealtheducation.org/training/learning-modules/. Accessed 10 Mar 2015.

National Survey of Physicians, Part I: Doctors on Disparities in Medical Care. Kaiser Family Foundation. https://www.kff.org/uninsured/national-survey-of-physicians-part-i-doctors/. Published 2002. Accessed 22 Jan 2019.

Nelson JA. Disclosure of lesbian, gay, and bisexual identity by adolescents and young adults to health care providers and its relationship to sexual orientation victimization [dissertation]. New York, NY: New York University; 2006.

Obedin-Maliver J, Goldsmith ES, Stewart L, et al. Lesbian, gay, bisexual, and transgender-related content in medical education. JAMA. 2011;306(9):971–7. https://doi.org/10.1001/jama.2011.1255.

One Colorado Education Fund. Invisible: the state of LGBT health in Colorado. Denver, CO: One Colorado; 2011.

Pathela P, Hajat A, Schillinger J, Blank S, Sell R, Mostashari F. Discordance between sexual behavior and self-reported sexual identity: a population-based survey of New York City men. Ann Intern Med. 2006;145:416–25.

Polek C, Hardia TL, Crowley EM. Lesbians' disclosure of sexual orientation and satisfaction with care. J Transcult Nurs. 2008;19(3):243–9.

Primary Care Protocol for Transgender Patient Care. Center of Excellence for Transgender Health. Primary Care Protocol for Transgender Patient Care. Published 2016. Accessed 22 Jan 2019.

Questions about Sexual Orientation and Gender Identity in Clinical Settings: A Study in Four Health Centers. Fenway Institute and the Center for American Progress. http://thefenwayinstitute.org/wp-content/uploads/COM228_SOGI_CHARN_WhitePaper.pdf. Published 2013. Accessed 22 Jan 2019.

Senreich E. Are specialized LGBT program components helpful for gay and bisexual men in substance abuse treatment? Subst Use Misuse. 2010;45(7–8):1077–96. https://doi.org/10.3109/10826080903483855.

Sexual Minority Assessment Research Team (SMART). Best practices for asking questions about sexual orientation on surveys. Williams Institute. https://williamsinstitute.law.ucla.edu/wp-content/uploads/SMART-FINAL-Nov-2009.pdf. Published 2009. Accessed 22 Jan 2019.

Sherman MD, Kauth MR, Shipherd JC, Street RL Jr. Communication between VA providers and sexual and gender minority veterans: a pilot study. Psychol Serv. 2014;11(2):235–42. https://doi.org/10.1037/a0035840.

Speak Up Against Bias. Teaching Tolerance. http://www.tolerance.org/sites/default/files/general/speak_up_pocket_card_2up.pdf. Accessed 10 Nov 2014.

Stanley CL. Correction of military records following repeal of Section 654 of Title 10, United States Code. sldn.3cdn.net/8b5bfaa11d5854c9e5_k2m6b382s.pdf. Published 2011. Accessed 5 Jun 2017.

Statement of HHS Secretary Kathleen Sebelius on LGBT Pride Month. US Department of Health and Human Services.http://www.hhs.gov/news/press/2013pres/06/20130603a.html. Published 2013. Accessed 04 Sept 2014.

Stevens P. Lesbian health care research: a review of the literature from 1970 to 1990. Health Care Women Int. 1992;13(2):91–120. https://doi.org/10.1080/07399339209515984.

Szalacha LA. Safer sexual diversity climates: lessons learned from an evaluation of Massachusetts Safe Schools Program for gay and lesbian students. Am J Educ. 2003;110(1):55–88.

Understanding Issues Facing Transgender Americans. GLAAD. www.glaad.org/sites/default/files/understanding-issues-facing-transgender-americans.pdf. Published 2015. Accessed 13 Mar 2015.

The Joint Commission. Advancing effective communication, cultural competence, and patient- and family-centered care for the Lesbian, Gay, Bisexual, and Transgender (LGBT) community: a field guide. Oak Brook, IL; October 2011.

Which states allow gay marriage? Mother Jones; May 19, 2014; updated June 6, 2015. http://www.motherjones.com/politics/2014/05/gay-marriage-states-legal-map. Accessed 04 Sept 2014.

White JC, Levinson W. Lesbian health care: what a primary care physician needs to know. West J Med. 1995;162:463–6.

Whittle S, Turner L, Al-Alami M. Endangered penalties: transgender and transsexual people's experiences of inequality and discrimination. London: The Equalities Review; 2007.

Wilkerson JM, Rybicki S, Barber CA, Smolenski DJ. Creating a culturally competent clinical environment for LGBT patients. J Gay Lesbian Soc Serv. 2011;23(3):376–94.

Zhao Y, Montoro R, Igartua K, Thombs BD. Suicidal ideation and attempt among adolescents reporting "unsure" sexual identity or heterosexual identity plus same-sex attraction or behavior: forgotten groups? J Am Acad Child Adolesc Psychiatr. 2010;49(2):104–13.

Interdisciplinary Approach to Care

Brian A. Nuyen, Jason D. Domogauer,
Laura Jennings, Julie Kinzel, and Michele J. Eliason

Enhancing LBGT Health Care Through an Interdisciplinary Approach

Interdisciplinary Collaborative Practice in Health Care

A patient-centered, interdisciplinary team–based approach to care is now the model used in many health care institutions. Such teams encompass a range of health professions, including physicians, nurse practitioners (NPs), physician assistants

The first listed author is the chapter's associate editor from The Equal Curriculum Project. The chapter authors are otherwise ordered according to their preference.

B. A. Nuyen (✉)
Stanford University School of Medicine,
Stanford, CA, USA

J. D. Domogauer
Rutgers New Jersey Medical School,
Newark, NJ, USA

L. Jennings
University of Pennsylvania Health System,
Philadelphia, PA, USA

J. Kinzel
Drexel University Physician Assistant Program,
Philadelphia, PA, USA
e-mail: jjk28@drexel.edu

M. J. Eliason
San Francisco State University,
San Francisco, CA, USA
e-mail: meliason@sfsu.edu

(PAs), nurses, health care students, social workers, and representatives of community programs. An Institute of Medicine 2003 report lists teamwork—focused on improving safety outcomes, increasing communication, and enhancing collaboration skills—as a core principle for students and professionals in the health care system. Research has also demonstrated the positive impact of this care model on patient outcomes. In a retrospective population-based study, medical intensive care unit patients who were cared for by an interdisciplinary team had a significantly lower mortality rate than did patients who were not. Another study documented significant improvements in patient perceptions of health, self-efficacy, and well-being when care was delivered by an interdisciplinary team. Finally, the medical home, a team-based interdisciplinary approach developed in 1967, has been shown to lead to positive patient outcomes, increased patient satisfaction, reduction in medical errors, and improved quality of care.

Unfortunately, not every health care institution is equipped to provide interdisciplinary team–based care, and the transition to such a model requires training of health professionals and administrators. It is fortunate that team-based interdisciplinary education and training is becoming a focus of many health care training institutions, giving students and young professionals the knowledge and skills to work effectively in such teams. As a means of developing a successful team and minimizing obstacles, each member should be informed of each health professional's specific role and responsibility. It is also important to allow team members numerous opportunities, on a consistent basis, to express concerns or ideas while ensuring an open, judgment-free environment. Research has found that such an environment fosters stronger bonds among team members and a deeper commitment to helping one another improve patient care.

Barriers to Development of an Interdisciplinary Team Approach to LGBTQ Care

Unfortunately, knowledge and understanding of patient-centered, interdisciplinary team–based care for LGBTQ patients is lacking. This deficiency stems from a deficiency of research on LGBTQ individuals' general health and wellness. For instance, a 2011 study reported that nearly one-third of all articles related to LGBT health published between 1950 and 2007 were specifically focused on HIV/AIDS and other sexually transmitted infections. A 2014 study found that only 12 National Institutes of Health–funded studies between 1989 and 2011 were focused on LGBT health care services. Also, few health care training programs (e.g., medical, dental, nursing, PA) incorporate more than a just a few hours of LGBTQ health education/training into their general curricula. Such shortcomings within the literature and health professional training may contribute to the fragmented and ineffective delivery of care for many LGBTQ individuals. Last, many of the known prevalent health concerns affecting the LGBTQ population (e.g., tobacco use, cancer risk, alcohol use/abuse) are medical concerns that benefit from an interdisciplinary care approach.

Fortunately, advocacy has helped change this lack of knowledge and training. *Healthy People 2020* highlights the health care needs of sexual and gender minorities, encouraging institutional research efforts focused on this population. Furthermore, in 2011, President Barack Obama instituted a new rule mandating that Medicare- and Medicaid-participating hospitals grant access to individuals regardless of their sexual orientation or gender identity. One of the most important efforts has come from the Joint Commission, which, in an effort to improve patient outcomes and overall patient satisfaction, produced a field guide (discussed thoroughly in Chap. 3) for providers to improve communication, cultural competence, and patient- and family-centered care of the LGBT patient population. It is recommended that one provider be identified within each organization to focus on education and advocacy efforts. The Joint Commission also encourages the creation of an advisory board consisting of representatives from the LGBT community and organizations to provide feedback and resources to both hospital administration and health care providers regarding the care they provide as a team.

Culturally Competent Team-Based Care for LGBTQ Patients: Examples

Despite a lack of readily available resources for and research on interdisciplinary patient-centered care of LGBTQ patients, many institutions apply generalized practices to train their health professionals in LGBTQ care. To encourage busy health professionals to attend training on LGBTQ health and cultural competency, many institutions opt for incentives such as continuing medical education credits. Training is often provided in seminars, during which professionals learn about the disparities faced by LGBTQ patients, as well as how an interdisciplinary team can meet their needs. Often there is emphasis on the importance of the responsibility of all caregivers to seek training in cultural competence. By providing such training, the institution can promote itself as a welcoming place for LGBTQ patients searching for service providers with a compassionate understanding of sexual and gender minority health concerns.

Some health care institutions have demonstrated strong efforts to cultivate cultural competency and interdisciplinary team–based care. Wynia and Matiasek identified eight hospitals across the United States with innovative practices that effectively worked across cultures, languages, and varying health literacy levels to

Table 4.1 Successful culturally competent practices

Serving as champions of communication programs
Collecting information on patient needs
Engaging communities
Developing a diverse and skilled workforce
Involving patients
Spreading awareness of cultural diversity
Providing effective language assistance services
Addressing low health literacy

achieve advanced patient-centered communication with vulnerable patient populations in their institutions (Table 4.1).

The premier example of an LGBTQ culturally competent interdisciplinary team–based approach is the Fenway Community Health Center, established in 1971 as a primary care center. After 1980, the center expanded the focus of its programming from infectious diseases (HIV/AIDS) to include such areas as substance use and parenting. The interdisciplinary collaboration has now expanded further, with primary medical care, HIV/AIDs, gynecology, gerontology, podiatry, nutritional counseling, mental health, addiction services, and pharmacy, as well as complementary methodologies such as chiropractic, massage, acupuncture, and health promotion. Fenway also provides community education, domestic and homophobic violence prevention programs, parenting programs, family planning services, and same-sex marriage clinics. This expansion clearly required the commitment and continued training of all staff, with a focus on cultural competency for all health professionals and ancillary staff to improve LGBTQ health. The Fenway Community Health Center has identified the needs of the community and provides resources to address them under one roof.

Many other organizations offer successful examples of LGBTQ patient–centered interdisciplinary cultural competency training and resources. The Downstate Team Building Initiative is a multicultural interdisciplinary group working to unite various health professions students through a multisession team-building curriculum. PFLAG, which is most famous for supporting the families of LGB persons, has widened its focus to improvement of LGBTQ

patient care, producing a guide for allied health care professionals addressing the care required to fulfill the increasingly visible needs of the LGBTQ patient population. The guide leads the reader through several case scenarios illustrating LGBTQ patients' needs and the strategies with which to properly and sensitively render care to these patients.

Key Points

- Interdisciplinary health care teams are most successful when their members receive proper LGBTQ patient care training and are provided with opportunities for open discussions on patient care and problem-solving.
- Proper training of interdisciplinary teams in culturally competent team-based care is crucial to provide optimal care for LGBTQ patients.
- Successful interdisciplinary health care facilities focus on LGBTQ patients' overall health and needs.

Roles of Health Professionals in Providing Quality Comprehensive Care

As the health systems continue to evolve, it is important to consider the unique roles various health professionals play in providing quality comprehensive care for LGBTQ individuals over their lifespans. There is no rubric for the type or number of health professionals in the creation of an interdisciplinary team. Rather, the team is fluid and situation-dependent, varying with the demands on a given institution and the needs of an individual or population. This section focuses on several health professionals in addition to physicians and discusses the roles of some less frequently considered team members. It is impossible for every potential team member to be identified and described in this book—therefore, any exclusion is not reflective of that position's lack of importance.

With the forecasted primary physician shortage, many more midlevel providers—PAs and NPs—will be required to assume the care of greater numbers of patients. This need will be further exacerbated in various lower socioeconomic and otherwise underserved communities, which generally struggle to attract physicians. Research suggests that NPs bring an alternative perspective and skill base in addressing patient care, leading to reduced cost, increased patient satisfaction, and positive patient outcomes. Similarly, PAs have organizationally endorsed interdisciplinary team–based care. Larry Herman, past president of the American Academy of Physician Assistants (AAPA) said, "Physician assistants were team before team was cool. We've always practiced this model." The group emphasizes the importance of educating all PAs to reach out to communities where patients lack health care or are marginalized and to use a team-based interdisciplinary approach to fill gaps in care.

Nursing practice encompasses many crucial and diverse roles, from initial patient evaluation to end-of-life care. Nurses have a unique opportunity to establish a welcoming and safe foundation by using inclusive language: they may gather important information during an LGBTQ patient's encounter that can be circulated to the rest of the interdisciplinary team. Research has shown that nurses who set a welcoming, nonjudgmental tone during the initial patient interview are able better facilitate disclosure of patient's self-identity, potentially leading to an improved patient experience. Through proper training, nurses are primed to act as key members of many interdisciplinary teams by addressing the needs of LGBTQ individuals in a variety of scenarios.

Social workers, psychologists, and counselors are often overlooked as members of an interdisciplinary team, but they bring a unique focus on emotional and social resources for LGBTQ patients and their families. These clinicians help individuals explore their emotions, develop coping strategies, and identify ways to adapt to their environment. In addition to facilitating personal development, social workers focus on adapting the environment to the patient (e.g., coordination with community resources, discharge planning, securing housing). Counselors have worked to incorporate LGBTQ-inclusive language to affirm the patient and the patient's family. As members of the interdisciplinary health team, effective counselors apply constant reflection and checking of privilege to their work to yield a valuable patient-provider relationship and improve patient outcomes.

Similarly, social workers seek patient self-determination and place importance on the dignity and worth of the patient and family. The social worker's assessment permits a thorough evaluation of the family structure and the patient's role within it. The National Association of Social Workers recently evaluated hospital social workers and their approaches to cultural sensitivity and found that a proactive approach, rather than a reactive or inactive one, was the most effective means of self-educating on LGBT needs and collaborating with the health care team. Such proactive education allows accurate assessment and linking of care management services. An effective social worker assesses a patient's health care support and is sensitive to each stage of a patient's coming-out journey. The counselor and social worker can each play a key role in identifying and responding to patient needs and thus improve the quality and efficacy of services provided.

With fluctuating legal and political discrimination as a critical social determinant of health, legal assistance has often become a necessary component of the LGBTQ person's care team. Legal issues such as visitation, adoption, custody and visitation, marriage and domestic partnership, transgender/gender identity, domestic violence, harassment and discrimination, and health care inequalities cause considerable stress and may play a critical role in health outcomes. At the time of this writing the question of federal protections for LGBTQ individuals to prevent loss of employment resulting from sexual orientation or gender identity is unsettled. Many LGBTQ persons are at risk of losing health care coverage if they lose their jobs. Some organizations (e.g., Lambda Legal,

American Civil Liberties Union, Amnesty International) are working toward full legal equality and protection of LGBTQ individuals; some work specifically to bridge the gap between law and health care. Although not often thought of as members of the interdisciplinary care team, patient relations workers, lawyers, and legal consultants have played an important role in ensuring LGBTQ patients' equal access to health care and their constitutional rights of equality, privacy, and expression. Attorneys have often been at the forefront of legal battles to ensure that health care institutions and providers are not allowed to deny visitation by same-sex partners or withhold care on the basis of sexual orientation or gender identity. Janice Langbehn was not allowed to visit her partner who had collapsed while on a family vacation, despite her holding a durable health care power of attorney. The subsequent lawsuit, *Langbehn v. Jackson Memorial Hospital*, led to the release of new regulations by the Department of Health and Human Services requiring federally funded hospitals to have written visitation policies; to inform patients of their right to designate visitors, including same-sex spouses and domestic partners; and to not discriminate by granting visitation rights on the basis of sexual orientation or gender identity. Although prominent legal cases regarding LGBTQ health care show care providers and institutions in a negative light, other health care professionals work with legal teams, providing their expert opinions to help secure the equal treatment and optimal health of LGBTQ individuals.

The ideal team composition and prominence of various roles are likely to change at different points over a patient's lifespan. For instance, LGBTQ youth often require specialized services. The CDC reports that LGBT youth are four times more likely to have attempted suicide than their heterosexual peers. Transgender youth report worse general health and a lack of social support. Furthermore, although family acceptance has been shown to be protective of mental health and linked to less substance use and lower sexual risk, family rejection is extremely common for LGBT youth. Therefore mental health professionals play a particularly strong role in the interdisciplinary team of an LGBTQ youth.

Support organizations vary with a patient's phase of life. Many agencies and programs are focused on addressing the health gaps of LGBTQ youth, empowering LGBTQ youth to engage in advocacy, leadership, and policy reform. School-based health centers are crucial in reducing disparities in health access and child health status by providing a consistent source of primary care in an accessible context. They have been shown to be a well-placed resource in reducing both financial and nonfinancial barriers to care. Chap. 6 describes the significance of gay-straight alliances (GSAs) in supporting adolescents' overall well-being.

LGBTQ elders also benefit from special services. As LGBTQ people age, **family choice**—the aging person's desire to grow old in the company of partners, spouses, LGBTQ friends, or family—is a central topic of concern. A 2011 Joint Commission field report revealed that LGBT elders are less likely than their cisgender heterosexual counterparts to have children as a primary support, and isolation is a major concern. Residential retirement facilities have historically been unwelcoming of LGBTQ patients, leading to the separation of LGBTQ elders from friends or partners and even homelessness. Perhaps because of this, some LGBTQ elders have had to reshape their communities, drawing support from a larger pool of individuals (e.g., friends, community agencies, partners) than their heterosexual peers do. In 2010, Services and Advocacy for LGBT Elders (SAGE) launched a National Resource Center on LGBT Aging for all providers to better address elders' concerns. Chap. 7 discusses the role of SAGE in navigating housing difficulties experienced by LGBT elders. The necessity of additional health and community services (e.g., home health care, physical or occupational therapy, Meals on Wheels, senior activity programs, hospice care) speaks to the importance of interdisciplinary care for LGBTQ seniors. These services address the **social determinants of health**, which have a more profound effect on overall health than health care alone.

Key Points

- Physician assistants and nurse practitioners may fill an important access-to-care niche for LGBTQ persons who are also members of other underserved communities.
- Nurses who set a welcoming, nonjudgmental tone during the initial patient interview are able better facilitate disclosure of patient's self-identity.
- Social workers have diverse roles from elucidating family structures and roles to identifying appropriate community-based resources for LGBTQ persons.
- It is important to anticipate legal concerns when working with LGBTQ patients.
- LGBTQ youth and elders are special populations who benefit from specific community-based resources.
- Elderly LGBTQ people often experience discrimination and isolation in retirement facilities.

Case-Based Examination of Interdisciplinary Care

Case 4.1

Jerry, a transgender man, desires a hysterectomy to align his body with his gender identity. After much searching, he finds a gynecologist who is willing to treat transgender men and goes to the large university hospital/clinic setting where the provider is located. The first challenge he faces comes at the reception desk, where the receptionist looks shocked when Jerry announces that he is there to see a gynecologist and asks him, "Are you sure?" When he says that he is sure, she hands him the admission forms. The demographic section of the forms asks only whether the patient is male or female, so Jerry writes in "Transgender."

The receptionist asks for Jerry's insurance card. Jerry hands it over, wondering whether he should tell her that his insurance company has already denied his request for hysterectomy. He knows that he will have to pay for it himself. Next he checks in at the gynecology clinic, which is crowded with women. All of the posters on the wall show feminine-looking women holding babies. He finds a seat, and the woman next to him asks, "Is your wife seeing Dr. Link?" Before he can decide how to answer, the nurse, also a woman, comes to the door and calls for Jerry. She also looks shocked when he stands up, and repeats, "Are you Jerry ___?" "Yes," he responds, hearing the women in the waiting room go suddenly quiet, all their eyes on him. The nurse recovers her composure and escorts him to the exam room. She asks him to disrobe and put on the hospital gown. She leaves, and Jerry immediately hears excited whispering in the hallway. He is obviously the source of much gossip. Finally Dr. Link arrives, greets him warmly, says that she has worked with other transgender men, and treats him respectfully. However, as Jerry leaves he wonders why she did not bother to educate her staff. He likes Dr. Link but does not feel inclined to return to her clinic.

What changes can be made to improve Jerry's next visit?

Advice about LGBTQ patient care is often focused on physicians and overlooks other members of the health care team, including receptionists and unit clerks, who may serve as the first line of interaction with a patient. As a means of ensuring a welcoming environment for LGBTQ patients, all employees, including maintenance staff, should undergo LGBTQ competency training. The physical climate (e.g., posters on the wall, magazines in the waiting room) of a clinic or other health care institution should reflect the diverse identities of the patient population, regardless of whether a physician or institution believes that the patient population includes LGBTQ-identifying patients. Documentation and use of preferred names and pronouns is important. It is also appropriate for staff to move away from using gender-presumptive titles such as Mr., Mrs., and Ms. unless a preference is declared by a patient. Dr. Link, as the leader of her health care team, should have ensured that all members of the office received proper training. If an LGBTQ-identifying patient expresses concern(s) about interactions with the staff, Dr. Link must immediately address the issue and consider education of the staff to prevent any such situations in the future.

Case 4.2
Darius, a 28-year-old African-American man, presents to the emergency department after a bicycle accident. He found to have a badly sprained ankle. Sarah, a physical therapist, comes to the ED with a pair of crutches to give Darius directions for their use and instructions for home care. She first stops by the nurses' station to review his chart. The nurse who is caring for Darius tells Sarah that he is a pleasant man, that he is married, and that his spouse arrived at the ED shortly after Darius was brought in. On entering the curtained area Sarah finds Darius sitting on the bed and another man sitting in a chair beside him. Sarah asks Darius whether he would like to wait for his wife to return and whether it is ok for his friend to remain in the room as they discuss the next steps in his care. The other young man erupts in anger: "What do you mean, his wife? Why do you assume that we're just friends? We're married! The

nurse and the front desk know this!" Sarah is taken aback. She simply did not know that the two men were a couple and assumed that the second man was a friend.

What steps could Sarah have taken to have avoided offending Darius and his partner?
*Sarah, like many health care professionals, approached her patient with a heteronormative viewpoint and her own assumptions—in this case, she assumed that "married" meant a relationship with someone of the opposite gender. This is an example of **heterosexual assumption**. Sarah's experience speaks to the lesson that providers should never assume a patient's sexual orientation or gender identity; rather, the provider should engage the patient in discussion to allow the patient to share his or her identity. This practice not only lets the provider better understand the patient and his or her unique needs but also facilitates an improved patient/provider relationship, which may lead to improved care and patient outcomes. Darius's case also highlights a missed opportunity for the practice of interdisciplinary care by Darius's nurse and Sarah, his physical therapist. Sarah would likely have avoided the situation described in the case study if she had engaged the nurse in subsequent questions about Darius and his significant other. Not only would such discussion have provided information on Darius's identity; it might also have provided insight into the degree of care support he could expect at home.*

Case 4.3
Maria is a 48-year-old lesbian-identifying cis-woman who has been with her partner, Carmen, for 16 years. Maria has colon cancer and is being admitted to the hospital for

surgery. For financial reasons, they are not married and have been unable to consult a lawyer about legal documents to protect their relationship. They are an "open secret" in their families, tolerated as long as they do not talk about their relationship or show any intimacy around family members. For this reason, neither woman is close to her family of origin, but fortunately the two do have the support of friends during this difficult time.

When Maria is admitted to the surgical unit, Carmen is asked to leave so the nurses can go through the admissions process. This upsets both Maria and Carmen, but they oblige. Carmen returns to Maria's room and is holding her hand when the anesthesiologist comes in. This time Maria indicates that she wants Carmen to stay with her, and the physician allows it. After Maria is taken to surgery, Carmen meets two close friends, who join her in the surgery waiting area. When the surgeon comes to the door and asks for Maria's family, Carmen steps forward. "Are you the sister?" the surgeon asks. Carmen is unsure how to respond and simply says that she is Maria's roommate. "I'm sorry, but I can only give information to spouses or family members," the surgeon replies. Carmen's friends are visibly angry, but they know that Maria and Carmen are afraid to disclose their relationship. There is nothing they can do but be supportive of Carmen and try to find some way to get around the system and get information.

Which health care professionals might have helped Maria and Carmen? In what ways could these health professionals have provided assistance to the couple?

It is critically important for health care institutions and professionals to address any fears of disclosure and to make the health care environment welcoming and safe for LGBTQ patients and their families. Today many health care institutions, especially those that participate in Medicare and Medicaid, have established policies that prohibit same-sex partner discrimination in hospital visitation, regardless of whether a couple has a legally recognized relationship. Unfortunately, situations such as Maria and Carmen's still occur, even when the federal government has mandated policies that should prevent this discrimination in the first place.

The case also highlights a lack of interdisciplinary care. Maria and Carmen's experience could have been better facilitated through the inclusion of hospital caseworkers, counselors, psychologists, or others who would have been able to engage the couple and better understand their needs. Also, had an interdisciplinary approach been taken, the status of the women's relationship could have been shared with the entire health care team to ensure that Maria and Carmen's needs were addressed.

Case 4.4 A woman found lying in the street, bleeding from knife wounds, is brought to the emergency department. The driver's license in her wallet identifies her as Stephanie Johnson, a 36-year-old woman, but when the paramedics remove her bloody clothing they see that Stephanie has a penis and testes. One of the paramedics sees three police officers pointing and laughing, and one of them comments, "That explains why it got knifed." When the ambulance arrives at the hospital, the paramedics do not know whether to report that the patient is male or female and feel uncomfortable about giving report of the case. When Stephanie is transferred to the intensive care unit, the nurses wonder how they should address the patient. One resident announces that he will refuse to take care of that "freak." Stephanie dies of her injuries before regaining consciousness.

What can be done to ensure that a transgender or gender-nonconforming individual does not encounter this type of treatment in the future?

This case illustrates the dehumanizing language ("it," "freak") that is often used in regard to transgender patients, as well as some ethical and moral issues involved in caring for LGBTQ-identifying individuals. It was extremely inappropriate for the police officers to be making public comments/jokes about Stephanie and even worse for them to suggest that her trans identity was justification for the violence that ended up claiming her life. The refusal of the resident to care for the patient reflects an ethical and moral failure of the health care system to provide nondiscriminatory care, especially lifesaving care, to all individuals, regardless of sexual orientation or gender identity.

This case also provides insight into the numerous but often overlooked professionals who contribute to an interdisciplinary care team. In trauma situations, interdisciplinary care may begin with law enforcement and paramedics. Therefore it is important that these individuals also receive proper training on engaging, working with, and caring for LGBTQ individuals. This case shows what can happen when such professionals and institutions do not supply proper training. The paramedic's reluctance to provide critical details about Stephanie and the resident's refusal to treat her may have contributed to delayed or suboptimal care and, as a result, to Stephanie's death. Institutions and interdisciplinary teams must ensure that all members are properly trained in the provision of care to LGBTQ patients and are knowledgeable about federal, local, and institutional nondiscriminatory policies. Any member of a properly functioning interdisciplinary team would have been able to step forward and serve as an advocate for Stephanie to ensure that she received the most compassionate, knowledgeable care possible.

Conclusion

This chapter discussed how numerous health care professionals and services, including community resources, play a critical role in fulfilling the diverse, complex needs of the LGBTQ population. Because of the system's lack of understanding of these needs, patients may not seek medical attention and may be mistreated or misunderstood when they do. Many health professions training programs lack adequate curricular time or cultural competency content on LGBTQ people. Members of interdisciplinary teams should work collaboratively to achieve improved patient-centered health outcomes for LGBTQ people. This means not only that health professions training programs must prepare trainees to work on interdisciplinary teams but also that they must improve their curricula to help newer generations of providers become sensitive to the needs of *all* the patients they serve.

Boards-Style Application Questions

Question 1. A 78-year-old man with advanced Alzheimer disease presents to the emergency department, accompanied by a slightly younger man. After introducing yourself and eliciting a history of present illness (HPI), you discover that the two men have been partners for more than 40 years and have come to the ED because the older man has fallen down a flight of stairs. Physical examination reveals minor contusions but no serious injuries. You are preparing to discharge the patient when the patient's partner pulls you aside and tells you that he no longer feels capable of caring for the patient alone in their home.

What is the proper response to this man's concern?

A. Discharging the patient to a nursing facility
B. Sympathetically telling him that there is nothing you can do

C. Telling him that you understand and encouraging him to keep trying
D. Requesting the assistance of a social worker who can discuss the available options

Question 2. A 34-year-old woman presents to an LGBTQ community health center that is focused on providing care to the uninsured. She appears anxious and apprehensive, shifting in her chair and nervously tugging at her sleeves. The staff is worried for the patient and fears that she may leave before being seen by a physician. Unfortunately, the clinic is very busy, and all of the physicians are with other patients.

Who is the next best individual to talk with this patient at this time?

A. A culturally competent nurse
B. A first-year nursing student
C. A first-year medical student
D. A front desk clinic staff member

Question 3. A 75-year-old transwoman presents to a Veterans Affairs hospital with diabetic complications. During the history of present illness it is discovered that she lives alone and has no family or other support system. The patient says she frequently forgets to check her glucose level and states that she does not see the point. She mentions that she used to be much better about taking care of her diabetes when she had a stronger support system but notes that many of her friends have died.

To which agency should this patient be referred for additional assistance as she undergoes care for her illness?

A. Lambda Legal
B. Services and Advocacy for GLBT Elders (SAGE)
C. Parents and Friends of Lesbians and Gays (PFLAG)
D. GLMA: Health Professionals Advancing LGBT Equality

Question 4. Dr. Dellini runs a primary care office in a midsized urban city. She sees a mixed population of patients, including a relatively large LGBTQ population. During a well visit, one of her lesbian-identifying patients says to her, "If it wasn't for you I wouldn't come back to your office." Further questioning by Dr. Dellini reveals that her front desk staff has been making rude comments to her LGBTQ patients.

Which of the following staff members should be trained in LGBTQ care?

A. Nurses
B. Physicians
C. Office staff
D. Nurse practitioners
E. Physician assistants
F. All of the above

Question 5. A small inpatient rehabilitation hospital is focused on improving its care to the LGBTQ community. The health care team consists of nurses, physicians, physical therapists, physician assistants, and other hospital staff. So far, everyone appears committed to providing a welcoming environment.

What is best next step in ensuring successful LGBTQ care at the hospital?

A. Creating a list of LGBTQ-friendly providers at the hospital
B. Advertising the hospital in the community as an LGBTQ-welcoming facility
C. Creating an advisory board consisting of representatives from the LGBTQ community
D. Highlighting LGBTQ-identified staff at the hospital as role models to showcase workplace diversity

Question 6. Lina, 58-year-old cisgender lesbian-identifying woman, is admitted to the intensive care unit of the local hospital. She has late-stage terminal breast cancer and has therefore been receiving hospice care for the past five months. Her partner, Jane, accompanies her. They have been together for 20 years and married for the past three years. Palliative comfort measures, discussed previously discussed by Lina and Jane, are started. While talking with a nurse, Jane begins to cry. She states that she is afraid of losing Lina and of being alone. The two never had children, and both were estranged from their families because of their sexual orientation.

What can be done for Jane as you care for Lina during this difficult time?

A. Unfortunately, nothing, because Lina, not Jane, is your patient
B. Referring Jane to a general cancer spouse survivor support group
C. Sympathetically apologizing but informing Jane that there is nothing you can do
D. Contacting Lina's hospice case manager and discussing the current situation, taking Jane's unique needs into consideration

Boards-Style Application Questions Answer Key

Question 1. Option D is the best available option. An LGBTQ-friendly social worker who is knowledgeable of the available resources is the person best equipped to determine the desires of both men and assist them in making a realistic and healthy decision. Discharging the patient to a nursing facility (A) may not be the best option for the couple; in fact, it may actually result in unintended negative consequences. Research has found that the great majority of LGBTQ seniors prefer to stay in their homes and feel forced to reenter the closet when they are placed in potentially unwelcoming nursing care facilities. It is important to fully understand the desires of both men before making such a decision. If a nursing facility is the desired option, try to ensure that the facility is welcoming to LGBTQ patients and actively trains staff to care for LGBTQ patients. It is not appropriate to tell the partner that there is nothing else to be done (option B) when there are local, state, and national resources that may provide the two with assistance. If you are unsure of what those resources might be, conduct a Web-based search or consult someone who does know.

Although it is good to acknowledge the partner's concerns, it is not a good idea to leave the man in a situation of increasing concern that has already resulted in injury to his partner (option C).

Question 2. On the basis of the limited information presented, option A is the best choice: One must not assume that the patient identifies as part of the LGBTQ community simply because she has presented to the clinic, but in light of her presentation at this clinic, a health care provider trained in caring for members of the LGBTQ community should be one of the first members of the health care team to meet with the woman.

Question 3. Option B is correct. SAGE is the country's largest and oldest organization dedicated to improving the lives of older LGBT adults through various innovative services and programs. Because the patient appears to be in need of an active support system that is sensitive to her personal and medical needs, SAGE is the best option. Lambda Legal is an organization focused on achieving full recognition of the civil rights of LGBT individuals and those with HIV, but the patient is not presenting with a legal issue, so option A is not the best option. Although PFLAG (option C) is a national organization that promotes the health and well-being of LGBT individuals, it is not the best option because it not specifically focused on LGBT elders. The Gay and Lesbian Medical Association: Health Professionals Advancing LGBT Equality is focused on ensuring equality in the health care professions for LGBTQ people; because the patient is not a health care professional, this is not the best option.

Question 4. Option F is correct. Any member of a health care team who interacts with patients, in either an administrative or a health care–providing capacity, should be trained in the sensitive, culturally competent care of LGBTQ individuals. It should not matter whether a practice knowingly treats LGBTQ individuals, because many patients are LGBTQ-identifying but choose not to disclose this information. Additionally, office and hospital forms should be reviewed for sexual orientation and gender identity inclusiveness.

Question 5. It has been shown that LGBTQ individuals seek health care from providers who promote an understanding of sexual and gender minority health concerns and from those who are identified within the LGBTQ community as someone to be trusted. Involving invested LGBTQ-identifying members of the community by establishing an advisory board (option B) is the best next step at this time. An advisory board or committee should be developed during the early stages of the project as a source of feedback, resources, and advice to both hospital administration and health care providers. The advisory board can provide advice, from the type of training to provide to which unique services might be needed by the community. Creating a provider list (option A) is a great step in assisting LGBTQ individuals in identifying providers. However, to be on such a list, the provider should first demonstrate some degree of knowledge or training to confirm that he or she is capable of properly caring for LGBTQ patients. Therefore this would not be the best next step at this time. Option C is similar to option B; a hospital should first develop an advisory board and provide proper training to its staff before promoting itself as a welcoming environment. Although the intention of showcasing real workplace diversity described in option D is admirable, outing LGBTQ-identified staff is inappropriate without their consent and will not be effective in ensuring successful LGBTQ care.

Question 6. As a health care provider, you should acknowledge that a disease does not define an individual and that it is not isolated to a single person. Chronic diseases, especially cancer, affect the individual's family and community. It is important to recognize this and take steps to ensure the health and needs of the patient's family. Situations such as Lina and Jane's are prime opportunities to engage other health care providers and community resources and ensure that care does not end when the patient and family leave the hospital or office or after a loved one has died (option D). Telling Jane that there is nothing you can do (option A) is not the correct choice, because it is not true. Because

Lina is in hospice care, Jane will be provided support and bereavement services for one year after Lina's death. Services may take a variety of forms, including phone calls, print resources, and support groups. However, when you are recommending bereavement support it is important to take Jane's unique needs into consideration. Referring Jane to a survivor support group that consists mainly of heterosexual individuals (option B) may or may not allow Jane to feel welcomed, comfortable, or understood. For this reason it is important to identify LGBTQ-targeted support groups and make these options known to Jane. As with option A, it is not appropriate to tell Jane that there is nothing else to be done (option C) when there are actually local, state, and national resources that might serve her. If you are unsure of what those resources might be, conduct a Web search or refer to someone who might know. Again, this is a great opportunity to reach out to other providers, in this case, the hospice case manager, and work with that individual to ensure Jane's unique needs are identified and properly met.

Sources

Advancing Effective Communication, Cultural Competence, and Patient- and Family-Centered Care for Lesbian, Gay, Bisexual, and Transgender (LGBT) Community: A Field Guide. Oakbrook Terrace, IL: The Joint Commission; 2011.

Bergh N, Crisp C. Defining culturally competent practice with sexual minorities: implications for social work education and practice. J Soc Work Educ. 2004;40(2):221–38.

Betancourt J, Green AR, Carrillo E. Cultural competence in health care: emerging frameworks and practical approaches. Washington, DC: The Commonwealth Fund; 2002.

Boehmer U. Twenty years of public health research: inclusion of lesbian, gay, bisexual and transgender population. Am J Public Health. 2002;92(7):1125–30.

Cashman S, Reidy P, Cody K, Lemary C. Developing and measuring progress toward collaborative, integrated, interdisciplinary health care teams. J Interprof Care. 2004;18(2):183–96. https://doi.org/10.1080/1356182 0410001686936.

Chrisman NJ. Extending cultural competence through systems change: academic, hospital, and community partnerships. J Transcult Nurs. 2007;18(1 Suppl):68S–76S; discussion 77S-85S

Conlon A, Aldredge P. Department of health and human services: implications for hospital social workers. Health Soc Work. 2013;38(1):19–27. https://doi.org/10.1093/hsw/hls063.

Eliason MJ, Dibble SL, De Joseph JF, Chinn P. LGBTQ cultures: what healthcare professionals need to know about sexual and gender diversity. Philadelphia, PA: Lippincott; 2009.

Engum S, Jeffries P. Interdisciplinary collisions: bringing healthcare professionals together. Collegian. 2012;19(3):145–51.

Gilbert MJ. Principles and recommended standards for cultural competence education of health care professionals. Los Angeles, CA: California Endowment; 2003.

Hoffman N, Freeman K, Swann S. Healthcare preferences of lesbian, gay, bisexual, transgender and questioning youth. J Adolesc Health. 2003;45(3):222–9.

Hooker R, Cipher D, Sekscenski E. Patient satisfaction with physician assistant, nurse practitioner, physician care: a national survey of medicare beneficiaries. J Clin Outcomes Manag. 2005;12(2):88–92.

Hope J, Lugassy D, Meyer R, Jeanty F, Myers S, Jones S, et al. Bringing interdisciplinary and multicultural team building to health care education: the downstate team-building initiative. Acad Med. 2005;80(1):74–83.

Hughes M, Kentlyn S. Older LGBT people's care networks and communities of practice: a brief note. Int Soc Work. 2011;54:436–44. https://doi.org/10.1177/0020872810396254.

Iandoli E. New chair of physician assistant studies: PAs are key team players in healthcare. New York, NY: New York Institute of Technology; 2013. http://www.nyit.edu/about_nyit/news/new_chair_of_physician_assistant_studies. Accessed July 1, 2015.

Kane-Lee E, Bayer C. Meeting the needs of LGBT patients and families. Nurs Manag. 2012;43:42–6. https://doi.org/10.1097/01.NUMA.0000410866.26051.ff.

Kutash K, Duchnowski AJ, Lynn N. School-based mental health: an empirical guide for decision-makers. Tampa, FL: Research & Training Center for Children's Mental Health, Louis de la Parte Florida Mental Health Institute, University of Florida; 2006.

Langbehn v Jackson Memorial Hospital. http://www.lambdalegal.org/in-court/cases/langbehn-v-jackson-memorial.

Lambda Legal. http://www.lambdalegal.org.

LGBT Movement Advancement Project & Services and Advocacy for Gay, Lesbian, Bisexual and Transgender Elders (SAGE). Improving the lives of LGBT older adults. 2010 [cited 2015 February 23]. Available from: http://www.sageusa.org/files/Improving the Lives of LGBT Older Adults - Large Font.pdf.

LBGT PA Caucus. http://www.lbgpa.org.

Lesbian, Gay, Bisexual, and Transgender Health. Retrieved from www.healthypeople.gov.

LGBT Health Care Education Center. http://www.lgbthealtheducation.org.

Martin J, Bedimo A. Nurse practitioner, nurse midwife, and physician assistant attitudes and care practices related to persons with HIV/AIDs. J Am Acad Nurs Pract. 2000;12(2):35–41.

Mayer K, Bradford J, Makadon HJ, Stall R, Goldhammer H, Landers S. Sexual and gender minority health: what we know and what needs to be done. Am J Public Health. 2012;98(8)

Mayer K, Mimiaga MJ, VanDerwarker R, Goldhammer H, JBl B. Fenway Community Health's model of integrated community-based LGBT care, education, and research. In: Meyer IH, Northridge ME, editors. The health of sexual minorities: public health perspectives on lesbian, gay, bisexual, and transgender populations. New York, NY: Springer; 2011. p. 693–715.

Michon K. Health care antidiscrimination laws protecting gays and lesbians: can doctors withhold treatment because of a patient's sexual orientation or gender identity? Legal Topics. http://www.nolo.com/legal-encyclopedia/health-care-antidiscrimination-laws-protecting-32296.html. Accessed 23 Feb 2015.

Neville S, Henrickson M. Perceptions of lesbian, gay, and bisexual people of primary healthcare services. J Adv Nurs. 2006;55(4):407–15.

Obedin-Maliver J, Goldsmith E, Stewart L, White W, Tran E, Brenman S, et al. LGBT-related content in undergraduate medical education. JAMA. 2011;306:971–7.

Straight for Equality in Health Care. Washington, DC: PFLAG National; 2009.

Pies C. Improving health of LGBT people: how being counted counts. National Women's Health Network; 2011.

Rosenthal T. The medical home: growing evidence to support a new approach to primary care. J Am Board Fam Med. 2008;21(5):427–40.

Russell S, Muraco A, Subramaniam A, Laub C. Youth empowerment and high school gay-straight alliances. J Youth Adolesc. 2009;38:891–903.

Ryan C, Russell S, Huebner D, Diaz R, Sanchez J. Family acceptance in adolescence and the health of LGBT young adults. J Child Adolesc Psychiatr Nurs. 2010;23(4):205–13.

Saha S, Beach MC, Cooper LA. Patient centeredness, cultural competence and healthcare quality. J Natl Med Assoc. 2008;100(11):1275–85.

Saulnier C. Deciding who to see: lesbians discuss their preferences in health and mental health care providers. Soc Work. 2002;47(4):355–65.

Sequeira GM, Chakraborti C, Panunti BA. Integrating lesbian, gay, bisexual, and transgender (LGBT) content into undergraduate medical school curricula: a qualitative study. Ochsner J. 2012;12:379–82.

Silow-Carroll S, Alteras T., Stepnick L, Patient-centered care for underserved populations: definition and best oractices; 2006.

Smith L, Shin R, Officer L. Moving counseling forward on LGB and transgender issues: speaking queerly on discourses and microaggressions. Couns Psychol. 2012;40(3):385–408.

Synder J. Trend analysis of medical publications about LGBT persons. J Homosex. 2011;58(2):164–88.

The Healthcare Executive's Role in Fostering Inclusion of LGBT Patients and Employees. Chicago, IL: American College of Healthcare Executives. http://www.ache.org/policy/inclusion-lgbt.cfm. Published March 8, 2013. Accessed 23 Feb 2015.

Wynia M, Matiasek J. Promising practices for patient-centered communication with vulnerable populations: examples from eight hospitals, 2006, The Commonwealth Fund.

Prevention

5

Brian A. Nuyen, Florence Doo, Philipp Hannan, and Ronni Hayon

Introduction

Prevention of disease takes numerous forms. Environmental regulations, traffic safety, water sanitation, nutrition programs, immunizations, health education campaigns, bicycle helmet give-aways, and tobacco cessation programs are all meaningful examples of disease prevention. Because most of the variability in the population's health status is attributable to **social determinants of health** other than health care, non-clinical prevention programs have powerful impacts. For LGBTQ people, the greatest improvements in health status may come from changes in the social determinants and development of more inclusive or targeted prevention programs.

The first listed author is the chapter's associate editor from The Equal Curriculum Project. The chapter authors are otherwise ordered according to their preference.

B. A. Nuyen (✉)
Stanford University School of Medicine,
Stanford, CA, USA

F. Doo
Mount Sinai West, New York, NY, USA

P. Hannan
University of Arizona, Tucson, AZ, USA
e-mail: philipp.hannan@ucdenver.edu

R. Hayon
University of Wisconsin School of Medicine and
Public Health, Madison, WI, USA
e-mail: ronni.hayon@fammed.wisc.edu

It is important to understand the scope of different prevention strategies. The Institute of Medicine (IOM) created classifications for this purpose. Universal prevention strategies are designed to reach the entire population, without regard to individual risk factors. Classic examples are water sanitation or addition of folate to grain products in the US to prevent neural tube defects in fetuses. **Selective prevention strategies** target subgroups of the general population that have biological, psychological, social, or environmental risk factors that are greater than the general population. Some examples are education programs on binge drinking for college students or screening of blood lead levels in children who live in older homes. **Indicated prevention strategies** target individuals who show signs of being at risk or have early manifestations of disease. Some indicated interventions are prescribing a statin to a patient with high cholesterol or frequent testing for HIV in a patient who has unprotected sex. Other frequently used prevention classifications are **primary, secondary, tertiary prevention**. These are defined in Table 5.1.

Clinical screening tests vary from questionnaires to laboratory assays. Results of screening tests must be interpreted carefully. The **sensitivity** and **specificity** tests are biological properties of laboratory tests or psychometric properties of questionnaires. Sensitivity is the probability that a test will be positive when disease is in fact present in an individual. Specificity is the probability that a test will be nega-

Table 5.1 Categories of prevention

Primary prevention	Intervening before health effects occur, through measures such as vaccinations, altering risky behaviors (e.g., poor eating habits, tobacco use), and banning substances known to be associated with a disease or health condition
Secondary prevention	Screening to identify diseases in the earliest stages, before the onset of signs and symptoms, through measures such as mammography and regular blood pressure testing
Tertiary prevention	Managing disease post-diagnosis to slow or stop disease progression through measures such as chemotherapy, rehabilitation, and screening for complications

Table 5.2 United States preventive services task force grade definitions

Grade	Definition
A	The USPSTF recommends the service. There is high certainty that the net benefit is substantial. *Suggestion for Practice: Offer or provide this service.*
B	The USPSTF recommends the service. There is high certainty that the net benefit is moderate or there is moderate certainty that the net benefit is moderate to substantial. *Suggestion for Practice: Offer or provide this service.*
C	The USPSTF recommends selectively offering or providing this service to individual patients based on professional judgment and patient preferences. There is at least moderate certainty that the net benefit is small. *Suggestion for Practice: Offer or provide this service for selected patients depending on individual circumstances.*
D	The USPSTF recommends against the service. There is moderate or high certainty that the service has no net benefit or that the harms outweigh the benefits. *Suggestion for Practice: Discourage the use of this service.*
I	The USPSTF concludes that the current evidence is insufficient to assess the balance of benefits and harms of the service. Evidence is lacking, of poor quality, or conflicting, and the balance of benefits and harms cannot be determined. *Suggestion for Practice: Read the clinical considerations section of USPSTF Recommendation Statement. If the service is offered, patients should understand the uncertainty about the balance of benefits and harms.*

tive when disease is not present. Ideal screening tests are rapid, inexpensive, and minimally invasive. If necessary, screening tests favor high sensitivity over high specificity. False positives are subsequently weeded out with confirmatory tests that have high specificity. Two other important properties of tests are the **positive predictive value** and **negative predictive value**. The positive predictive value is the probability that an individual has disease when the test result is positive. If a disease is rare in a population of people tested, false positive tests may greatly outnumber true positive tests, making the positive predictive value low. Negative predictive value is the probability that an individual does not have a disease when the test result is negative.

The United States Preventive Services Task Force (USPSTF) is the most significant US organization for clinical prevention guidelines. They assess the quality of evidence for a prevention practice with respect to a defined population. A favorable recommendation requires evidence that the practice changes health outcomes (i.e., decreases morbidity and/or mortality) and that the practice itself does not introduce excessive risk to patients. The quality of any given practice is assigned a grade (Table 5.2). Major medical organizations like the American College of Obstetricians and Gynecologists and the Infectious Disease Society of America conduct their own reviews and produce their own guidelines, which may differ. Of special note is the Center of Excellence for Transgender Health at the University of California, San Francisco.

External Resource 5.1
The Center of Excellence for Transgender Health is the leading expert organization providing guidelines for the primary care of transgender and nonbinary people. http://transhealth.ucsf.edu

Key Points
- Prevention strategies range from broad to targeted. The Institute of Medicine classifies the scopes of prevention strategies as universal, selective, and indicated.

- Prevention can also be considered primary, secondary, or tertiary, depending on where in the disease course an intervention is initiated.
- The United States Preventive Services Task Force (USPSTF) is the most significant organization promulgating clinical prevention guidelines in the US.

Challenges and Limitations of LGBTQ Health Research

The complex and overlapping array of definitions used to describe **sexual identity**, **sexual behavior**, **sexual desire**, **sex assigned at birth**, and **gender identity** pose a significant challenge when identifying sexual and gender minority subpopulations for study. The list of questions needed to allow an LGBTQ research participant to accurately describe oneself is long, and researchers struggle to find the appropriate balance between thoroughness and pragmatism when asking these questions. Further complicating this array of possibilities is the fluidity of sexuality and gender identity over time—e.g., a lesbian who does not **come out** until later in life; a man who has same-sex sexual experiences in adolescence but not as an adult; or a transgender woman whose ultimate gender identity is not expressed until middle age. Racial, ethnic, socioeconomic, and other factors further impact an individual's responses to these questions. Different researchers have used different questions to assess sexual minority status and different definitions of what constitutes a sexual minority.

Consider the case of a patient whose sexual identity is queer pansexual, but when given the limited options of gay, lesbian, and bisexual within one study, she chooses bisexual. When she participates in a different study, she has the option to supply her own sexual identity in a free-response field. While the second study is more affirming of her right to self-identification, she becomes lumped into an "other" category that is heterogeneous and that lacks statistical power for comparisons.

It should come as no surprise that many LGBTQ people are reluctant to identify themselves as members of this stigmatized group for research. We have previously discussed internalized stigma, in which individuals "accept the legitimacy of society's negative regard for the stigmatized group." The more specific terms *internalized homophobia* and *internalized transphobia* are more commonly used. In health care, it is suggested that internalized stigma may manifest in the belief "that [LGBTQ patients] do not deserve respect from their health care provider or the same access to health care as heterosexuals." A similar sentiment may extend to participating in health research.

Fear of mistreatment and stigmatization is a significant barrier for many **sexual and gender minority (SGM)** people considering participation in research. In a 2001 supplement to the journal *AIDS*, McFarland and Caceres postulated that "marginalization engenders suspicion on the part of MSM [men who have sex with men] towards governmental institutions, researchers, and service providers that in turn produces barriers to social research, public health surveillance, and HIV prevention programs." The Institute of Medicine described the consequences of this suspicion: "Challenges include nonparticipation and item nonresponse (which occurs when a respondent provides some of the requested information, but certain questions are left unanswered, or certain responses are inadequate for use). Nonparticipation and nonresponse threaten the generalizability of research data to the extent that those who do not disclose their sexual orientation or transgender identity accurately, or decline to participate altogether, differ in relevant ways from those who do disclose and participate." In research terms, this is a form of selection bias.

SGM research has also been hindered by reliance on convenience and non-probability samples. For example, a convenience sample of MSM from urban night clubs may help identify an association between drug use and condomless sex, but the prevalence of these behaviors in MSM in the general population cannot be estimated from a convenience sample. Furthermore, this finding may not otherwise be generalizable to MSM.

LGBTQ people have not often been studied in terms of their unique risk factors for disease (e.g., homophobic stigma, use of cross-gender hormone therapy), nor have they been reliably included in studies that form the basis of major recommendations from organizations like the USPSTF. Some recommendations, such as colorectal cancer screening, can be translated easily to LGBTQ populations. In contrast, intimate partner violence guidelines and resources may not translate well to LGBTQ people due to heteronormative conceptualizations. LGBTQ-focused tobacco cessation campaigns may be more effective than conventional campaigns.

Chap. 13 is a more comprehensive discussion of data collection and research regarding LGBTQ health. Intentional, coordinated efforts are necessary to establish scientifically meaningful categorizations for research, to ensure inclusion in research, and to determine which areas of LGBTQ health need more study.

Key Points

- The flexibility of terms used to describe sexuality and gender and inconsistency among researchers about the best way to define and assess sexual minority status have made research with LGBTQ populations challenging.
- LGBTQ people have throughout modern history been stigmatized by the medical community, complicating their relationships with health care providers and health researchers.
- Health care providers do not receive adequate training in health issues affecting LGBTQ populations.

Violence

Introduction and Epidemiology

One manifestation of prejudice and discrimination against sexual and gender minorities is that they face disproportionate violence. Due to the protected status of LGBTQ people in the US, such violence may be classified as a **hate crime** if its motivation is governed by intentional prejudice against the group. Approximately 2000 acts of violence are reported annually against LGBT individuals, varying only slightly from year to year. However, violence affects certain LGBTQ sub-groups more heavily, placing them at greater risk of victimization by hate crimes. The highest risk LGBTQ groups are transgender people, people of color, and gay men.

Violent acts can be physical, sexual, and/or psychological. Risk factors for victimization by and perpetration of violence include substance use, acceptance of violence and dominance, hypermasculinity, and empathic deficits. Additional risk factors for LGBTQ people include facing discrimination and stigmatization from both internal and external sources and unfavorable socioeconomic factors.

Screening for violence is obviously more subjective and more influenced by contextual factors than a test for HIV or a urine drug screen. Though the health care provider may strive to maximize safety, ensure confidentiality, build rapport, ask questions without assumption or judgment, and offer appropriate resources, the patient may not be ready or able to disclose at a given time. Additionally, there are many reasons to ask about violence: to understand the patient's social context, to identify modifiable risks such as substance use, to involve law enforcement, to offer treatment for related biomedical issues (e.g., post-exposure prophylaxis for HIV), to provide trauma-informed care (including modifying the exam for comfort, referring for mental health care), and most critically, to prevent injury and homicide.

Physical Violence
Physical violence describes unwanted physical activity of a perpetrator against a victim. Risk factors for increased likelihood of violence–both perpetration and experience–correlate with experiencing maltreatment as a child, unfavorable family characteristics (e.g., substance use, mental health problems, criminal backgrounds), and

poor family relationships. Several of these risk factors are more prevalent in LGBTQ populations, and studies have demonstrated increased risk of victimization by violence amongst this population. For example, studies show that sexual minority students are 2.29 times more likely than heterosexual students to report instances of physical violence in the last 6 months.

Sexual Violence

Sexual violence is sexual activity in which consent is absent or expressed only under coercion by physical, verbal, or psychological means. LGBT individuals have been repeatedly shown to have an increased risk of experiencing sexual violence secondary to a variety of factors. Risk factors independent of sexual orientation or gender identity that increase one's risk for victimization by sexual violence include exposures to family violence, peer attitudes towards forced sex and aggression, hypermasculine environments, and multiple sexual partners. While direct causative agents for same-sex sexual violence remain unclear, several plausible contributory factors have been identified, including homophobic bullying and higher prevalence of unfavorable socioeconomic factors among LGBTQ individuals, such as homelessness.

Intimate Partner Violence

Intimate partner violence (IPV) is any type of violence—including physical and sexual—directed at an individual's partner. In the whole US population, nearly one in four adult women and approximately one in seven adult men report having experienced severe physical violence from an intimate partner in their lifetime. This abuse has significant detrimental effects on the victim, with lifelong risk of both death and disability. The CDC has developed a comprehensive list of risk factors for IPV, which are organized into four categories: individual (such as low self-esteem), relationship (such as marital conflict and instability), community (such as poverty and associated factors), and societal (such as traditional gender roles).

Recent efforts to focus on IPV among LGBTQ communities have revealed significant disparities in recognition, prevention, and support. Among LGBT individuals, risk of IPV has been shown to be as high if not higher than the US general population. Barriers to support include: legal definitions of domestic violence that exclude same-sex couples, risk of "outing" oneself when seeking help, lack of LGBT-specific or LGBT-friendly assistance resources, and discrimination from staff of service providers, law enforcement officials, and courts. In general, IPV is underreported, poorly studied, and lacks an adequate and specific public support system.

While IPV among LGBTQ individuals has similar issues with power dynamics, cycles of abuse and escalation of aggression, there are some unique factors to consider. Notably, forcing a closeted partner "out" may represent either an abuse tactic or a reason why the victim may not seek support. Intimate partners of persons with HIV have an added potential method for abuse, with threats from the partner to disclose HIV status or even withhold medications. In addition, previous experiences with psychological or physical trauma, along with violence and discrimination, hinder LGBTQ victims from seeking help when suffering from IPV. Lesbians and bisexual women in same-sex relationships also report elevated levels of rape, assault, or stalking by their partners. While poorly described in the literature, transgender persons typically face higher levels of violence throughout their lives. Clinicians should maintain a low threshold to investigate potential IPV among LGBTQ patients and be prepared to refer patients to available resources.

It is important to note that sexual and gender minority patients may fear being "outed" by the provider during the discussion of violence to authorities or other providers. Depending on the provider's state, reporting laws may complicate confidentiality. Patients should be informed of the extent to which the law limits confidentiality or obligate reporting.

Symptoms

Symptoms of violent victimization vary from person to person and may be subtle and nonspecific. Indicators of victimization vary just as widely, including any or multiple of the following depending on the type and frequency of violence:

- Injuries to the head, neck, chest, breasts, abdomen, and/or genitals
- Injuries inconsistent with the medical history or presenting symptoms
- Injuries consistent with abuse, like bilateral or multiple injuries in varying stages of healing
- Repeated visits to the provider for vague complaints, such as fatigue
- Somatic symptoms
- Secrecy and discomfort when asked about a relationship
- Controlling or possessive partners
- High frequency of sexually transmitted infections, pregnancies, miscarriages, and abortions
- Missed appointments
- Social isolation

The diagnosis of victimization by violence is clinical and depends on appropriate assessment of risk factors and screening questions.

Screening

For ethical and methodological reasons, screening tools are difficult to study. Screening tools vary in their focus (e.g., past sexual assault versus very recent intimate partner violence), in the target population (e.g., white women in the emergency department), and in the administration method (e.g., self-report on paper). No single tool stands out as best in comparative studies. Evidence of improved outcomes is not sufficiently robust for the USPSTF to recommend universal screening (Table 5.3). However, the American Medical Association recommends that physicians "routinely inquire about physical, sexual, and psychological abuse as part of the medical history," and most major specialty organizations recommend improving physician awareness of and response to IPV.

Generic questions about physical violence can set the stage for more sensitive questions and can also identify interpersonal violence by persons who are not intimate partners:

Table 5.3 Recommendation for intimate partner violence screening

Population	Organization	Recommendation
Women of reproductive age	USPSTF 2018	The USPSTF recommends that clinicians screen for intimate partner violence (IPV) in women of reproductive age and provide or refer women who screen positive to ongoing support services.

- "In the last 12 months, has anyone hit, kicked, pushed, or otherwise threatened you?"
- "Do you worry about your physical safety in your neighborhood?"
- "Are there any weapons in your home, including guns?"
- "When you are upset, do you ever want to harm or injure somebody? Has that happened?"
- "When was the last time anyone threatened or hurt you because of your sexual orientation [or gender identity]?"

GLMA: Health Professionals Advancing LGBTQ Equality recommends that screening for sexual violence should involve the following questions:

- "Have you ever been hurt (physically or sexually) by someone you are close to or involved with, or by a stranger?"
- "Are you currently being hurt by someone you are close to or involved with?"
- "Have you ever experienced violence or abuse?"
- "Have you ever been sexually assaulted or raped?"

Screening for physical and psychological abuse can involve additional questioning to assess for abuse or **bullying**. Consider asking patients—especially youth and adolescents—about the following:

- Interactions with peers and possible exposure to bullying
- New onset of phobias (of school, work environment), psychosomatic conditions, or attention problems

- Safety at the home or workplace
- New onset of depression, anxiety, or other psychiatric problems

Regarding screening for IPV, research indicates that the question "Do you feel safe at home?" is ineffective. This question has been shown to have a false negative rate of 80%, with most women who experienced violent victimization answering "yes" to this screening question. Instead, it is suggested to ask specific questions about IPV. The HITS screen is a validated tool for asking a patient how often their partner Hits, Insults, Threatens, or Screams at them.

In summary, major organizations vary in the degree to which they support universal screening for IPV. Screening of all reproductive-aged (presumably cisgender) women is not controversial. In other populations, there is currently neither substantial evidence of harm nor benefit for universal screening. However, **patients presenting with signs, symptoms, or other red flags potentially related to IPV should be evaluated**, either with validated tools or in-depth interview. In this situation, the evaluation is an indicated prevention strategy. Providers must take care not to apply stereotypic or heteronormative thinking when possible signs or symptoms of IPV are present.

Tools that have high sensitivity, that make no assumptions about gender, and that have been validated in both men and women are probably suitable for LGBTQ people. Providers should also be mindful of the scope of questionnaires; they vary significantly for range of time assessed, validation in other languages, and content about sexual assault, sexual violence, access to guns, and perpetration history.

Treatment

Treating injuries associated with violence is only the first step in helping a victim of violence. While providing medications and treatment for acute or emergent needs is necessary, it is also important to minimize the probability of a repeat incident. Patients should be queried regarding extent of violence, injuries sustained, sexual health concerns, reproductive health concerns, mental health concerns including suicidal ideation, homicide treats, patient or partner use of alcohol or illicit drug use, access to guns, attempts to leave, and the involvement of any children (possibly triggering a mandatory Child Protective Services report). The physical exam should include an injury survey, pregnancy test if applicable, and STI checks. In cases of rape, post-exposure prophylaxis for STIs and HIV is indicated. Management of these concerns can be challenging due to partner-patient dynamics and power imbalances.

Recommending that the patient avoid returning to the same environment is insufficient. The patient's safety in the current situation should be maximized, including developing a safety plan and escape plan in case of emergency. The patient's should be discreetly informed of resources, including IPV organizations and shelters. Health care providers can assist in identifying cycles of power and control in relationships but should avoid taking unilateral actions when the patient is otherwise competent to make personal decisions. There is considerable potential for health care providers to aid their patients.

Readers may find more information by consulting the National Center on Domestic and Sexual Violence (NCDSV), the National Coalition of Anti-Violence Programs (NCAVP), and the National LGBTQ Institute on IPV.

Key Points
- Violence against LGBTQ individuals is a real threat and most commonly takes the form of physical, sexual, and intimate partner violence.
- Providers should be aware of symptoms of violence and perform screens of patients they suspect to be at risk.
- If a provider identifies a victim of violence, it is appropriate to offer additional care to the victim.

Mental Health

Universal screening is recommended for depression but not for suicide risk (Table 5.4). Assessing suicidality (suicidal ideations and suicidal behaviors) is appropriate in persons with symptomatic mental illness. Criteria for major depressive disorder and warning signs for suicide are presented in Tables 12.2 and 12.4, respectively. Epidemiology of mental illness in SGM people is discussed in Chap. 12.

The most commonly used instrument for screening for depression in primary care environments is the Patient Health Questionaire-2 (PHQ-2). The patient is queried:

Over the past 2 weeks, how often have you been bothered by any of the following problems?

Table 5.4 Recommendations for screening of depression and suicide risk

Population	Organization	Recommendation
General adult population, including pregnant and postpartum [persons]	USPSTF 2016	The USPSTF recommends screening for depression in the general adult population, including pregnant and postpartum [persons]. Screening should be implemented with adequate systems in place to ensure accurate diagnosis, effective treatment, and appropriate follow-up.
Adolescents aged 12–18 years	USPSTF 2016	The USPSTF recommends screening for major depressive disorder (MDD) in adolescents aged 12–18 years. Screening should be implemented with adequate systems in place to ensure accurate diagnosis, effective treatment, and appropriate follow-up (category B).
Adolescents, adults, and older adults	USPSTF 2014	The USPSTF concludes that the current evidence is insufficient to assess the balance of benefits and harms of screening for suicide risk in adolescents, adults, and older adults in primary care (category I).

- *Little interest or pleasure in doing things*
- *Feeling down, depressed or hopeless*

The patient answers not at all (0), several days (1), more than half the days (2), or nearly every day (3) to each question. A total score of three or greater triggers completing the longer PHQ-9. If suicidal ideations or significant depression are reported, further evaluation by a mental health professional, safety planning, and/or a follow-up plan should be considered. SAD PERSONS (Table 10.11) is a useful tool for evaluating the need for hospitalization. However, it is not a substitute for a safety evaluation by a trained professional. Available screening tools for suicide risk are poor. In the LGBTQ patient—especially adolescents—abuse, bullying, family rejection, and homelessness should be included in the evaluation. Family acceptance in LGBTQ adolescents is the most important protective factor. The clinician should maintain a somewhat higher index of suspicion for suicide risk in LGBTQ patients than patients in general.

Other commonly used screening tools are the GAD-7 for generalized anxiety disorder, PC-PTSD for post-traumatic stress disorder in the primary care environment, and the Geriatric Depression Scale (GDS) for depression in persons over 60. These screening tools are employed as selective prevention strategies in selected settings or populations or as an indicated strategy for individuals at the discretion of a health care professional.

Substance Use

Introduction and Epidemiology

LGBT individuals experience higher prevalence of smoking, alcohol use, and other substance use than the general population. The potential cause of this disparity has been studied, and the most significant and most universal risk factor remains increased social stress in the context of discrimination. Additionally, decreased family support and socioeconomic stability contribute to significant increase in substance use.

Smoking prevalence is significantly increased among LGBTQ individuals. Gay, bisexual, and transgender men have been shown to smoke an average of 50% more than other men, and lesbian, bisexual, and transgender women have been shown to smoke nearly 200% more than other women. Recent data show that self-reported smoking prevalence has reached 20.5% among lesbian and gay individuals, 28.6% among bisexual individuals, and 15.3% among straight individuals. The high prevalence has been linked to deliberate targeting of LGBTQ youth by tobacco advertisement, which has caused LGBTQ individuals to continue smoking into adulthood more often than the general population. In addition to smoking more frequently at a younger age, additional risk factors specific to smoking include lower educational attainment, low socioeconomic status, depression, stress, victimization by violence, and concurrent alcohol use.

Compared to the data regarding smoking, data about alcohol use among LGBT individuals is more heterogeneous. Mixed results among surveys have shown adult LGBT populations to have drinking prevalence either equivalent to or higher drinking than the general population. LGBT youth, however, consistently show higher prevalence of alcohol use than the general population, with surveys showing 72.2% alcohol use prevalence among some populations of LGBT youth when compared to 60.9% in comparable non-LGBT populations. Interestingly, this disparity may not impact long-term alcohol use habits, and alcohol use prevalence normalizes after 18 years of age. The risks factors predisposing LGBTQ individuals to alcohol use are hypothesized to include peer modeling, minority group stigmatization, and experiencing homophobia.

The descriptive epidemiology of recreational drug use is covered in Chap. 12.

Symptoms

Substance use disorder is defined by motivation—cognitive, behavioral, and physiological—towards a substance despite harm caused by the substance. Usually, substance use disorders are associated with both an intoxication effect and a withdrawal syndrome, although only one or neither may be seen.

Screening

It is up to the provider's clinical reasoning to assess potential benefits and harms of evaluating a patient for illicit drug use (Table 5.5). The most common method for screening for illicit substances is toxicology of the urine, although questionnaires are useful under many circumstances. Urine drug screening is usually performed with the patient's knowledge.

Assessment of tobacco use is now the standard of care in virtually all health care settings (Table 5.6). For tobacco, both the form of tobacco and the cumulative exposure (e.g., cigarettes in pack-years based on 20 cigarettes per pack) should be documented. A significant threshold used in research is whether a patient has smoked 100 or more cigarettes. If so, the patient is a current smoker or former smoker rather than a nonsmoker. Conversion factors can be used when patients use cigarillos, cigars, or pipe tobacco.

Screening for unhealthy alcohol use is also the standard of care in virtually all health care settings for patients 18 and older (Table 5.7). Various brief questionnaires can be used in the primary care setting, such as the abbreviated Alcohol Use Disorders Identification Test–Consumption (AUDIT-C). The Cut Down, Annoyed, Guilty, Eye-Opener (CAGE) questionnaire is a tool used to screen for alcohol dependence, but it does not capture the full spectrum of unhealthy alcohol use. AUDIT-C and CAGE

Table 5.5 Recommendation for screening for illicit drug use

Population	Organization	Recommendation
Adolescents, adults, and pregnant [persons]	USPSTF 2008	The USPSTF concludes that the current evidence is insufficient to assess the balance of benefits and harms of screening adolescents, adults, and pregnant [persons] for illicit drug use (grade I).

Table 5.6 Recommendations for tobacco evaluation, counseling, and treatment

Population	Organization	Recommendation
Adults who are not pregnant	USPSTF 2015	The USPSTF recommends that clinicians ask all adults about tobacco use, advise them to stop using tobacco, and provide behavioral interventions and US Food and Drug Administration (FDA)–approved pharmacotherapy for cessation to adults who use tobacco (category A).
Pregnant [persons]	USPSTF 2015	The USPSTF recommends that clinicians ask all pregnant [persons] about tobacco use, advise them to stop using tobacco, and provide behavioral interventions for cessation to pregnant [persons] who use tobacco (category A).
School-aged children and adolescents	USPSTF 2013	The USPSTF recommends that primary care clinicians provide interventions, including education or brief counseling, to prevent initiation of tobacco use among school-aged children and adolescents (category B).

Table 5.7 Recommendation for screening and brief intervention of alcohol use

Population	Organization	Recommendation
Adults 18 years or older, including pregnant [persons]	USPSTF 2018	The USPSTF recommends screening for unhealthy alcohol use in primary care settings in adults 18 years or older, including pregnant [persons], and providing persons engaged in risky or hazardous drinking with brief behavioral counseling interventions to reduce unhealthy alcohol use (category B).

sometimes use lower cut-offs for women. For transgender and nonbinary people, it is reasonable to score congruent with gender identity or by using the more conservative (more sensitive,

less specific) cut-off. A questionnaire for identifying risky substance use in adolescents ages 12–18 is Car, Relax, Alone, Forget, Family, Friends, Trouble (CRAFFT).

> **External Resource 5.2**
> The Substance Abuse and Mental Health Services Administration (SAMHSA) and Health Resources Services Administration (HRSA) manage the **Center for Integrated Health Solutions**, a national training and technical assistance center that promotes the development of integrated primary and behavioral health services and related workforce development. They have aggregated some of the best available screening tools for mental health and substance use. http://bit.ly/TECe1ch05_01

Moderate drinking under *US Dietary Guidelines for Americans 2015–2020* is considered as no more than one drink per day for women and two drinks per day for men. Binge drinking is a pattern of drinking that results in a blood alcohol concentration of 0.08 g or higher, typically when men consume five or more drinks or women consume four or more drinks in about two hours. A 2018 systematic review of alcohol research found that sex assigned at birth and gender identity are poorly operationalized in alcohol exposures studies, making current recommendations difficult to translate to transgender people. Whatever the threshold, the most significant short-term issue is whether alcohol interferes with the patient's normal functioning, increases risk-taking, or results in harm. Longer-term biomedical risks include cirrhosis, cardiovascular disease, cognitive impairment, and various cancers should also be discussed when providing patient education about drinking guidelines.

Treatment

The treatment of intoxication or withdrawal syndromes for illicit drugs is beyond the scope of this text. However, it is important to recognize that both pharmacological and behavioral methods may be required to achieve remission and decrease probability of relapse. For example, a person recovering from opioid addiction may benefit from drugs such as naltrexone, buprenorphine-naloxone, or methadone; individual psychotherapy such as cognitive behavioral therapy or motivational enhancement; and therapy or peer groups such as Narcotics Anonymous.

1-800-QUIT-NOW is the nation's tobacco cessation hotline. Patients attempting to quit tobacco can receive limited supplies of nicotine replacement therapy like patches, gum, and lozenges for free. Some health systems also have specialized tobacco cessation clinics. Prescriptions approved for tobacco cessation are bupropion and varenicline. Evidence supports developing a quit plan and setting a quit date. When multiple strategies are used together, the likelihood of success greatly increases.

> **External Resource 5.3**
> Smokefree.gov and the **truth initiative** also include special outreach campaigns for LGBTQ people. https://smokefree.gov/; https://truthinitiative.org

After acute alcohol detoxification is safely completed, alcohol addiction can be treated with medications such as naltrexone (oral or long-acting injectable), acamprosate, or disulfiram; individual or group therapy; and 12-step peer support programs such as Alcoholics Anonymous, SMART Recovery, or Double Trouble in Recovery for dual diagnosis. Peer support groups typically have lists of regional meetings, some of which are intended for LGBTQ people.

> **Key Points**
> • LGBTQ individuals are at a significant risk for substance use disorders, including tobacco, alcohol, and illicit substances.

> • The provider should rely on clinical reasoning when deciding when and how to screen for illicit substances.
> • Alcohol and tobacco use should be assessed in every adult patient periodically.
> • It is appropriate to treat any individual with a substance use disorder for the addiction and to counsel for cessation.

Cancer

In general, unless otherwise noted, the LGBTQ population and non-LGBTQ population should be screened according to already existing age-appropriate guidelines. Transgender individuals with natal parts remaining (e.g., FtM individuals who have a cervix) should have age-appropriate screenings that reflect **anatomic inventory**. As discussed at the beginning of this chapter, sexual orientation and gender identity questions have typically not been included as a variable in research for screening guidelines.

Although the tendency is to group LGBTQ people together for the purposes of discussion, research suggests that screening guidelines for cancer should be better aligned with each subpopulation. Studies including lesbians, gay men, bisexuals, and transgender people suggest distinct and dense clusters of risk factors that significantly raise their risk for developing certain cancers. Coupled with already-lower screening frequency in LGBTQ people, cancers are detected at later stages, resulting in poor prognosis and exacerbating health disparities.

Colorectal and Lung Cancer

Colorectal and lung cancers are the leading causes of cancer-related deaths. Screening guidelines for colorectal and lung cancer can be applied to LGBTQ people without modification, especially given that cumulative tobacco exposure is a condition for low-dose computed tomography

Table 5.8 Recommendations for colorectal and lung cancer screening

Population	Organization	Recommendation
Adults aged 50–75 years	USPSTF 2016	The USPSTF recommends screening for colorectal cancer starting at age 50 years and continuing until age 75 years (category A).
Adults aged 55–80 with a history of smoking	USPSTF 2013	The USPSTF recommends annual screening for lung cancer with low-dose computed tomography (LDCT) in adults aged 55–80 years who have a 30 pack-year smoking history and currently smoke or have quit within the past 15 years. Screening should be discontinued once a person has not smoked for 15 years or develops a health problem that substantially limits life expectancy or the ability or willingness to have curative lung surgery (category B).

Table 5.9 Recommendations for cervical cancer screening

Population	Organization	Recommendation
Women aged 21–65 years	USPSTF 2018	The USPSTF recommends screening for cervical cancer every 3 years with cervical cytology alone in women aged 21–29 years. For women aged 30–65 years, the USPSTF recommends screening every 3 years with cervical cytology alone, every 5 years with high-risk human papillomavirus (hrHPV) testing alone, or every 5 years with hrHPV testing in combination with cytology (cotesting) (category A).
Persons aged 21–65 years with a cervix, including transgender and nonbinary persons	Center of Excellence for Transgender Health	As above, not limited to cisgender woman.

screening for lung cancer (Table 5.8). Frequency of colorectal cancer screening depends on the method. Stool-based tests are typically annual; colonoscopy every 10 years; CT colonography every five years; and flexible sigmoidoscopy every five years or, when paired with a fecal immunochemical test, every 10 years. Availability of flexible sigmoidoscopy is declining in the US.

Cervical Cancer

Despite being at risk for exposure to HPV and cervical dysplasia, lesbians and bisexual women have been shown to get routine screening Pap exams less often than heterosexual women. Routine screening guidelines should be followed for all women (Table 5.9). Women with HIV are at increased risk of cervical dysplasia, and consequently, screening recommendations differ for this population. Women should have two Pap smears 6 months apart in the first year following diagnosis with HIV. If the results of these initial two tests are normal, yearly Pap smears should be obtained thereafter. Any abnormal results should be managed according to guidelines published elsewhere.

Female-to-male (FtM) transgender patients present a unique challenge to the clinician. There are case reports of gynecologic cancers in FtM patients, though they are few in number. FtM patients who have not undergone hysterectomy or who still have a cervix should be advised that routine Pap tests are recommended. Exogenous testosterone can induce changes to the cervical cells, so FtM patients have a high unsatisfactory sample prevalence compared to cis-gender females. In addition, gynecological exams can be extremely uncomfortable and distressing for FtM patients not only because of gender dysphoria, but also because exogenous testosterone can cause decreased vaginal secretions and contribute to vaginal atrophy. Providers can increase comfort for these patients in several ways, the most important of which is asking the patient what would make the exam more tolerable. Providers should consider allowing patients to have a support person present, using the smallest speculum possible, using sufficient lubricant, and using neutral language (e.g., "I'm separating your tissue" vs. "I'm separating the labia") or patient-preferred alternative language for their anatomy.

In general, Pap smears in MtF transgender persons are not indicated in a surgically constructed neovagina. For transwomen who have had gender confirmation surgery, it is appropriate, however, to do periodic speculum exams to inspect the neovagina and vulva for lesions.

External Resource 5.4
Sherbourne Health Centre in southeast Toronto launched a campaign to improve Pap screening in trans men called **Check It Out Guys**. http://www.checkitoutguys.ca

Breast and Ovarian Cancer

Recent systematic reviews conclude that no published data support a higher incidence of breast cancer among lesbians and bisexual women. Population density estimates, however, do suggest higher incidence of breast cancer among lesbians and lower incidence among bisexual women. Given the discrepancy among data and the overall prevalence and mortality of breast cancer, recommending that lesbians and bisexual women receive routine screening remains paramount. Lesbians and bisexual women have more risk factors for developing breast cancer. Nulliparity and obesity are both associated with development of breast cancer and are common in lesbian and bisexual women. Greater tobacco use and alcohol consumption may contribute as well. While poor access to health care may be another risk factor, some studies show that there is no significant difference in mammography utilization between lesbian and bisexual women and their heterosexual counterparts.

While limited data are available, there does not appear to be an increased risk of breast cancer among transgender individuals using testosterone or estrogen. That being said, MtF persons should

be offered mammography at age 50 and older after they have at least five years of exposure to feminizing hormones. With a positive family history, the age requirement may be lowered based on clinical judgment. FtM patients should have routine breast cancer screening per recommendations if they have not had complete chest reconstruction or if they have only had breast reduction. These are recommendations from the Center of Excellence for Transgender Health. The USPSTF has not promulgated any clear guidelines on this issue yet (Table 5.10).

While many factors that are risks for ovarian cancer (obesity, less frequent and delayed parity, tobacco use, etc.) are more prevalent in lesbians, there are very limited data on whether the incidence of ovarian cancer is higher in lesbians. The USPSTF recommends against routine screening for ovarian cancer.

Table 5.10 Recommendations for breast cancer screening

Population	Organization	Recommendation
Women aged 50–74 years	USPSTF 2016	The USPSTF recommends biennial screening mammography for women aged 50–74 years (category B).
Women aged 40–49 years	USPSTF 2016	The decision to start screening mammography in women prior to age 50 years should be an individual one. Women who place a higher value on the potential benefit than the potential harms may choose to begin biennial screening between the ages of 40 and 49 years (category C).
Natal females including transgender men and nonbinary persons	Center of Excellence for Transgender Health	Biennial screening mammography is appropriate for natal females 50–74 who have breasts, even after breast reduction. Persons with total mastectomy or complete chest reconstruction do not require screening mammography. With improved evidence, persons on testosterone for many years could be excluded.

Anal Cancer

Incidence of anal cancer has been steadily climbing in the US over the past few decades. Factors associated with increased risk of anal cancer include tobacco use, receptive anal sex (in females or males), history of cervical or vulvar dysplasia, and immunocompromised state due to organ transplants or HIV. Incidence of anal cancer is particularly high in HIV-positive MSM. A thorough history is an essential part of early detection of anal cancer. Health care providers should ask individuals about anorectal symptoms (discomfort, lesions, rectal bleeding, pain, itching, etc.) and risk factors (history of STI infection, HPV-related malignancies, tobacco use, receptive intercourse, etc.) as part of a routine screening visit.

Human papillomaviruses (HPV), notably HPV-16 and 18, are known to cause dysplastic changes in the squamocolumnar junction (the transformation zone) between the rectum and anus and at the uterine cervix. Given the tremendous success of cervical cancer screenings since the advent of the Papanicolau smear, new focus has been placed on anal cancer. Those most at risk include MSM and those with immunosuppression, notably HIV infection. Most estimates show that anal HPV is quite prevalent among MSM: nearly 65% of men without HIV and 90% of those with HIV have tested positive for anal HPV. HPV causes approximately 80% of anal cancers. HPV vaccination may eventually obviate the need for screening programs for women and perhaps men.

While there are some data that anal Pap testing is a cost-effective screening test for men and women who are at an increased risk of squamous cell carcinoma of the anus (SCCA), currently there are no published consensus guidelines that recommend routine screening anal cancer screening. Neither the USPSTF, nor the Infectious Diseases Society of America, nor the American Cancer Society recommends routine anal Pap smears. The Department of Veterans Affairs recommends that "all at-risk men and women should be screened for anal cancer at baseline and annually thereafter by digital rectal examination (DRE)." In their guidelines for screening and management of anal squamous neoplasms, the American Society of Colon and Rectal Surgeons acknowledges that the quality of evidence for screening is low but still makes a recommendation that anal Pap tests may be useful in the detection of precursor lesions (low grade and high grade anal intraepithelial neoplasia). The New York State Department of Health AIDS Institute also recommends routine anal cancer screening as a targeted intervention for persons with HIV. Those recommendations include a yearly review of anogenital symptoms, a visual inspection of the anogenital region and a digital rectal exam for all HIV-positive adults regardless of age. They also recommend yearly anal cytology for HIV-positive MSM, any patient with a history of anogenital condyloma and for women who have a history of cervical or vaginal dysplasia.

If an anal Pap is abnormal, or if there is a visible or palpable lesion on exam, referral for high resolution anoscopy is warranted. However, inexperienced anoscopists may not provide adequate sensitivity to produce improved results. While the slow progression of AIN to anal cancer suggests that aggressive management may be unnecessary, further investigation is required.

> **Key Points**
> - In general, the LGB population should be offered cancer screenings according to already-existing age-appropriate guidelines.
> - Transgender individuals should be offered age-appropriate cancer screenings for their current anatomy.
> - While there are no published consensus guidelines for anal cancer screenings, it is reasonable to offer anal Pap smears to individuals at increased risk of anal cancer (tobacco use, receptive anal sex, history of cervical or vulvar dysplasia, and immunocompromised state due to organ transplant or HIV).

Infectious Disease

See Chap. 8 for an in-depth discussion of STIs and Chap. 11 for an in-depth discussion of HIV/AIDS. Chap. 8 discusses screening criteria and testing intervals for STIs in terms of SGM subpopulations. Here, it is useful to consider infectious disease prevention in terms of identifying infected individuals, treating infected individuals, and mitigating risk in uninfected persons using behavioral and biomedical methods.

The USPSTF recommends HIV testing during every pregnancy and at least one lifetime HIV test for persons aged 15–65 (category A). Depending on risk factors, HIV tests can be given a few times yearly. Treatment of HIV is also prevention. A person with undetectable viral load is extremely unlikely to transmit the virus.

Barrier methods, prophylactic medication, immunization, and behavior modification are broadly applicable preventive strategies for pathogens. A relatively recent development is the prophylactic use of antiretrovirals in persons without HIV, called pre-exposure prophylaxis (PrEP). As of 2018, the USPSTF has produced a draft recommendation for PrEP and solicited feedback (Table 5.11). PrEP and high-risk classifications are discussed further in Chap. 11.

Table 5.11 HPV vaccines

Vaccine formulation	Population	Schedule
HPV Bivalent Strains 16, 18	Females 9 through 25 years old	3 doses at 0, 1, 6 months
HPV Quadrivalent Strains 6, 18, 16, 18	Girls, women, boys, and men 9 through 26 years old	3 doses at 0, 2, and 6 months
HPV 9-valent Strains 6, 11, 16, 18, 31, 33, 45, 52, 58	Females and males 9 through 45 years old	2 doses at 0, 6–12 months between 9 and 14 years old *or* 3 doses at 0, 2, 6 months between 9 and 45 years old

Package inserts refer to sex assigned at birth. Bivalent vaccine is for persons with a cervix. Quadrivalent and 9-valent vaccines are for all genders

Table 5.12 Draft recommendation for pre-exposure prophylaxis for HIV

Population	Organization	Draft recommendation
Persons at high risk of HIV acquisition	USPSTF	The USPSTF recommends that clinicians offer pre-exposure prophylaxis (PrEP) with effective antiretroviral therapy to persons who are at high risk of HIV acquisition (category A).

Persons with HIV, injection drug users, persons living with or having sex with someone with hepatitis B, MSM, and some foreign-born groups are recommended for serologic screening of hepatitis B by the USPSTF (category B). Data are limited in transgender people. Immunization against hepatitis A and B is universally recommended in infancy for everyone but also in adulthood for MSM, injection and noninjection drug users, persons with HIV, some travelers, and some medically vulnerable groups.

Vaccines for human papillomavirus (HPV) have covered progressively more strains of HPV and wider age ranges. The 9-valent vaccine covers HPV strains 16 and 18 (high risk strains accounting for over 70% of cervical cancers); 31, 33, 45, 52, and 58 (other high-risk strains); and 6 and 11 (low risk strains causing genital warts). The 9-valent vaccine is approved for the prevention of cervical, vulvar, vaginal, and anal cancers caused by HPV. HPV is thought to account for 70% of oropharyngeal cancers in the US, suggesting another potential benefit of immunization. Table 5.12 summarizes the coverage and approved populations for HPV immunizations.

Bone Density Screening

Sex steroids are physiologically important for bone health and prevention of fractures. Both estrogen and testosterone at physiologic levels are known to have a net effect of decreasing bone resorption (the relative contribution of each to both bone formation and resorption is beyond the scope of this text). Consequently, lower levels of

Table 5.13 Recommendations for bone density screening

Population	Organization	Recommendation
Women 65 years and older	USPSTF 2018	The USPSTF recommends screening for osteoporosis with bone measurement testing to prevent osteoporotic fractures in women 65 years and older (category B).
Postmenopausal women younger than 65 years at increased risk of osteoporosis	USPSTF 2018	The USPSTF recommends screening for osteoporosis with bone measurement testing to prevent osteoporotic fractures in postmenopausal women younger than 65 years who are at increased risk of osteoporosis, as determined by a formal clinical risk assessment tool (category B).
Transgender people	Center of Excellence for Transgender Health	Transgender people (regardless of birth-assigned sex) should begin bone density screening at age 65. Screening between ages 50 and 64 should be considered for those with established risk factors for osteoporosis. Transgender people (regardless of birth assigned sex) who have undergone gonadectomy and have a history of at least 5 years without hormone replacement should also be considered for bone density testing, regardless of age.
Transgender people without gonads and without hormone therapy	Center of Excellence for Transgender Health	Transgender people without gonads, and who are not using hormone replacement, should follow screening and prevention guidelines for agonadal or postmenopausal women, regardless of birth-assigned sex or gender identity.

sex steroids due to menopause and gonadectomy result in decreasing bone mineral density. Therefore, there are parallels between bone density screening recommendations in cisgender women and transgender people (Table 5.13).

Conclusions

Prevention recommendations that do not specify gender or sex are almost always applicable sexual and gender minorities as well. Closer scrutiny to recommendations is needed when reproductive physiology, sexual behaviors, and personal anatomy are more variable, or in conditions that are sensitive to the effects of marginalization and discrimination (e.g., depression, substance use). The future is likely to bring more evidence-based recommendations that apply to specific subgroups of sexual and gender minorities.

This chapter has given significant attention to clinical prevention guidelines, but some of the most significant prevention opportunities lie outside of the walls of hospitals and clinics, addressing broader social determinants of health in LGBTQ populations. Effective interventions are likely to reverse or mitigate root causes of LGBTQ health inequities with diverse public health approaches.

Boards-Style Application Questions

Question 1. A 22-year-old male named Greg presents to clinic for a wellness exam. As part of a thorough history, you ask about sexual history, sexual orientation, gender identity, partners, and exposures. He initially identifies as a straight cisgender male. Upon further questioning, he has a history of exclusively male sexual partners and says that he's "probably bisexual." He is in a nonmonogamous relationship with a cisgender male and uses condoms infrequently. How would you classify this patient's sexual behavior?

A. MSM
B. MSF
C. Bisexual
D. Gay
E. Straight

Question 2. How would you classify Greg's sexual identity?

A. MSM
B. MSF
C. Bisexual
D. Gay
E. Straight

Question 3. Which of the following questions would be most appropriate to screen for intimate partner violence (IPV)?

A. Do you feel safe at home?
B. Have you ever been hurt by someone close to you?
C. Have you lost interest in things you usually enjoy?
D. All of the above
E. B & C only

Question 4. A 35-year-old female-to-male (FtM) patient named Erick presents to your office to establish care with you. During introductions, you ascertain by asking that this patient uses the pronouns *he*, *him,* and *his*. He has been on testosterone for about five years and is happy with his physical changes, but has not yet been able to afford hysterectomy or chest reconstruction. He has never had a Pap smear since "that kind of checkup freaks me out." He smokes about a half pack of cigarettes per day but has smoked as much as two packs per day at some point in his life. He identifies as pansexual and has had multiple sexual partners in the past year which include transmen, cis women, and cis men. What screening tests should he be offered?

A. Cervical cancer screening (Pap smear)
B. Lung cancer screening
C. Mammogram
D. STI testing
E. All of the above
F. A and D only

Question 5. After some discussion, Erick agrees to have a cervical cancer screen. What are some techniques that you can use to make this exam more comfortable for your patient?

A. Asking him if there are certain words he prefer that you use or avoid
B. Scheduling the exam on a different day when he can bring a support person
C. Using the smallest speculum available
D. All of the above

Question 6. Your next patient is a 50-year-old transgender woman who is coming in for her routine complete physical. She had gender affirmation surgery many years ago and has been on stable doses of estrogen for over a decade. Her only medical issue is obesity, with a BMI of 41. She is in a long-term monogamous relationship with her cisgender female partner of many years. What routine screening tests should you offer this patient?

A. Colon cancer screening
B. Mammogram
C. Pap smear of the neovagina
D. STI screening
E. All of the above
F. A and B only
G. A, B, and C only

Boards-Style Application Questions Answer Key

Question 1. The correct answer is A. Sexual orientation (options C, D, and E) does not indicate sexual behavior, or vice versa. It can only be said regarding sexual behavior that Greg is man who has sex with men. MSF (option B) is not used to refer to any sexual behavior.

Question 2. The correct answer is C. *Bisexual* is his self-identification. His sexual history lacking contact with women is irrelevant, so it would be inappropriate to call him gay both because the word does not describe sexual behaviors and because it is not the identification he used for himself (option D). A person's current sexual identity or sexual orientation could be straight even without history of romantic or attraction to women (E). MSF (B) is not used to refer to any sexual behavior.

Question 3. The correct answer is E. Despite its continuing popularity, (A) has been demonstrated to have very low sensitivity. Option B would be correct on its. It is a good question because it is objective and is on the HITS screening, which has been validated in men and women. Option C is a question about anhedonia, which is a common depression symptom in abused persons that is reasonable to ask about, but it is non-specific to intimate partner violence.

Question 4. The correct answer is F. STI testing is indicated based on his recent sexual history (option D). Erick does not require mammograms at his age (C) unless less there is breast cancer in a first degree relative occurring at a young age. If he gets total chest reconstruction, he will never need mammograms, but they are still indicated after breast reduction. Low-dose computed tomography (B) for lung cancer screening applies only to those who have accumulated enough pack-years of smoking and who are between 55 and 88 years old. Everyone with a cervix between ages 21 and 65 needs Pap smears, though the frequency may vary.

Question 5. The correct answer is D. In the long term, it is best to prevent adverse experiences that will dissuade Erick from future screenings. It is clear that (A) and (B) demonstrate personal respect by not using invalidating vocabulary and minimizing anxiety, respectively. It is particularly important to use small specula in trans men using hormones due to vaginal changes from testosterone therapy (C).

Question 6. The correct answer is F. Colon cancer screening (option A) is indicated in all persons starting at 50, or younger depending on family history. Mammograms (B) are recommended in transgender women if they are at least 50 *and* have had at least five years estrogen and progesterone use. High-risk clinical factors like family history suggest considering younger starting age. Surgically constructed neovaginas do not require Paps (C). Her sexual history is very low risk, obviating the need for STI screening (D).

Sources

American Medical Association. Opinion 2.02: physicians' obligations in preventing, identifying, and treating violence and abuse. Chicago: American Medical Association; 2008. http://www.ama-assn.org/ama/pub/physician-resources/medical-ethics/code-medical-ethics/opinion202.page. Accessed 21 Jan 2019.

Arroll B, Goodyear-Smith F, Crengle S, et al. Validation of PHQ-2 and PHQ-9 to screen for major depression in the primary care population. Ann Fam Med. 2010;8(4):348–53. https://doi.org/10.1370/afm.1139.

Buchmueller T, Carpenter CS. Disparities in health insurance coverage, access, and outcomes for individuals in same-sex versus different-sex relationships, 2000-2007. Am J Public Health. 2010;100(3):489–95. https://doi.org/10.2105/AJPH.2009.160804.

Centers for Disease Control and Prevention. Intimate partner violence: risk and protective factors. http://www.cdc.gov/ViolencePrevention/intimatepartnerviolence/riskprotectivefactors.html. Accessed 20 Dec 2012.

Centers for Disease Control and Prevention. Current cigarette smoking among adults—United States, 2016. MMWR Morb Mortal Wkly Rep. 2018;67(2):53–9.

Centers for Disease Control. Recommended immunization schedule for adults aged 19 or older, United States; 2018. https://www.cdc.gov/vaccines/schedules/hcp/imz/adult.html. Accessed 21 Jan 2019.

Chen PH, Rovi S, Vega M, Jacobs A, Johnson MS. Screening for domestic violence in predominantly Hispanic clinical settings. Fam Pract. 2005;22(6):617–23.

Cochran SD, Mays VM, Bowen D, et al. Cancer-related risk indicators and preventive screening behaviors among lesbians and bisexual women. Am J Public Health. 2001;91(4):591–7.

Coulter RWS, Jun HJ, Calzo JP, et al. Sexual-orientation differences in alcohol use trajectories and disorders in emerging adulthood: results from a longitudinal cohort study in the United States. Addiction. 2018; 113(9):1619–32. https://doi.org/10.1111/add.14251.

Daley AE, Macdonnell JA. Gender, sexuality and the discursive representation of access and equity in health services literature: implications for LGBT communities. Int J Equity Health. 2011;10:40. https://doi.org/10.1186/1475-9276-10-40.

Deutsch M. Guidelines for the primary and gender-affirming care of transgender and gender nonbinary people. 2nd ed. San Francisco: UCSF; 2019. http://transhealth.ucsf.edu/pdf/Transgender-PGACG-6-17-16.pdf. Accessed 19 Jan 2019.

Gatos KC. A literature review of cervical cancer screening in transgender men. Nurs Womens Health. 2018;22(1):52–62. https://doi.org/10.1016/j.nwh.2017.12.008.

Gilbert PA, Pass LE, Keuroghlian AS, Greenfield TK, Reisner SL. Alcohol research with transgender populations: a systematic review and recommendations to strengthen future studies. Drug Alcohol Depend. 2018;186(1):138–46.

Green DP, Mcfalls LH, Smith JK. Hate Crime: an emergent research agenda. Annu Rev Sociol. 2001;27:479–504.

Grulich AE, Poynten IM, Machalek DA, Jin F, Templeton DJ, Hillman RJ. The epidemiology of anal cancer. Sex Health. 2012;9(6):504–8. https://doi.org/10.1071/SH12070.

Herrmann N, Mittmann N, Silver IL, et al. A validation study of the geriatric depression scale short form. Int J Geriatr Psychiatry. 1996;11:457–60. https://doi.org/10.1002/(SICI)1099-1166(199605)11:5<457::AID-GPS325>3.0.CO;2-2.

http://www.agencymeddirectors.wa.gov/Files/AssessmentTools/9-cageform.pdf. Accessed 21 Jan 2019.

http://www.coloradohealthpartnerships.com/provider/care/CRAFFT.pdf. Accessed 21 Jan 2019.

http://www.ncdsv.org/ncd_about.html.

https://avp.org/ncavp/.

https://lgbtqipv.org/.

https://pubs.niaaa.nih.gov/publications/Newsletter/winter2004/Newsletter_Number3.htm. Accessed 21 Jan 2019.

https://www.cdc.gov/nchs/nhis/tobacco/tobacco_glossary.htm. Accessed 21 Jan 2019.

Institute for Work and Health. Primary, Secondary, and Tertiary Prevention; 2014. https://www.iwh.on.ca/what-researchers-mean-by/primary-secondary-and-tertiary-prevention. Accessed 21 Jan 2019.

Institute of Medicine (US) committee on lesbian, gay, bisexual, and transgender health issues and research gaps and opportunities. The health of lesbian, gay, bisexual, and transgender people: building a foundation for better understanding. Washington, DC: National Academies Press; 2011. https://www.ncbi.nlm.nih.gov/books/NBK64806/. https://doi.org/10.17226/13128.

Kann L, McManus T, Harris WA, et al. Youth risk behavior surveillance—United States, 2017. MMWR Surveill Summ. 2018;67(8):1–479.

Liszewski W, Ananth AT, Ploch LE, Rogers NE. Anal Pap smears and anal cancer: what dermatologists should know. J Am Acad Dermatol. 2014;71(5):985–92. https://doi.org/10.1016/j.jaad.2014.06.045.

McFarland W, Caceres CF. HIV surveillance among men who have sex with men. AIDS. 2001;15(3):S23–32.

Meads C, Moore D. Breast cancer in lesbians and bisexual women: systematic review of incidence, prevalence and risk studies. BMC Public Health. 2013;13:1127. https://doi.org/10.1186/1471-2458-13-1127.

Muller EE, Rebe K, Chirwa TF, Struthers H, McIntyre J, Lewis DA. The prevalence of Human Papillomavirus infections and associated risk factors in men-who-have-sex-with-men in Cape Town, South Africa. BMC Infect Dis. 2016;16(1):440. https://doi.org/10.1186/s12879-016-1706-9.

Mohamad NV, Soelaiman IN, Chin KY. A concise review of testosterone and bone health. Clin Interv Aging. 2016;11:1317–24.

National Institute on Alcohol Abuse and Alcoholism. Alcohol's effects on the body. https://www.niaaa.nih.gov/alcohol-health/alcohols-effects-body. Accessed 21 Jan 2019.

Nelson HD, Bougatsos C, Blazina I. Screening women for intimate partner violence: a systematic review to update the U.S. Preventive Services Task Force recommendation. Ann Intern Med. 2012;156(11):796. Epub 2012 May 7.

New York State Department of Health AIDS Institute. Anal dysplasia and cancer guideline. https://www.hivguidelines.org/hiv-care/anal-dysplasia-cancer/. Accessed 21 Jan 2019.

Newcomb ME, Heinz AJ, Mustanski B. Examining risk and protective factors for alcohol use in lesbian, gay, bisexual, and transgender youth: a longitudinal multilevel analysis. J Stud Alcohol Drugs. 2012;73(5):783–93.

O'Connell M, Boat T, Warner K. Preventing mental, emotional, and behavioral disorders among young people. Washington, DC: National Academies Press; 2009.

Patel P, Bush T, Kojic EM, et al. Prevalence, incidence, and clearance of anal high-risk Human Papillomavirus infection among HIV-infected men in the SUN study. J Infect Dis. 2018;217(6):953–63. https://doi.org/10.1093/infdis/jix607.

Patterson WM, Dohn HH, Bird J, Patterson GA. Evaluation of suicidal patients: the SAD PERSONS scale. Psychosomatics. 1983;24(4):343–5, 348–9. https://doi.org/10.1016/S0033-3182(83)73213-5.

Peralta RL, Fleming MF. Screening for intimate partner violence in a primary care setting: the validity of "feeling safe at home" and prevalence results. J Am Board Fam Pract. 2003;16(6):525–32.

Prins A, Ouimette P, Kimerling R, et al. The primary care PTSD screen (PC-PTSD): development and operating characteristics. Prim Care Psychiatry. 2003;9:9–14.

Punukollu M. Domestic violence: screening made practical. J Fam Pract. 2003;52(7):537–43.

Roberts SJ, Patsdaughter CA, Grindel CG, Tarmina MS. Health related behaviors and cancer screening of lesbians: results of the Boston Lesbian Health Project II. Women Health. 2004;39(4):41–55. https://doi.org/10.1300/J013v39n04_03.

Rollè L, Giardina G, Caldarera AM, Gerino E, Brustia P. When intimate partner violence meets same sex couples: a review of same sex intimate partner violence. Front Psychol. 2018;9:1506. https://doi.org/10.3389/fpsyg.2018.01506.

Shakil A, Donald S, Sinacore JM, Krepcho M. Validation of the HITS domestic violence screening tool with males. Fam Med. 2005;37(3):193–8.

Sherin KM, Sinacore JM, Li XQ, Zitter RE, Shakil A. HITS: a short domestic violence screening tool for use in a family practice setting. Fam Med. 1998;30(7):508–12.

Shiels MS, Kreimer AR, Coghill AE, Darragh TM, Devesa SS. Anal cancer incidence in the United States, 1977-2011: distinct patterns by histology and behavior. Cancer Epidemiol Biomark Prev. 2014;24(10):1548–56. https://doi.org/10.1158/1055-9965.EPI-15-0044.

Smith S, Chen J, Basile KC, Gilbert LK, Merrick MT, Patel N, et al. National intimate partner and sexual violence survey (NISVS): 2010–2012 state report. National Center for Injury Prevention and Control, Centers for Disease Control and Prevention: Atlanta, GA; 2017. https://www.cdc.gov/violenceprevention/pdf/NISVS-StateReportBook.pdf. Accessed 19 Jan 2019.

Spitzer RL, Kroenke K, Williams JB, Lowe B. A brief measure for assessing Generalized Anxiety Disorder: the GAD-7. Arch Int Med. 2006;166(10):1092–7.

Steele SR, Varma MG, Melton GB, Ross HM, Rafferty JF, Buie WD. Practice parameters for anal squamous neoplasms. Dis Colon Rectum. 2012;55(7):735–49.

Stop Bullying.gov. Understanding the roles of health and safety professionals in community-wide bullying prevention efforts. https://www.stopbullying.gov/sites/default/files/2017-09/hrsa_guide_health-and-safety-professionals_508v2.pdf. Accessed 21 Jan 2019.

Substance Abuse and Mental Health Services Administration. AUDIT-C Overview. https://www.integration.samhsa.gov/images/res/tool_auditc.pdf. Accessed 21 Jan 2019.

Taft A, O'Doherty L, Hegarty K, Ramsay J, Davidson L, Feder G. Screening women for intimate partner violence in healthcare settings. Cochrane Database Syst Rev. 2013, 2013;(4):CD007007. https://doi.org/10.1002/14651858.CD007007.pub2.

Tharp AT, DeGue S, Valle LA, Brookmeyer KA, Massetti GM, Matjasko JL. A systematic qualitative review of risk and protective factors for sexual violence perpetration. Trauma Violence Abuse. 2013;14(2):133–67. https://doi.org/10.1177/1524838012470031.

The Williams Institute. Intimate partner violence and sexual abuse among LGBT people: a review of existing research. November 2015. https://williamsinstitute.law.ucla.edu/wp-content/uploads/Intimate-Partner-Violence-and-Sexual-Abuse-among-LGBT-People.pdf. Accessed 21 Jan 2019.

U.S. Preventive Services Task Force. Screening for intimate partner violence and abuse of elderly and vulnerable adults. http://www.uspreventiveservicestaskforce.org/uspstf/uspsipv.htm. Accessed 20 Dec 2012.

United States Preventive Services Task Force. Final recommendation statement on HIV Infection: screening. https://www.uspreventiveservicestaskforce.org/Page/Document/RecommendationStatementFinal/human-immunodeficiency-virus-hiv-infection-screening#copyright-and-source-information. Accessed 21 Jan 2019.

US Department of Health and Human Services. Alcohol alert. https://pubs.niaaa.nih.gov/publications/aa63/aa63.htm. Accessed 21 Jan 2019.

US Department of Veterans Affairs. Primary care of veterans with HIV: anal dysplasia. https://www.hiv.va.gov/provider/manual-primary-care/anal-dysplasia.asp. Accessed 24 Feb 2015.

US Preventive Services Task Force. Screening for colorectal cancer: US preventive services task force recommendation statement. JAMA. 2016;315(23):2564–75. https://doi.org/10.1001/jama.2016.5989.

Child and Adolescent Medicine

Jeremy Connors, Laura Irastorza, Aron Janssen, and Bobby Kelly

Psychosocial Development and Self-Awareness in LGBTQ Youth

Despite the greater availability of information to youth and overall cultural shift toward visibility and acceptance of LGBTQ people, LGBTQ youth are not guaranteed acceptance or affirmation in the family, school, or social milieu. The challenges of identity formation are greatly magnified for many LGBTQ youth, who must contend with damaging influences from a largely **heteronormative** society. Consequently, at critical periods of development, LGBTQ youth may cope with harmful influences that in turn drive risky health behaviors. However, there are many opportunities in the school, community, and clinic to create a more positive environment for LGBTQ youth.

The first listed author is the chapter's associate editor from The Equal Curriculum Project. The chapter authors are otherwise ordered according to their preference.

J. Connors (✉)
Rutgers New Jersey Medical School, Department of Medicine, Newark, NJ, USA

L. Irastorza
Arnold Palmer Children's Hospital, Orlando, FL, USA

A. Janssen
New York University, New York, NY, USA

B. Kelly
Geisel School of Medicine at Dartmouth, Hanover, NH, USA

This section touches briefly on what is known about the development of sexual orientation and gender identity in children through the main stages of childhood and adolescence. Understanding how children develop concepts of their own sexuality can help health professionals better support not just sexual and gender minority youth but all youth. Because of the developmental focus of this chapter, it includes content on **differences of sex development** (DSDs, sometimes referred to as *disorders of sex development*). Though DSDs are not a focus of this book, a discussion of the development of sexuality and sexual identity would be incomplete without it.

Development of Concept of Sexuality, Orientation, and Identity

Childhood (Birth to 7 Years)
Capacity for sexual response is present from birth, as evidenced by erections in newborn boys and vaginal secretions in girls. However, a sense of sexuality does not develop until later, with the awareness of one's sexual organs and physical differences between sexes usually occurring between the ages one and two years. By the time children are four years old they typically grasp the concepts of "boy" and "girl" and can often identify themselves as one or the other. Children engage in a range of sensual and sexual play, such as fondling their genitals or sucking on

fingers and toes. Although children begin to show some interest in the genitals of others at this stage, their sexual play becomes more private and covert as they become familiar with cultural norms and expectations. As children move from childhood to preadolescence, their perception of sexuality and orientation typically involves a natural curiosity combined with a sense of covertness, resulting in many unanswered questions.

Preadolescence (8–12 Years)

These unanswered questions come at a time when most children are either in school or otherwise frequently interacting with other children their age. Sex is discussed by preadolescent youth, with peers providing both accurate and inaccurate information. At this stage, many youth experience the hormonal changes of early puberty. Youth not only start to exhibit secondary sexual characteristics but also begin to experience sexual attraction. Youth who have not already engaged in masturbation are likely to begin exploration at this time. Sexual attraction and fantasies become more common. According to early studies exploring sexual identity of sexual minority youth, including more than 200 LGB youth, same-sex attraction was identified by gay boys around age nine and in lesbian girls around age 10.

Several models for the development of a homosexual identity have been proposed. Early models put forth by Cass (1979) and Troiden (1989) suggested a staged process involving recognition of the stigma associated with a homosexual identity, with eventual self-acceptance and disclosure to others. These models eventually fell into disfavor, in part because of limited study populations and changing perceptions of homosexuality by the mainstream culture. Current investigations of the development of sexual orientation identity are focused on milestones, including awareness of sexual attraction, potential self-labeling of one's sexual identity, disclosure to others, and early sexual encounters.

Adolescence (13–19 Years)

As youth move from preadolescence to adolescence, sexual identity and fantasies continue to develop, resulting in a desire for sexual exploration. Masturbation continues to be common, but teens become much more likely to engage in sexual contact with others. At this stage, sexual desire is high and risk-taking increases. According to the Centers for Disease Control and Prevention (CDC), 47% of American high school students surveyed had engaged in sex, and 15% had had sex with four or more people during their lives. Notably, 41% of these teens who had had sex in the preceding three months did not use a condom.

Data indicating what percentages of this sexual contact are opposite-gender and same-gender are limited. One study from 1998 showed that 5–10% of adolescent boys and 6% of adolescent girls reported having sexual experiences with people of the same gender. The CDC has been conducting the Youth Risk Behavior Surveillance survey (YRBS) for many years and published the report *Sexual Identity, Sex of Sexual Contacts, and Health-Risk Behaviors Among Students in Grades 9–12*. The conclusion of this report was that sexual minority students are more likely to engage in health-risk behaviors than other students are. The report has subsequently sparked much research in this area.

It is not implied that sexual minority youth have sexual identities and sexual behaviors that are strictly congruent (e.g., if one is a woman who has sex with women, one also identifies as lesbian or bisexual). Many people, whether because of internal struggle, competing desires, bisexuality, evolving identity, or other reasons, do not experience complete concordance of their identity, attractions, and behavior. This is certainly the case with youth, who increasingly adopt more fluid and more nuanced sexual identities.

Sexual minority youth may often be victimized or feel judged because of their newly identified sexual orientations. As a result, many hide their true feelings, withdraw socially, and ultimately engage in unhealthy and risky behaviors. Fortunately, with the ubiquity of the internet, youth have a new way to gain access to diverse and personally relevant resources. Studies suggest that creating and maintaining high-quality comprehensive online resources—with links to offline adjunct resources—can help develop and support the sexual health of sexual minority youth.

Office-Based Care for LGBTQ Youth

Any clinician who participates in the preventive health care of children and adolescents should be familiar with the American Academy of Pediatrics (AAP) publication *Bright Futures Guidelines*. A joint effort by the AAP and the Federal Maternal Child Health Bureau (MCHB) of the Health Resources and Services Administration (HRSA), *Bright Futures Guidelines* is "a set of principles, strategies, and tools that are theory-based, evidence-driven, and systems-oriented that can be used to improve the health and well-being of all children through culturally appropriate interventions."

In recent years, the AAP and the Institute of Medicine have published materials addressing the ever-growing field of research sexual minority youth, providing tools to augment the *Bright Futures Guidelines*. However, these tools are limited in number and quality, and there remains much to be learned about sexual and gender minority youth. Further cross-sectional and longitudinal research is essential, and many organizations, including the National Institutes of Health (NIH), the Department of Health and Human Services (HHS), and HRSA have made it a priority by creating steering committees to direct such research.

Chap. 3 covers strategies to make care environments welcoming. The remainder of this section emphasizes the same principles but with an emphasis on LGBTQ youth. Existing recommendations for office-based care of LGBTQ youth are distilled into six major principles (see Table 6.1).

Table 6.1   Six principles of office-based care for LGBTQ youth

Create a welcoming environment
Use gender-neutral language
Ask genuine, open-ended questions
Provide affirmation
Understand health risks and appropriate recommendations
Be familiar with quality resources, including local experts
Advocate

Creating a Welcoming Environment

First and foremost, it is essential to create a culture of support and respect in the office, which will foster culturally competent care. It is the healthcare provider's responsibility to deliver quality health care, tailored to meet each patient's needs. Trust is vital as children transition into their teenage years. If an adolescent patient does not sense that a clinician can be trusted, it is extremely unlikely that the patient will disclose details about sexuality.

The entire office staff must exhibit cultural competency and respect. Nurses, medical assistants, registration staff, and secretaries should all be aware of and use non-presumptive and non-judgmental language and behaviors in their interactions with patients. This can be accomplished through the implementation of office-wide professional development programs, the development of a specific vocabulary, the production of registration forms with inclusive language, or even the display of visual symbols of diversity such as rainbow stickers in the office.

A critical element is informing youth of the principle of confidentiality and its few exceptions. Youth are more willing to open up to clinicians if they understand that, for most topics, confidentiality is respected and that clinicians are required to share very few things with parents and guardians. It is good practice from early adolescence onward to plan a portion of the encounter in which parents and guardians and others accompanying a young patient step away so more sensitive issues may be raised. Finally, it is important to be aware of state and federal laws that allow minors (depending on age) to seek and consent to specific kinds of care independently and confidentially, including special exceptions that apply to sexual health and family planning. However, it is ideal to encourage youth to be open and honest with their parents or guardians whenever possible.

Using Gender-Neutral Language and Asking Genuine, Open-Ended Questions

Especially in discussions of relationships with patients starting in early adolescence, the use of gender-neutral language is important. Some clinicians find it useful to use both pronouns, whereas others use the generic plural *they*. Replacing presumptive or uninclusive questions such as "Do you have a boyfriend?" with "Are you dating anybody?" or "Are you and your girlfriend sexually active?" with "Tell me about your sexual partner" can mean the world to sexual and gender minority youth. With this principle in mind, providers can use the "5 P's of sexual health" recommended by the CDC—Partners, Practices, Protection from STIs, Past history of sexually transmitted infections (STIs), and Prevention of pregnancy—more effectively (see Tables 8.1 and 10.3). Other mnemonics, such as the HEEADSSS (Home, Education, Eating, Activities, Drugs and Alcohol, Depression, Suicide, Sexuality, and Safety) should be refined to be inclusive of the experiences of sexual and gender minority youth.

Providing Affirmation

With youth of all genders and sexual orientations, affirmation serves as the foundation for rapport and trust. It is crucial when working with sexual and gender minority youth: *Ensure that the patient feels heard and that you are in fact listening!* Clinicians should be ready to affirm the feelings of transgender or questioning youth, letting them know that they are not alone in their dysphoric feelings and that you can help get them connected with appropriate resources and support.

Understanding Health Risks and Appropriate Recommendations

The CDC's most recent recommendations regarding screening for STIs are based on the patient's STI risk which is informed by the sexual behaviors identified during the sexual history. Identifying details regarding sexual behavior—including the number, genders, and anatomies of partners, as well as the use of any appropriate STI protection—will help guide the clinician in STI screening and risk estimation. For the most current details, care providers may access the guideline on the CDC website. The 2015 guidelines are incorporated into Chap. 8.

External Resource 6.1
Centers for Disease Control and Prevention: 2015 Sexually Transmitted Diseases Treatment Guidelines. http://bit.ly/TECe1ch06_01

There are several ways to obtain a sexual history from an adolescent while maximizing comfort. Some clinicians use computer- or tablet-based programs to help teens answer sensitive questions regarding sexual behavior; others use paper questionnaires. Responses should be used to tailor anticipatory guidance and preventive health recommendations, including discussion of STI screening, birth control, mental health, and substance use. Chap. 8 discusses components of the high-quality sexual history and discusses some linguistic pitfalls of the sexual history for adolescents.

Becoming Familiar with Quality Resources and Local Experts

Though it is unreasonable to expect health professionals to be experts in all areas, it a clinician's responsibility to provide patients with quality resources, including referrals to local experts. Every office should have an up-to-date list of local resources, including pediatricians proficient in transgender health, local chapters of PFLAG (formerly Parents, Friends and Family of Lesbians and Gays), GSAs (Gay-Straight Alliances), and updated online resources for LGBTQ teen patients and their parents. GSAs encompass support groups and counseling opportunities, covering topics ranging from substance use and gender nondiscrimination to political action and safety concerns. GSAs are powerful resources for psychological empowerment and can provide LGBTQ youth with essential mental health support through a time that some begin the coming-out process. Accessing and partnering with community organizations to support LGBT youth can be an opportunity to positively influence health outcomes both inside and outside the clinic. Clinicians should play an active role in the community, supporting their patients and identifying and seeking to improve any systemic problems at the school level that could affect the health of their patients.

Health professionals must be aware of the limitations of their expertise and, on identifying deficits in knowledge, seek development opportunities. There are multitudes of high-quality resources available online, including modules published through the National LGBT Health Education Center.

External Resource 6.2

The **National LGBT Health Education Center** provides educational programs, resources, and consultation to health care organizations with the goal of optimizing quality, cost-effective health care for lesbian, gay, bisexual, and transgender people. https://www.lgbthealtheducation.org

---

Advocating

All pediatric patients are at risk for **bullying**, but sexual and gender minority youth, or those who are deemed by their classmates to be so, are at increased risk of experiencing violence at school, including bullying. According to a 2009 survey of more than 7000 LGBT youth, eight in 10 students were verbally harassed at school, four in 10 were physically harassed at school, six in 10 felt unsafe at school, and one in five had been the victim of a physical assault at school. These figures are much higher than those in the general population.

Clearly, providers who care for youth must be aware of these increased risks. These youth are not only at increased risk of physical harm but also of mental health problems, including suicidal ideation and suicidal behavior. Health professionals can play active roles in their community, serving as community experts to advocate for victims of bullying, and helping establish anti-bullying programs. Clinicians can also act as advocates for their sexual and gender minority patients with parents or guardians who are not fully supportive by referring parents and caregivers to PFLAG and offering educational information and support.

Key Points
- Stage of development has a critical impact on a child or adolescent's concept of sex, gender, sexuality, orientation, and identity. It is therefore important for healthcare providers to understand how all children develop a concept of their own sexuality.
- The American Academy of Pediatrics and the Institute of Medicine have published materials to help clinicians foster a supportive environment and healthy life for sexual minority youth (Table 6.1).

Case 6.1

A 17-year-old natal male named DeShawn is in his primary care provider's office for a routine preventive visit. The provider notes that DeShawn uses the pronouns *he*, *him*, and *his*. The provider conducts a sexual history that encompasses the routine CDC-recommended format of the "5 P's," including numbers of male and female partners, specific questions about the sites of sexual contact (including receptive/insertive, oral, anal, etc.), and condom use. DeShawn confides that he has had two male sexual partners, with whom he has had insertive anal and receptive oral sex without any condom use. He says that he and his partners have never had any STI screening tests performed.

- **Where can the PCP find information about appropriate screening tests for DeShawn?**
- **What are the current recommendations regarding screening tests?**
- **What anticipatory guidance is appropriate for DeShawn during this preventive visit?**

Because DeShawn has never had any screening tests, he should certainly have some done today. A list of recommended tests can be found on the CDC website. He should undergo screening blood tests for HIV and syphilis, an oropharygneal swab nucleic amplification test (NAAT) for gonorrhea, and urine NAATs for gonorrhea and chlamydia. According to the CDC website, "CDC recommends the NAAT for gonorrhea and chlamydia screening at nongenital sites. Although NAATs are more sensitive and superior to culture at these sites, these tests are not US Food and Drug Administration cleared for these indications. However, they can be used by laboratories that have met all regulatory requirements for an off-label procedure. The National Network of Prevention Training Centers' Website has a list of laboratories that are Clinical Laboratory Improvement Amendments (CLIA)–verified to test rectal and pharyngeal specimens for gonorrhea and chlamydia using NAATs."

In addition to the recommended anticipatory guidance that is published in the Bright Futures Guideline, DeShawn should be offered counseling regarding the proper use of condoms and other barriers to help prevent the spread of STIs. The provider should use gender-neutral language in any anticipatory guidance provided and pose genuine, open-ended questions when exploring gender identity and sexuality but specific questions when assessing risk.

Sexual Anatomy, Gender Identity and Expression, and Differences of Sex Development

As discussed earlier in this text, gender and sexuality are comprised of multiple components that are not necessarily binary. Everyone proceeds through their own individual developmental process, influenced by biological, psychological, and sociocultural factors, and these processes define how each of us identifies. Gender itself can be broken into anatomic sex, gender identity, and gender expression. **Anatomic sex** can be defined as the sum of the structures that differentiate male from female. **Gender identity** is the self-defined and subjective internal experience of one's own gender. **Gender expression** consists of physical characteristics and behaviors presented by an individual, directed outward to others. Each of these domains has its own process.

In medicine, discoveries about typical development often come from an understanding of what happens in atypical development. The same can be said of gender development. Understanding the experiences of those with variations in the multiple domains of gender and sexuality increases awareness about how gender and sexual development occur and what impact they have on individuals and families.

Before fetal development, an individual spermatocyte, with either its X or Y chromosome, is paired with an individual oocyte, with its X chromosome, to form the zygote, which later develops into an embryo. Before week six of development, genetically male (XY) and female (XX) embryos demonstrate no significant anatomical differences. Each embryo has the capacity to form either a typical male or female reproductive system, or some combination or intermediary of both. After week 6, anatomic and hormonal changes begin. The development of internal genitalia and the external genitalia are independently mediated, both beginning in a multipotent state and differentiating in response to genetic and hormonal factors. By week eight of development, the testes begin to secrete Müllerian inhibiting substance (MIS), which promotes the development of the male internal reproductive system and regression of the female internal reproductive system. In the absence of MIS, regardless of the chromosomal makeup of the embryo, the female internal reproductive system is formed. In a separate process, the development of the external genitalia is primarily mediated by the presence or absence of usable testosterone. In the presence of usable testosterone (and its by-products), the genitalia are masculinized, and the penis and scrotum are formed. In the absence of these hormones, the clitoris, labia and external portion of the vagina are formed.

Development of the internal genitalia depends on the presence or absence of MIS. The development course of external genitalia depends on the presence or absence of testosterone. Usually these processes are aligned. An XY embryo will most often make MIS and testosterone and develop male internal and external genitalia, but this is not always the case. In roughly one of every 50 births, there is a **difference of sexual development** (DSD, also previously known as *disorders of sexual development*). This means that 2% of the population have genitalia that are neither stereotypically male nor stereotypically female. Though gender and sexuality are more often described as falling on a spectrum, natal sex also exhibits wide variation of expression. Much understanding of the biological influences on gender identity and sexual development came initially from the study of persons with variant developmental processes.

In a study of natal females with classic congenital adrenal hyperplasia (CAH), which masculinizes the external genitalia because of high prenatal androgens, most subjects maintained a female gender identity. However, there were significant increases in all domains of gendered behavior that are typically different between boys and girls, including childhood play, affiliation with male/female peers, physical activity level, strength, and aggression. Individuals with complete androgen insensitivity syndrome, a condition in which 46XY individuals are unable to utilize androgens because of a genetic defect in the androgen receptor, are born with testes but female external genitalia. Unlike people with CAH, they show no differences in gendered behavior from healthy female controls.

Physiologic and endocrinologic explanations of the many origins, ranges of presentation, and medical and surgical management of DSDs are beyond the scope of this discussion. In addition to classic CAH and androgen insensitivity syndrome, the reader may want to independently explore 5α-reductase deficiency and SRY gene mutations. At the other end of the anatomic spectrum, DSDs include such conditions as epispadias and hypospadias.

Biological factors are intertwined with cognitive, psychosocial, and cultural effects. By the age of two to three years, most children have begun to label themselves as boys or girls, in a stage called *basic gender identity*. As children develop cognitively they begin to understand that their gender is stable over time. For example, a boy can identify his own gender at age three but may still believe that he could grow up to be a woman. By four to five years, most children understand that their own gender is fixed, but it is not until five to seven years that they understand that gender is fixed for others as well.

Though basic gender identity develops during toddlerhood, a deeper understanding of gender identity—awareness of one's gender and its implications—continues to evolve, and so the meaning and salience of one's gender evolves throughout the preschool years, latency, adolescence, and adulthood. Gender becomes more than just biology: boys and girls are expected to behave in certain ways that are congruent with expected roles in a given culture. Boys tend to prefer more rough-and-tumble play, girls more imaginative and social/relational play. Clearly there are children for whom this does not hold true. Many people can recall being "tomboys" or "girly boys" growing up, despite the absence of any DSD.

Experiences of people with DSD have clearly demonstrated that identity development is not equal to the sum of its parts. One's genitals and the balance of hormones do not define identity, but they certainly influence it. Practically speaking, this means that for any child who is born, gender identity cannot be accurately predicted based on the appearance of the genitals. For parents of children born with DSD, or for parents of children that demonstrate gender nonconformity, the uncertainty that surrounds gender can be stressful.

Optimal care for children with DSD requires a multidisciplinary team that may include subspecialists in endocrinology, surgery and/or urology, psychiatry/psychology, gynecology, genetics, neonatology, social work, nursing, and medical ethics, depending on the extremity of need. Teams with experience treating DSDs recommend a thorough diagnostic assessment as an important first step. As noted earlier, trends of gender identification vary with the underlying diagnosis and can help guide recommendations regarding how (or whether) to provide a child's initial gender assignment. Diagnosis, genital appearance, surgical options, need for lifelong replacement therapy, potential for fertility, views of the family, and, sometimes, circumstances relating to cultural practices are all factors that influence initial gender assignment.

It is important to be sensitive and make a good impression with the families of children with DSDs. Parents often have gender-based ideas of what their children will become, and it can be challenging to confront those ideas unexpectedly. The clinician should emphasize that a child with a DSD has great potential to succeed in life. Although the patient and family's privacy must be respected, a DSD is not shameful. The health-care team should discuss with the parents what information to share with family members and friends in the early stages. Parents must be informed about sexual development, and web-based information may be helpful, provided the content and focus of the information is balanced and sound. **Increasingly, it is recommended that surgical intervention be delayed until the child can participate in decision-making.** However, at the other extreme, early surgical management may be required to establish or preserve basic genitourinary function.

Although gender nonconformity is an entity separate from DSD, there is higher frequency of gender nonconformity among people with DSD. Families of children in both groups benefit from clear anticipatory guidance. From the beginning, this means that parents should be educated on the developmental processes discussed in this chapter. There is no evidence to suggest that reinforcement (either positive or negative) of any early gender role–based behavior has an impact on later gender identity consolidation. For instance, encouraging a natal male who likes dolls to instead play with toy trucks is not likely to influence his ultimate gender identity. Similarly, there is no evidence

to indicate that one can change sexual orientation, and, in fact, attempts to do so are harmful. However, there is clear evidence that family acceptance of variations in gender and sexuality is protective against negative psychosocial outcomes, including suicide. For this reason, parents must understand that their love and encouragement of their child, regardless of the ultimate outcome, is not just good parenting but a vital part of building resilience and protecting their child from harm.

> **Key Points**
> - Parents and health professionals should maintain distinct concepts of anatomic sex, gender identity, and gender expression.
> - One of every 50 births is marked by a difference of sexual development (DSD). That is, 2% of the population have genitalia that are neither stereotypically male nor stereotypically female.
> - Gender identity cannot be accurately predicted for any child based on genitals. Persons with DSD are more likely to be transgender or gender nonconforming.
> - In more and more circumstances, it is recommended that surgical reconstruction not be undertaken until the child can participate in decision-making.

Psychosocial Vulnerabilities and Resilience

Health care professionals are responsible for treating the whole patient. To properly screen, evaluate, and care for LGBTQ patients, the health care professional must be cognizant of psychosocial factors that affect a patient's health. LGBTQ youth are especially vulnerable during this time of transition between childhood and adolescence. Significant risk factors and related outcomes are described below and summarized in Fig. 6.1.

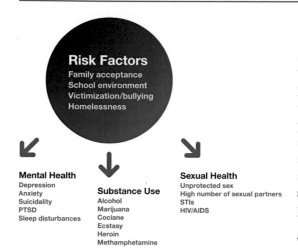

Fig. 6.1 Key risk factors and negative outcomes affecting LGBTQ youth

Risk Factors

Family Acceptance

Family acceptance is related to positive health outcomes in sexual minority youth and is essential for healthy adolescent development. It is ideal for families to be aware of their child's sexual orientation and/or gender identity because this knowledge allows parents to become sensitive to their child's needs and well-being. Although parents may have a negative reaction to a child's disclosure of identity, research has shown that parental knowledge of a child's orientation can lead to better understanding and an open, trusting relationship. In one study, LGB adolescents who reported high levels of family rejection during adolescence were 8.4 times more likely to attempt suicide, 5.9 times more likely to have depression, 3.4 times more likely to use illegal drugs, and 3.4 times more likely to engage in unprotected sexual sex than were their peers from families who reported no or low levels of family rejection. Sexual and gender minority youth who reported family acceptance during adolescence showed better general health and well-being than did peers who were not accepted by their families. Family acceptance is associated with higher levels of self-esteem, social support, and general health and is protective against depression, substance use, and suicidal ideation and suicide attempts in young adulthood.

Clinicians should screen patients for family acceptance during childhood and adolescence office visits. Confidentiality must be emphasized because many sexual and gender minority youth have already experienced rejection and may be unwilling to disclose such information. Health professionals may offer to help facilitate disclosure by youth to their families and should emphasize to the parents the importance of providing support to their children. **However, a clinician should never push for disclosure if doing so places the patient in danger.**

Victimization and Bullying

Sexual and gender minority youth often face bullying, harassment, and physical violence as a result of their actual or perceived sexual orientation or gender expression. Most research has been conducted in school settings, but bullying may occur in any social setting, including online. **Cyber-bullying** is the use of information technology to harm or harass other people in a deliberate, repeated, and hostile manner. This relatively new form of harassment is especially prevalent among adolescent youth, and resultant suicides by sexual and gender minority youth have been reported. In a recent national community survey of middle and high school LGBT students, more than 85% of respondents reported having been victims of verbal harassment, 40% had experienced physical harassment, and 19% had been physically assaulted at school in the previous year. In the same survey, nearly two-thirds of these students reported feeling unsafe in school because of their sexual orientation.

The results of this victimization may include post-traumatic stress disorder, sleep disturbances, anxiety, depression, nightmares, somatization, drug abuse, and suicide attempts. Care providers must engage sexual and gender minority youth in discussions of their school, home, and other social settings, including social media and potential for cyberbullying. Many victimized youth are afraid to disclose abuse, fearing further victimization and bullying, but it is important to encourage them to talk about incidences of bullying and report them to the proper authorities. Health professionals should also provide education to schools about the adverse health effects of bullying and the importance of intervening to stop harassment. One good resource is StopBullying.gov, which has information for both educators and youth on the various forms of bullying.

Homelessness

Sexual and gender minority youth are disproportionately overrepresented in both the foster care system and juvenile detention centers. Many such youth end up in foster care as a result of family neglect, abuse, or conflict resulting from their identity. These youth are at higher risk of harassment by other children and providers in the foster system, and they have an increased risk of depression, suicide, and substance use compared with heterosexual youth in the system. LGBT youth are less likely to find permanent homes and are often bounced around the system. Homeless youth who do not enter the foster system may have to rely on other means to survive, which can put them at risk for sexual and substance abuse. Some turn to survival sex as a means of supporting themselves.

Very little research has been conducted on sexual and gender minority youth in detention facilities, but LGBTQ youth tend to be viewed negatively by juvenile courts and juvenile correction staff. Their concerns put them at risk for physical isolation, or their concerns may be ignored altogether.

Health Outcomes

Mental Health

As seen in the discussion of risk factors above, screening of sexual and gender minority youth for mental health issues is crucial. LGB children are twice as likely to have depression and social anxiety than their heterosexual peers and are at increased risk for self-harm and suicide, with some research reporting a suicide attempt risk four times that of non–sexual minority youth. Transgender youth are at even higher risk for depression and suicide. Epidemiologic data on LGBTQ youth mental health are described in Chap. 12.

Substance Use

Substance use is another adverse health outcome related to the stressors of being a sexual minority youth. Studies on the use of legal and illegal substances have revealed significantly higher prevalence of use of tobacco, alcohol, marijuana, cocaine, ecstasy, methamphetamine, and heroin among sexual minority youth. The use of club drugs (e.g., cocaine, methamphetamine, ecstasy, ketamine, LSD) is especially worrisome because of its association with risky behaviors such as unprotected sex. Epidemiologic data on LGBT youth substance use are described in Chap. 12.

LGBTQ youth are also at risk for health complications associated with the use of these substances, including alcohol-related death, chronic obstructive pulmonary disease and lung cancer, and sudden death caused by drug overdose or toxicity. Healthcare providers should ask all youth about drug use, but sexual and gender minority youth are at especially high risk.

Sexual Health

Sexual and gender minority youth are more likely than their heterosexual peers to have sex, to have sex before 13 years of age, and to have sex with four or more people total. Gay or lesbian youth have been found to be about half as likely as heterosexual youth to have used a condom or other method of barrier protection. Sexual and gender minority youth are therefore at greater risk for sexually transmitted infections and the complications of those infections. One disparity is HIV infection. Data from the CDC show that HIV incidence continues to rise among young men who have sex with men (MSM) 13–24 years of age.

Clinicians should cover sexual health education at visits with all youth and tailor recommendations to sexual and gender minority youth. A thorough sexual history should be obtained. Refer to Chap. 8 for a thorough discussion of the sexual health history. Beware—youth vary in their concepts of what constitutes sex, sexual contact, and intercourse (e.g., sexual contact may be assumed to be only genital-genital contact, or penile-anal contact may not be considered a form of intercourse). Education on contraception and barrier methods is important, and information about STIs and their prevention should be discussed. Screening for STIs in patients who report high-risk behaviors may be performed. Vaccination against HPV should be offered to all patients starting at age 9. There are multiple formulations HPV vaccine (covering up to nine strains as of the writing of this chapter) with slightly different indications.

Key Points
- Health professionals should screen for risk factors such as family acceptance, bullying, and homelessness in LGBTQ youth.
- Adverse health outcomes, such as mental health issues, substance use, and increased risk of sexually transmitted infections, should be investigated during any routine visit with an LGBTQ youth.
- Resources should be provided to both the families and LGBTQ children/adolescents in anticipation of challenges these children may face in the future (anticipatory guidance).
- Most importantly, clinicians should always be open and offer a safe space for all youth. The development of sexual identity can be a very delicate and stressful time. A clinician may be the only person a child can talk to in confidence.

Conclusion

Any opportunity for a clinician to interact with a child or adolescent also represents an opportunity to foster the patient-provider relationship, identify potential health risks, conduct pertinent health screenings, and offer education.

Offices can be made LGBTQ-friendly by using gender-neutral questions, intake forms, and questionnaires. LGBTQ parents should be welcomed into the practice. Literature on sexual orientation and gender identity should be included in patient education materials offered. The clinician should obtain an appropriate and thorough history and assess risk factors in the patient's life. The information gathered can help guide the provider through the proper STI testing, immunizations, mental health referrals, and screenings.

Clinicians may also provide guidance for their young sexual and gender minority patients as they contemplate coming out to their parents. It is just as important to assist the parents of sexual and gender minority youth and provide resources to help guide the family through the LGBTQ child's adolescence and young adulthood.

External Resource 6.3
National Safe Place is a national youth outreach and prevention program for young people in need of immediate help and safety. https://www.nationalsafeplace.org

The **SafeZone Training Program** is a program created to promote and maintain culturally competent environments in workplaces, schools, and other social settings that are supportive of both LGBTQ and straight individuals. https://thesafezoneproject.com/

Boards-Style Application Questions

Question 1. During a routine well-adolescent exam, a 15-year-old patient tells the provider – after his mother has left the room – that he has been experimenting with sexual behaviors and has had two 15-year-old same-sex partners in the last year. He reports that he did not use condoms with either partner. The patient asks that this information be kept private from his parents and wonders whether he should be worried about anything. The most appropriate response to this adolescent is:

A. "That's something you need to talk to your counselor about. I can't help you here."
B. "I should ask your mother to come back in to discuss this before we go any further."
C. "Because your partners were same-sex, I'll have to contact their parents and let them know."

D. "Did you know that men who have sex with men are at increased risk for sexually transmitted infections, or STIs? You should get STI testing right now."

E. "I'm glad you felt comfortable sharing that with me. I do recommend that you get STI testing. We can talk about that and whether and how to include your parents."

Question 2. A 10-year-old boy who is well known to you has consistently told his parents that he identifies as female. He likes to wear dresses and asks his siblings to call him April. The child's parents ask whether this is normal and what to do. What is the most appropriate thing for the provider to say to this child's parents?

A. "This isn't normal. We need to call a psychiatrist right now so we can discuss the situation, because there's a chance of long-term repercussions."

B. "I'm a primary care doctor, and this isn't something that I should be discussing with parents. It's more appropriate for me to refer your child to a specialist before we go any further."

C. "It can be normal, but you shouldn't really encourage this behavior. You might want to hide the dresses, and I strongly discourage referring to him as 'she'; this can cause problems."

D. "Gender identity is complex. Although he may genetically be male, your child seems to identify as female. Counseling could be helpful, but above all it's most important that your child feels loved and is being heard."

E. "He's probably engaging in this behavior because he's lacking a male role model in his life. You should respond by providing masculine reinforcement and taking away any feminine reinforcement. Keep calling him by his male name."

Question 3. A 13-year-old girl has recently noticed that she is sexually attracted to one of her closest female friends, who is in same grade.

They have started dating. The school dance is a few months away, and she would like to ask her friend as her date, but she isn't sure how other students or teachers will react. She confides this concern to her school counselor, who is unsure how the school can help. Which of the following statements regarding the impact of school policies on the experiences of LGB students has been supported by research?

A. The only policies that exert any effect on the experiences of LGB students have been related to sexual education.

B. There is an association between LGB students who attend schools with gay-sensitive HIV instruction and increased sexual risk-taking.

C. Students at schools with antiharassment policies and gay-straight alliance clubs reported feeling safer and being less likely to be harassed.

D. The absence of studies exploring this topic suggests that there is no role for interventional research regarding school policies and safety.

E. Sexual minority youth in larger schools with more low-income and ethnically diverse students experience more frequent victimization and suicidality.

Question 4. What is the best approach to improving psychosocial outcomes in children with nonconforming gender roles or disorders of sex development (DSDs)?

A. It is important to emphasize that a child with gender variance or a DSD has great potential to succeed in life. As a health professional, you can help reduce the possibility of shame.

B. Parental acceptance is a primary factor in the development of resilience in these children. Efforts should be made to educate parents and children about gender and sexual development and to encourage parents to support their children's exploration of identity.

C. Optimal care for children with DSDs includes an interdisciplinary team comprising specialists in endocrinology, surgery and/or urology, psychiatry/psychology, gynecology, genetics, neonatology, social work, nursing, and medical ethics working together with the family and the child to make important medical decisions.

D. All of the above

Question 5. A child born with ambiguous genitalia is found to have a chromosomal makeup of 46XX. The clinical history and genetic evaluation findings are consistent with a diagnosis of congenital adrenal hyperplasia (CAH). What should the parents be told about this child's gender identity?

A. Genetic females with CAH identify as women in adulthood.
B. If the child is raised as a girl, she will identify as one; if the child is raised as a boy, he will identify as one.
C. The child's genitals are mismatched with her gender identity. Steps should be taken in infancy to align her gender identity with her genitalia.
D. Although there are trends of gender identification for children born with CAH, we cannot predict from birth how such a child will ultimately identify a gender.

Question 6. Twelve-year-old Lisa Adams is accompanied by her mother to your office for a well-child exam. The family moved to the area only recently, and this is her first visit with you. Lisa's mother poses most of the health-related questions, but Lisa interjects once and a while. Before moving on to the physical exam, you ask her mother to step outside the room while you ask Lisa some more specific questions. What should you discuss with Lisa after her mother leaves the room?

A. Her sexual attractions and sexual activity
B. Risky behaviors such as alcohol use, recreational drug use, and sexual activity
C. The meaning of confidentiality and how what will be discussed is between Lisa and the doctor only
D. All of the above

Question 7. After some further questions, Lisa opens up to you and begins to explain how she has recently started to question her sexual identity. She has been seeing another girl in school but has told no one about it. Lisa begs you not to tell her mother, fearing that she would be in a lot of trouble. She reports that she has seen two boys in school being bullied because they are gay and says that she does not want the same thing to happen to her. She tells you that she is not sexually active but would like to be soon. She does not drink alcohol or use any recreational drugs but has friends who have tried both. What should you do next?

A. Ask Lisa whether she has ever stolen anything or broken the law
B. Tell Lisa that her friends are wrong for drinking alcohol and using drugs
C. Screen Lisa for mental health issues and have a discussion about coming out to her family when she is ready
D. Tell Lisa it is okay to keep her sexual identity hidden and that it is best to do so because of the possibility of bullying

Boards-Style Application Questions Answer Key

Question 1. The correct answer is E: responding positively to the child's disclosure, recommending STI testing, and making it clear that disclosing this information to the parents is the child's call. It is important to ensure that youth feel comfortable sharing their health information openly and honestly, and one key way of doing this is creating a welcoming environment, including the use of supportive language and accurate information. Although providers should encourage youth to be honest with their parents, assuring the teen patient of confidentiality when it comes to their health is paramount because it also fosters trust in the provider. Asking the mother back into the exam room for the discussion, immediately warning the child of the dangers of STIs, telling the child that his partners' parents must be contacted, and telling the child that he needs to talk to a counselor instead are unhelpful and will not foster a trusting relationship with the provider. The sexual and reproductive health services that can be offered to a 15-year-old and the degree of confidentiality guaranteed vary depending on state laws.

Question 2. The correct answer is D: explaining that gender identity is complicated and stressing the need for parental support. Primary care providers should feel equipped to discuss the topic of gender with their patients, not necessarily as experts but at least to help direct the family to the appropriate resources. Specifically, when it comes to young patients struggling with gender identity, it is crucial that youth understand that they are not alone in their dysphoria and that there are resources out there. Providers should affirm their patients' feelings and help them get the assistance they need, be it counseling or an endocrinologist referral. Studies have *not* shown that gender identity is a consequence of a lack of role models, and reinforcement of cis-gender pronouns or norms does *not* help these patients.

Question 3. The correct answer is C. School policies can have a real impact on the experiences of sexual minority students. Although transgender health research is sorely lacking, published data do show that anti-harassment policies and GSAs improve students' perceived level of safety and decrease harassment prevalence. It is simply not true that sex education is the only policy exerting any effect on LGB students' experiences; that sexual risk-taking is more prevalent among LGB students who receive gay-sensitive instruction; that there is no role for interventional research regarding school policies and safety; or that victimization and suicidality are more common among sexual minority youth in larger schools with larger low-income and ethnically diverse student populations.

Question 4. The correct answer is D, all of the above. The best medical care for infants with DSDs comprises multiple facets, and an interdisciplinary approach is ideal. Family members should be into the care team whenever possible.

Making it clear to parents that the child with a DSD has the potential to lead a fulfilling life and supporting families to help them become accepting of their children with DSDs are important duties for the health professional.

Question 5. The correct answer is D. There are trends in gender identification for different origins of DSD, as well as a greater overall likelihood of gender nonconformity, but gender identity cannot be predicted with certainty. Many families opt to raise their children as the "expected" gender, but preparing families to be flexible and adaptive is an important part of cultivating family resilience.

Question 6. The correct answer is D, all of the above. It is important to establish confidentiality (and its few exceptions) early in the private interview, to ask Lisa about her sexual attractions and activity, and to screen for risky behaviors.

Question 7. The correct answer is C: screening Lisa for mental health issues and discussing how she can come out to her family when she is ready. Although it is important to provide anticipatory guidance and ensure her safety, advising Lisa to hide her sexuality could be damaging. It is appropriate to target mental health, sexual health, and substance use issues during the interview, but speaking judgmentally of her friends who have experimented with drugs and alcohol will not foster a good relationship with Lisa. Whether and when to come out to her family and community are up to Lisa, but it is often the case that sexual minority youth fare better once they do.

Sources

Birkett M, Espelage DL, Koenig B. LGB and questioning students in schools: the moderating effects of homophobic bullying and school climate on negative outcomes. J Youth Adolesc. 2009;38(7):989–1000.

Blackless M, Charuvastra A, Derryck A, Fausto-Sterling A, Lauzanne K, Lee E. How sexually dimorphic are we? Review and synthesis. Am J Hum Biol. 2000;12:151–66.

Cass V. Homosexuality identity formation: A theoretical model. J Homosex. 1979;4(3):219–35.

Centers for Disease Control and Prevention. *A guide to taking a sexual history*. Washington, DC: US Department of Health and Human Services. http://www.cdc.gov/std/treatment/sexualhistory.pdf. Accessed 31 Jan 2019.

Centers for Disease Control and Prevention. Trends in HIV/AIDS diagnoses among men who have sex with men—33 states, 2001-2006. MMWR Morb Mortal Wkly Rep. 2008;57(25):681–6.

Centers for Disease Control and Prevention. Youth risk behavior surveillance—United States, 2011. MMWR Morbid Mortal Wkly Rep. 2012;61(SS-4):1–162.

Currie S, Mayberry M, Chenneville T. Destabilizing anti-gay environments through gay-straight alliances: possibilities and limitations through shifting discourses. Clearing House: A Journal of Educational Strategies, Issues and Ideas. 2011;85(2):56–60. https://doi.org/10.1080/00098655.2011.611190.

DeHaan S, Kuper LE, Magee JC, Bigelow L, Mustanski BS. The interplay between online and offline explorations of identity, relationships, and sex: a mixed-methods study with LGBT youth. J Sex Res. 2013;50(5):421–34.

DeLamater J, Friedrich W. Human sexual development. J Sex Res. 2002;39(1):10–14.1.

DiPietro J. Rough-and-tumble play: a function of gender. Dev Psychol. 1981;17:50–8.

Friedman MS, Koeske GF, Silvestre AJ, Korr WS, Sites EW. The impact of gender-role nonconforming behavior, bullying, and social support on suicidality among gay male youth. J Adolesc Health. 2006;38(5):621–3.

Hagan JF, Shaw JS, Duncan P, editors. Bright futures: guidelines for health supervision of infants, children, and adolescents. 3rd ed. Elk Grove Village: American Academy of Pediatrics; 2008.

Institute of Medicine, Committee on Lesbian, Gay, Bisexual, and Transgender Health Issues and Research Gaps and Opportunities. The health of lesbian, gay, bisexual, and transgender people: building a foundation for better understanding. Washington, DC: National Academies Press; 2011.

Kohlberg L. A cognitive developmental analysis of children's sex role concepts and attitudes. In: Maccoby E, editor. The development of sex differences. Stanford, CA: Stanford University Press; 1966. p. 82–173.

Kosciw JG, Greytak EA, Diaz EM, Bartkiewicz MJ. The 2009 National School Climate Survey: the experiences of lesbian, gay, bisexual and transgender youth in our nation's schools. New York: Gay, Lesbian Straight Education Network; 2010.

Lee PA, Houk CP, Ahmed SF, Hughes IA. Consensus statement on management of intersex disorders. Pediatrics. 2006;118:e488–500.

Leeuwen JM, Boyle S, Salomonsen-Sautel S, et al. Lesbian, gay, and bisexual homeless youth: an eight-city public health perspective. Child Welfare. 2006;85:151.

Levine D and the Committee on Adolescence. Office-based care for lesbian, gay, bisexual, transgender, and questioning youth. Pediatrics. 2013;132:e297. https://doi.org/10.1542/peds.2013-12831.

Meyer-Bahlburg H. Sex steroids and variants of gender identity. Endocrinol Metab Clin. 2013;42(3):435–52.

National Research Council. The health of lesbian, gay, bisexual, and transgender people: building a foundation for better understanding. Washington, DC: The National Academies Press; 2011.

Needham BL, Austin EL. Sexual orientation, parental support and health during the transition to young adulthood. J Youth Adolesc. 2010;39:1189–98.

Pilkington NW, D'Augelli AR. Victimization of lesbian, gay, and bisexual youth in community settings. J Commun Pathol. 1995;21:34–56.

Ridner SL, Frost K, Lajoie AS. Health information and risk behaviors among lesbian, gay, and bisexual college students. J Am Acad Nurse Pract. 2006;18(8):374–8.

Ryan C, Huebner D, Diaz RM, Sanchez J. Family rejection as a predictor of negative health outcomes in white and Latino lesbian, gay and bisexual young adults. Pediatrics. 2009;123:346–52.

Ryan C, Russell S, Huebner D, Diaz R, Sanchez J. Family acceptance in adolescents and the health of LGBT young adults. J Child Adolesc Psychiatr Nurs. 2010;23:205–13.

Smith G, McGuinness T. Adolescent psychosocial assessment: the HEEADSSS. J Psychosoc Nurs Ment Health Serv. 2017;55(5):24–7.

Troiden R. The formation of homosexual identities. J Homosex. 1989;17(1–2):43–74. https://doi.org/10.1300/j082v17n01_02.

Wilber S, Ryan C, Marksamer J. CWLA best practice guidelines: serving LGBT youth in out-of-home care. Washington, DC: Child Welfare League of America; 2006.

Zucker KJ, Bradley SJ. Gender identity disorder and psychosexual problems in children and adolescents. New York City: Guilford Press; 1995.

Adult Primary Care

Carl G. Streed Jr., Melanie Adams,
Christopher Terndrup, and Andrew Petroll

Unique Role of the PCP

External Resource 7.1
"To Treat Me, You Have to Know Who I Am" is a video by New York City Health and Hospitals highlighting the importance of knowing, understanding, and advocating for LGBT patients. Total time 10:18. http://bit.ly/TECe1ch07_01

Patients often look to their primary care provider (PCP) for help navigating the health care system and for referrals to appropriate specialists. PCPs can be physicians (MDs and DOs),

The first listed author is the chapter's associate editor from The Equal Curriculum Project. The chapter authors are otherwise ordered according to their preference.

C. G. StreedJr. (✉)
Boston University School of Medicine, Center for Transgender Medicine & Surgery, Boston Medical Center, Boston, MA, USA
e-mail: carl.streed@bmc.org

M. Adams
Cape Breton Regional Hospital, Sydney, NS, Canada
e-mail: mmadams@mta.ca

C. Terndrup
Oregon Health & Science University, Portland, OR, USA
e-mail: terndrup@ohsu.edu

A. Petroll
Medical College of Wisconsin, Wauwatosa, WI, USA
e-mail: apetroll@mcw.edu

nurse practitioners (NPs), and physician assistant (PAs). (For more information regarding the roles various health care professionals play in providing LGBTQ patients with comprehensive care, see Chap. 4). The PCP fulfills multiple roles for the patient within the health care system in order to provide comprehensive care:

- An advocate for the patient within the health care system and advocate for systemic changes in health system practices, policy, and legislation
- A gateway into the health care system regardless of diagnosis, personhood, or circumstance
- A patient confidante who knows the patient narrative, sexual orientation, gender identity, support system, past medical history, and confidentiality concerns and who can see their connection to the big picture
- The facilitator of difficult conversations with family, friends, and coworkers
- A provider of appropriate counseling, patient education, and preventive medicine
- The care team leader and coordinator of referrals, management, and follow-up

The lack of formal instruction and education regarding the needs of the LGBTQ population throughout health professional training perpetuates development of providers without the knowledge and experience needed to care for LGBTQ patients. LGBTQ patients may be justifiably uncomfortable returning to a provider who does not have the knowledge or skills needed to address their concerns.

© Springer Nature Switzerland AG 2020
J. R. Lehman et al. (eds.), *The Equal Curriculum*, https://doi.org/10.1007/978-3-030-24025-7_7

General Principles for Primary Care

The LGBTQ-friendly clinical encounter is discussed at length in Chap. 3, but it is worth again emphasizing the importance of inclusive language, gender-neutral terms, and the use of open-ended questions when encountering any new patient. As discussed in Chap. 3, intake forms and electronic health records (EHRs) in health care offices play an important role in a patient's comfort level. Forms should be structured in a way that is inclusive of the entire spectrum of human sexuality and should not discriminate against those who are gender-nonconforming or who are in the process of transitioning. Every new patient encounter should begin with a comprehensive history and investigations should be based on a patient's particular risk factors, behaviors and concerns – not assumptions based on sexual orientation or gender identity. It is important for physicians to take a comprehensive sexual history when meeting with a new patient. The sexual history should be conducted in a non-discriminatory manner, with appropriate use of language, tone, and body language. LGBTQ patients who are asked about sexual orientation are far more likely to disclose this information. Therefore, questions regarding the sex or anatomy of a patient's sexual partner(s) should be included in the sexual history. Clinical guidelines on prevention are discussed in Chap. 5, and sexual health is discussed in Chap. 8.

Many members of LGBTQ communities fear that the disclosure of sexual orientation or gender identity to their PCP will negatively impact their health care. It is important for PCPs to remain mindful of the stress that may be associated with disclosing sexual orientation. PCPs should also initiate a discussion of family life with all LGBTQ patients. By taking this small step, the PCP is showing the patient that they support their personal relationships and can provide the information and resources needed regarding reproductive health, family building, and medico-legal issues. Summarizing the health concerns addressed throughout the patient encounter is an effective way of ensuring that the patients' health care needs and concerns have been appropriately

addressed. Before the patient leaves the office, a follow-up visit should be scheduled to ensure continuity of care.

Key Points
- The PCP fulfills a variety of roles and ensures that patients receive comprehensive health care from multiple specialties and disciplines.
- By understanding unique barriers to health care, PCPs can advocate for LGBTQ patients and improve access to health care for the LGBTQ community.
- Investigations and recommendations for all patients should be based on a patient's individual risk factors as opposed to assumptions based on a patient's sexual or gender identity.
- Establishing a trusting and open provider-patient relationship is crucial to ensuring LGBTQ patients feel comfortable, safe, and supported.

Case 7.1
Andy, a 24-year-old female, is presenting to your office to establish care. When going over her intake form, you notice that it is incomplete. Andy has not filled out her gender, relationship status, or any of the questions relating to her gynecological/reproductive health.

- **How should you approach Andy to collect the missing information?**
- **What kinds of questions would be most appropriate to ask?**
- **What kinds of behaviors or statements would be important to avoid?**

Although it may be possible that Andy simply forgot to fill in these parts of the intake form, it is much more likely that she intentionally left these questions blank because she either did not feel comfortable answering them or perhaps she hoped to prompt a discussion on gender and sexual/reproductive health. By asking Andy to fill in the missing sections of the form or by filling in the form based on observations and her medical chart, the PCP is ignoring how she felt about the questions on the intake form in the first place. If Andy is struggling with gender or her sexual/reproductive health, ignoring the subtle omissions on her intake form may make her feel as though she cannot discuss these things with you. It is also possible that Andy was mistreated by staff before beginning the encounter with you and/or the form may not be inclusive of her gender identity or sexual orientation -- both of which would imply that you as a provider may not be LGBTQ-friendly.

The PCP should have an open discussion about the intake form with Andy and address any of her concerns as they arise. Begin with open-ended questions to prompt Andy. A potential opening statement is, "I noticed that you left sections of the intake form blank. I understand that some of these questions may be personal and perhaps difficult to answer for you. Please understand that all information that you tell me will stay between you and me; that information will help me better care for you. In your own words, help me understand how you define yourself in terms of gender and sexuality." Remember to maintain eye contact and welcoming body language.

Discriminatory or judgmental remarks, unwelcoming body language, and abrupt conclusion of the discussion should be avoided. If you as a provider are unsure of what to answer or ask, it is fair to admit this to the patient with a promise to learn or research more. It is unfair to use defense mechanisms to hide one's lack of knowledge.

Advocacy

Being an advocate at the local or national level through policy work, public health efforts, or peer education can greatly impact the lives, health, and wellbeing of LGBTQ persons. By advocating for the rights of LGBTQ patients, the health care provider can express the needs and concerns of their patients, set a precedent of care for the LGBTQ community, and evoke positive, sustainable change. Advocacy in LGBTQ-patient centered health often involves raising awareness of special health concerns in the LGBTQ population and ensuring LGBTQ patients can access health care with ease.

As with many minority populations, LGBTQ individuals struggle with unique barriers to health care. By understanding these barriers, health care professionals can begin to take crucial steps towards improving access to health care in LGBTQ communities. Some barriers, such as lack of education regarding LGBTQ health concerns, research trends and stereotypes in the health care community, and failure to establish a trusting patient-provider relationship during clinical encounters, will be discussed here. Other barriers to care, including medicolegal issues and health insurance, are discussed in Chaps. 2 and 3.

From the federal government to states to smaller institutions, policy has a significant impact on LGBTQ health. Marriage equality, adoption rights, and equal opportunity for employment and housing lead to direct and indirect improvements in health care and quality of life. Marriage rights have been proven to protect against depression. Supporting public health efforts may lead to better screenings. For example, rural MSM have recommended the internet as the best way for HIV/AIDS outreach. Health professions educators should focus on LGBTQ health education for practitioners. Many studies have shown poor inclusion of LGBT education in medical curricula. Lastly, health professionals can work to implement and improve health-related guidelines for LGBTQ populations.

Facilitating Conversations

At times, patients may ask their PCP to facilitate difficult conversations with family members, friends, and intimate partners, including **coming out**. When facilitating these conversations, it is important to be sure of who the patient wants present, what the patient hopes to accomplish with the meeting, and information the patient would like to keep confidential (possibly with some but not others). Ultimately the PCP is only present to support the patient and ensure the conversation progresses in a way that is productive. Often, having their PCP present provides patients with a sense of reassurance and security during difficult conversations with loved ones.

Counseling, Patient Education and Health Concerns with Emphasis on Prevention

Counseling and Patient Education

Counseling and patient education are two very important aspects of primary care that often require some tailoring depending on the patient, their lifestyle, and their risk factors. Patient education should be a priority during every patient encounter. Opportunities for patient education include healthy eating, exercise, smoking cessation, safer sexual practices, and intimate partner violence (IPV) victim support. It is important that patients understand that they are responsible for their own health care. By educating patients and guiding them through tough decisions, health care providers can ensure that their patients can make evidence-based decisions regarding their health care.

There are many community resources and national organizations with comprehensive online resources available to PCPs looking for help effectively counseling/educating their LGBTQ patients. It is important to tap into the resources available to the patients within the community to provide patients with support that is readily accessible. Appendices 1 and 2 of this text may be of use when searching for patient resources.

Primary Care and Prevention Priorities

PCPs should provide preventive services for all patients, and LGBTQ populations face significant health disparities related to lack of access to care. An emphasis on anticipating disease processes and detecting those present can help to address many health disparities. Beyond focusing on prevention and risk reduction outlined in the last section, clinicians can utilize resources such as the US Preventive Services Task Force (USPSTF) to provide the correct screenings. Most screening recommendations do not change between non-LGBTQ and LGBTQ populations, but the wording of some recommendations is misleading (e.g., recommendations for cervical cancer screening that do not clearly acknowledge that many transgender men need screening). Chap. 5 addresses this problem thoroughly.

There are several specific topics that should be addressed when working with patients who self-identify as LGBTQ. GLMA: Health Professionals Advancing LGBTQ Equality has published very helpful lists that highlight the top ten health concerns health care providers have identified as being of utmost importance to LGBT populations.

> **External Resource 7.2**
> GLMA: Health Professionals Advancing LGBTQ Equality has created resources for both patients and health care professionals, including **Top Ten Health Issues** tip sheets for patients. http://glma.org/

Although there are subtle differences amongst the health care concerns of lesbians, gay men, bisexuals and those who self-identify as transgender, there are also many similarities. According to GLMA, the most important discussion to facilitate with LGBT patients revolves around their sexual orientation, sexual behavior, and gender identity. This includes a discussion on how accessible care is to the patient and how their family and friends feel about their sexual orientation and/or gender identity. (Distinguishing between biological family and **family of choice** is necessary.) Whether coming out has compromised a patient's support system is an important piece of information for primary care providers looking to provide patients with comprehensive health care.

In order to provide comprehensive care, PCPs for LGBTQ patients should focus on these key areas: sexual and reproductive health; body image, diet, and exercise; mental health, substance use, cardiovascular disease, cancer, and intimate partner violence.

Sexual and Reproductive Health

- **HIV/AIDS, STIs and Safer Sexual Practices.** STIs and safer sexual practices should be discussed with all LGBTQ patients. Patients should be taught how to properly protect themselves and their sexual partners from contracting or transmitting STIs, and they should be counseled regarding the need for consistent use of barrier methods to prevent the transmission of STIs. Accurate diagnosis of STIs is significantly lower compared to heterosexual women, likely secondary to presumptions made by providers. Counseling on safer sexual practices and screening recommendations should be specific to the patient's sexual behaviors. Please refer to Chap. 8 for further information on safer sex recommendations.
- **Reproductive Health and Family Planning.** Reproductive health concerns are specific to the patient and partner involved with consideration to anatomy of each partner and the couple's desires for building a family—this includes both contraception and family building options. Reproductive health and family planning options include but are not limited to surrogacy, artificial insemination, in vitro fertilization, and adoption. Medicolegal issues, such as legal guardianship, insurance coverage for children, and hospital visitation rights may arise for couples whose partnership is not recognized by laws and/or policy.

- **Immunizations.** Ensure patients are up to date with their immunizations. Of special importance to the LGBTQ population are the HPV vaccine and hepatitis B vaccine. The CDC recommends MSM be immunized against hepatitis A and B. Because of HPV's association with oropharyngeal and anal cancers, the CDC also recommended HPV vaccination for the following groups: young men who have sex with men, including young men who identify as gay or bisexual or who intend to have sex with men through age 26; young adults who are transgender through age 26; and, young adults with certain immunocompromising conditions (including HIV) through age 26. These guidelines are likely to be updated given the approval of the 9-valent HPV vaccine for persons up to age 45.

Mental Health

Mental health concerns, particularly depression, anxiety, and suicide, disproportionately affect LGBTQ people. LGBTQ persons often carry risk factors for development of depression, such as discrimination, violence, and lack of social or family support. PCPs provide the bulk of front-line medical therapy for depression and anxiety. When further treatment is required, PCPs can help identify LGBTQ-affirming psychiatrists and psychotherapists.

Information on screening for depression and suicide risk is found in Chap. 5. Diagnostic specifics and models of pathogenesis are in Chap. 12.

Body Image, Diet, and Exercise

Issues surrounding body image, diet, and exercise are also important things to address during an encounter with LGBTQ patients. Gay and bisexual men tend to have higher incidence of bulimia and clinical or subclinical anorexia than their heterosexual counterparts. As indicated per each patient, screen for body image concerns.

Body dysmorphia and gender dysphoria should both be considered in discussing body image concerns. Lesbian women have increased prevalence of obesity when compared to heterosexual women. The PCP can ensure that patients are exercising regularly—but not excessively—and eating a well-balanced diet.

Substance Use

Alcohol, tobacco, and illicit drug use have been reported at higher prevalence for LGBTQ patients compared to the general US population. The abuse of some of these substances predisposes LGBTQ people to increased risks of cardiovascular disease and various cancers. Smoking is very common across LGBTQ populations, with estimates of prevalence of more than twofold the general population. Use of alcohol and illicit drugs varies significantly based on sexual orientation and gender identity. Substance use is also linked to greater sexual risk-taking behaviors.

Consult Chap. 2 for information related to health disparities, Chap. 5 for screening recommendations, and Chap. 12 for the epidemiology of substance use in LGBTQ people.

Cardiovascular Disease

Cardiovascular disease is another important cause of mortality for all patients. LGBTQ people have approximately double the prevalence of smoking compared to the general population. Lesbian women are, on average, more often overweight or obese than heterosexual women, and so it is important to discuss how obesity impacts their risk of cardiovascular disease. Elevated alcohol consumption in LGBT persons may also contribute. Transgender populations using hormone therapy have additional cardiovascular risks, but the magnitude of these risks is not well estimated. Finally, persons with HIV have elevated cardiovascular risks for several reasons. These issues are discussed more thoroughly in Section "Cardiovascular Disease" of this chapter.

Cancer

The diagnosis, treatment, and prognosis of cancer in LGBT individuals unfortunately lack the investigative rigor of other areas of oncology. As in other medically underserved populations, health disparities result partly from lack of identification or inclusion in cancer prevention programs and clinical trials. Databases and registries for many cancer-related trials do not collect information on sexual orientation or gender identity. Similarly, a relative absence of educational campaigns and outreach to LGBT people about cancer has led to unawareness and misconceptions among both patients and health professionals.

Two more factors compound cancer disparities in this population: lack of access to health care (see Chap. 2) and lack of timely screening. Experts suggest that negative experiences in the health care system cause LGBT patients to avoid routine cancer evaluation. However, some studies show that this may not be the case: gay men may receive screening colonoscopies more frequently than heterosexual males, and women show no difference in screening rates for breast cancer in some studies. The second problem comes after diagnosis. Many LGBT patients fear the coming out process to their many providers during treatment, from medical and radiation oncologists to outpatient and inpatient practitioners. They may be reluctant to involve their **family of choice**. Fortunately, there are increasing numbers of support groups specific to LGBTQ patients fighting cancer. More resources regarding cancer support groups can be found at The National LGBT Cancer Network.

External Resource 7.3

The **National LGBT Cancer Network** works to improve the lives of LGBT cancer survivors and those at risk by education the LGBT community about their increased cancer risks and the importance of screening and early detection; training health care providers to offer more culturally-competent, safe and welcoming care; and advocating for LGBT survivors in mainstream cancer organizations, the media, and research. https://cancer-network.org/

Colon Cancer and Lung Cancer LGBTQ people get the most common cancers, lung and colorectal cancer. Prevalence data, using estimates of cancer and sexual minority status to extrapolate incidence of cancer among LGB patients, have shown elevated incidence of colorectal cancer. However, when stratifying by sexual orientation, the disparity disappears for gay men and lesbians but remains for bisexuals. The significance of this has yet to be explained, but it is theorized to be related to poorer access to health care among bisexuals. Regardless, all LGBTQ patients should receive routine colon cancer screening.

Despite far higher prevalence of smoking, research has so far failed to demonstrate a disparity regarding lung cancer among LGBTQ people. Nevertheless, providers should provide smoking cessation counseling for all LGBTQ smokers with LGBTQ-inclusive or LGBTQ-specific information and resources when available.

Breast and Cervical Cancer As a population, lesbians have a unique risk profile for cervical and breast cancers (nulliparity or having a first child over 30, obesity, lower use of oral combined contraceptives, higher alcohol use) compared to their heterosexual peers. Of note, many uninformed or misinformed health care professionals have counseled that LGB women do not need regular screening for early detection of cervical dysplasia. This belief is also common in these patient populations. Lesbian and bisexual women (and WSW, depending on the study design) appear less likely than heterosexual women to receive Pap testing according to guidelines.

Data are mixed about whether LGB women differ from heterosexual women in terms of accessing screening mammography. Some research has suggested that bisexual women are least likely of LGB women to get mammograms. Attitudes and priorities regarding breast reconstruction after cancer may be different from that of straight women.

Ovarian and Endometrial Cancer Routine screening or tests are not indicated in general. Risk is individualized. Nulliparity or delayed childbirth (first child after age 30), obesity, little or no use of progestin-containing contraceptives, and little or no history of breastfeeding increase risk. These factors may influence index of suspicion if history or physical exam findings suggest these cancers.

Anal Cancer For persons who have receptive anal sex, preventive measures may include anal Pap smears, although there is conflicting evidence for this practice in HIV-negative people. Routine anal Pap tests are indicated for HIV-positive persons who have had receptive anal sex. Based on Pap results, high resolution anoscopy may be required. PCPs can easily learn to perform anal Pap tests, but there may be challenges identifying and coordinating referrals for high resolution anoscopy.

Transgender Cancer Disparities Regardless of gender identity, providers must consider the **anatomic inventory** first and foremost. For example, a transgender man may still have a cervix and therefore require regular Pap smears. Transgender men should still receive screening mammography if they have not had complete mastectomy or total chest reconstruction. Organs that are not routinely screened, such as the prostate or ovaries, should not be neglected in differential diagnosis for possibly related complaints.

In addition to gender dysphoria and trauma history, biological factors may make cervical Pap tests more challenging for patient and provider. Exogenous testosterone may change cervical cells, leading to greater likelihood of an unsatisfactory cell sample. A decrease in vaginal secretions and vaginal atrophy may occur due to testosterone therapy. In addition to being responsive to the potential anxiety and dysphoria induced by an exam, good lubrication and use of the smallest speculum possible help to minimize discomfort.

External Resource 7.4

Sherbourne Health Centre in southeast Toronto launched a campaign to improve Pap screening in trans men called **Check It Out Guys**. http://www.checkitoutguys.ca

Their tip sheet **"Tips for Providing Paps to Trans Men"** provides valuable suggestions for performing Paps in a sensitive way. http://bit.ly/TECe1ch07_02

There are significant issues relating to cisgender assumptions in venues where transgender men or gender-nonconforming people may receive counseling and screening services. Here are some examples:

- A transgender woman, already struggling with the idea of having a prostate (a male organ), receives educational materials that use masculine pronouns or refer to men.
- A transgender man receives a results letter for a mammogram that uses his legal name (not preferred name) and incorrect pronouns
- A masculine-appearing nonbinary patient feels uncomfortable waiting in a gynecologist's waiting room with cisgender women for a cervical Pap after the receptionist becomes confused when he checks in for the appointment

Intimate Partner Violence (IPV)

Recent efforts to focus on violence in LGBTQ communities have revealed significant disparities in recognition, prevention, and supportive resources. Public health research has shown elevated risk of lifetime sexual assault and victimization among all sexual minorities. Data on IPV in the LGBT population are limited, but suggests at least equal, if not greater, rates compared to the US general population. Unfortunately, despite recent efforts to understand this issue further, little is known regarding effective methods to prevent and support LGBTQ victims of IPV.

Some care providers assume IPV does not occur in same-gender relationships. This is not the case. A history may be difficult to elicit in these cases, especially if the provider has employed the **heterosexual assumption** or the patient is afraid of disclosing sexual orientation or gender identity to the interviewer. Asking if the patient "feels safe at home" may not uncover abuse: the question has very low diagnostic sensitivity. Providers should maintain suspicion for IPV when indications are present, without heteronormative bias.

The clinician should ensure that the patient has access to appropriate resources within the community (i.e., shelter, counseling). Patients may not be able to leave the partner due to financial, insurance, housing, or emotional dependency. In these cases, the patient requires close follow-up. Where available, the care team should identify LGBTQ-specific or inclusive resources available locally. The care team may need to assist the patient in navigating resources and organizations that are not inclusive or unprepared for LGBTQ people, such as shelters that will not accept transgender people or cannot ensure their safety. LGBTQ patients may not be served well by support groups or group therapies with cisgender, straight people.

Key Points
- GLMA: Health Professionals Advancing LGBTQ Equality provides patients and health care providers with lists of the top ten health concerns for LGBT patients. PCPs should look over these lists and ensure that these topics are being discussed regularly with LGBTQ patients.
- HIV/AIDS, STIs, immunizations, and safer sexual practices should be discussed with all LGBTQ patients, accounting for the patients' sexual orientation, sexual behaviors, anatomic inventory, and sexual history.
- Depression, anxiety disorders, alcohol use, and tobacco use are all significantly elevated in LGBTQ people.

- Struggles with diet, exercise, and body image are common in LGBTQ people.
- Segments of the LGBTQ population have elevated cardiovascular disease risk.
- Some characteristics of LGBTQ sub-populations result in increased cancer risk, poorer screening adherence, and worse access to care. Carefully tailored approaches are needed for transgender persons based on their anatomic inventory and care preferences.
- IPV is overlooked in LGBTQ people, and the availability of LGBTQ-inclusive resources is inconsistent.

Gathering a History and Performing a Sensitive Physical Exam

Clinical environment, patient confidentiality, and inclusive language all play important roles in creating a welcoming environment for LGBTQ patients. The LGBTQ-friendly clinical encounter is discussed at length in Chap. 3. This section stresses the importance of performing a comprehensive history and a sensitive physical examination. As with all new patients, a comprehensive history is an important way of getting to know the health concerns and medical needs of LGBTQ patients. Be sure to cover the following:

- Chief complaint, history of present illness, associated symptoms
- Allergies and medications, including vitamins and/or supplements that have not been prescribed
- Past medical, psychiatric, surgical, and family medical history
- Current and past health care professionals (i.e., surgeons, endocrinologists, psychiatrists)
- Social history (which is crucial to assessing risk factors and behaviors)
- Past and present tobacco, alcohol and illicit drug use; testosterone and intravenous drug use to assess for blood-borne pathogen risk

- Employment, level of education, future educational or professional aspirations
- Living situation, support system, important relationships
- Sexual orientation and complete sexual history

If the patient self-identifies as LGBTQ, it is important to ascertain to whom the patient has **come out** and how this has affected the patient's personal relationships. The comprehensive sexual history is discussed in Chap. 8. An adequate sexual history covers the CDC's Five P's of Sexual Health—Partners, Practices, Protection from STDs, Past history of STDs, and Prevention of pregnancy.

With the ubiquity of electronic health records (EHRs) and these systems' potential for data analysis, it is important to ensure that every component of the history is appropriately transcribed to the degree the patient is willing. In this way, PCPs can facilitate data analysis on these patients and contribute to health care quality improvement for the LGBTQ population. The PCP should never document sexual orientation or gender identity terms that patients do not use for themselves. See Chap. 3 for more information on documentation of sexual orientation and gender identity in the clinical encounter and Chap. 13 for its deeper implications for health disparities and research.

Health care providers should perform a comprehensive physical examination when seeing a patient for the first time. At subsequent visits, a focused physical examination based on the chief complaint is appropriate. Before examination, the patient should be asked if they are reluctant to have certain body parts examined. If so, the PCP should initiate discussion about these feelings and how to accommodate the patient. Health care professionals should narrate the exam, explaining what part of the body is being examined and why. Proper draping is essential, exposing only the part of a patient's body being examined. The patient may wish to have a support person or staff of a certain gender in the room during the most sensitive parts or all of the exam.

Gender dysphoria can cause significant distress around physical examinations, especially of the chest and genitals. Any history of sexual abuse and sexual assault are also important, especially during genitourinary examinations, because it may contribute to emotional distress. Patients should be informed of the importance of the more invasive parts of the physical examination (e.g., Pap smear, pelvic exam, rectal exam). Any parts of the physical examination that are difficult for the patient should be approached with care and not be repeated unnecessarily. It is sometimes the case that the patient will use alternate terms for their anatomy; care providers should follow the patient's lead and use the same terms. Care providers can also use neutral language during exams (e.g., "I'm separating your tissue" vs. "I'm separating the labia").

Continuity of care can be improved by making patients feel comfortable, safe, and supported. By taking the time to educate patients and by ensuring the establishment of a trusting doctor-patient relationship, one can ensure that LGBTQ patients receive comprehensive, effective, and appropriate medical care.

Key Points
- Performing a comprehensive history is the most important aspect of establishing rapport and ascertaining the unique health care needs of every new patient.
- Be sure to ask every new patient questions relating to their social and sexual history; it is important to assess the patient's risk factors in order to address behaviors that may be contributing to morbidity and mortality.
- Perform a thorough physical examination on all new patients. Focused physical exams are appropriate for subsequent patient visits.
- Be mindful of the patient's comfort level throughout the physical examination.

Inpatient and Outpatient Management

LGBTQ populations confront special problems regarding their health care related to discrimination, social and behavioral risk factors, and some unique medical conditions. Specific aspects of the lives of LGBTQ patients and their interactions with the medico-legal system affect their needs in primary medical care, both in the inpatient and the outpatient setting.

Disclosure of Identity in the Health Care Setting

Sexual orientation and gender identity (SOGI) data are not yet routinely collected and documented in most health care settings, but providers should obtain this information from new patients. Disclosure of identity is dependent on many factors within the health care setting, including the patient's level of self-acceptance, other persons present, expectations of acceptance or rejection by others, the chief complaint, the pace of clinical care, and the setting of clinical care. For example, a trauma patient in the emergency department may resent being asked about their sexual orientation and gender identity due to perceived irrelevance and priority of the trauma. But in the case of a transgender patient facing repeated assault for her transgender identity, discussing identity and social history may elucidate underlying problems, leading to referral to community resources and improvements in the patient's safety. Chaps. 2 and 3 more fully discuss factors impacting disclosure in the clinical setting.

The greatest opportunities for improving LGBTQ health care lie in "traditional health care settings" and not in specialty clinics. Experts note that primary care is best suited to impact the intersectional nature of LGBTQ communities, their varied backgrounds, and their health. Chap. 3 addresses the concept of patient-centered care in more depth.

Previously this chapter discussed the PCP's role as a confidante, facilitator of discussions, and team leader of specialist and allied health professional care. Implicit in this role is the need for knowledge of appropriate specialists and resources. GLMA: Health Professionals Advancing LGBTQ Equality maintains a searchable database of LGBT-friendly physicians throughout the United States. This database can be an excellent tool for PCPs who are looking for specialist services for LGBTQ patients. Specific services may be difficult to find, particularly in rural areas.

Inpatient Medicine: Social Context of Admissions

Given discrimination and specific behavioral risk factors of LGBTQ patients, some inpatient admissions relate to their socioeconomic environment. Hospitalists and PCPs should be familiar with these issues and be able to address them when patients enter a complex hospital system. Homelessness and lack of access to health care exemplify the social context of inpatient admissions.

Many LGBTQ adolescents find themselves homeless because the home environment is unsafe or because they are rejected when they come out to their families. Subsequently, they suffer all the potential medical consequences of poor hygiene, violence, unsafe sexual practices, exposures to the elements, and substance use often seen in the homeless. **One-third or more of homeless youth are LGBTQ.** Homeless youth have high prevalence of mental illness and substance use problems; prevalence is even higher in racial or ethnic minorities due to **intersectionality**. These issues are clear risk factors for hospitalization. Obtaining social services and insurance coverage is significantly hampered by the lack of a stable location. For more information regarding health care for the homeless population, consult the National Health Care for the Homeless Council.

For transgender patients, there are additional reasons that lack of insurance and lack of access to care lead to hospital admissions. One study showed that in absence of access to care up to 25% turn to self-performed surgeries or non-prescribed hormone therapies. These unsupervised treatments can lead to serious consequences from blood loss or poor wound healing, as well as severe reactions to impure or incorrectly administered hormones.

Inpatient Medicine: Visitation Rights

In January 2011, the Obama Administration approved changes to the Center for Medicare-Medicaid Services (CMS) policy regarding visitation rights. This protects patients' right to declare which loved ones will be allowed to visit them in the hospital and requires hospitals receiving funds from Medicare or Medicaid to have policies assuring this right. LGBTQ patients often have a **family of choice** that does not match cultural or legal conceptions. Unfortunately, there are many documented instances in which family of choice – and even legal partners and legal guardians – have gone unrecognized in decision-making and visitation. PCPs can anticipate these and other medicolegal issues for their LGBTQ patients.

Key Points
- LGBTQ patients suffer significant risks for hospitalization based on social factors such as inadequate access to health care and social services.
- All patients reserve the right to designate who they would like to visit them in the hospital; LGBTQ people may prefer "chosen" families.
- PCPs are perfectly suited to provide patient-centered care, including risk reduction and preventive medicine.
- LGBTQ patients may require additional preventive care in addition to most of the routine screenings needed by heterosexual and cisgender patients.
- Health care providers can utilize many avenues to address LGBTQ disparities in health care, including community organizations, policy work, and peer education.

Health Concerns of LGBTQ Elders

There are approximately 1 million to 2.8 million
LGBT elders within the US with a projected
number of two million to six million by 2030.
While investigating LGBTQ health disparities,
many researchers have noticed a paucity of information about LGBTQ elders (65 years of age or
older). As more LGBTQ people come out,
LGBTQ elders also have become increasingly
visible in health care. Health care providers generally have a poor understanding of the experiences of LGBTQ elders. This population is
marginalized by society, by health care systems,
and sometimes even by LGBTQ communities.

Sociologists note the importance of temporal
context for LGBTQ identities. LGBTQ elders
experienced a different era of LGBTQ rights,
which was more oppressive and unaccepting of
LGBTQ identities. This experience colors
LGBTQ elders' perceptions and interactions
with the contemporary health care system.
Additionally, LGBTQ elders experienced semi-
nal events such as the 1969 **Stonewall Riots** that
led to the formation of some of the first advocacy
organizations dedicated to decriminalization of
male same-sex sexual behaviors. In 1973, the
American Psychiatric Association declassified
homosexuality as a mental disorder. Elders also
experienced early AIDS activism, and many suffered great personal losses of loved ones to
HIV. Some lost entire social circles. Chap. 1 summarizes landmark historical events in the LGBTQ
community.

As a function of the prevailing societal
homophobia and transphobia earlier in life,
LGBTQ elders have suffered a different degree
of social stressors, including stigmatization, dis-

crimination, violence, and internalized
homophobia. This degree of stress may lead to
adverse health outcomes, particularly mental
health and substance use concerns. In addition,
long-term psychological distress caused by isolation and discrimination has been associated
with more chronic conditions and health care
limitations.

Coming Out

Coming out may be a difficult process for
LGBTQ elders due to the negative and homopho-
bic/transphobic culture they experienced.
Primary care providers should not assume that
elders who have been seemingly heterosexual
their whole lives cannot be LGBTQ. LGBTQ
elders face a heightened sense of fear and anticipated discrimination – whether personal, social,
or institutional – compared to younger generations. Fear of disclosure may lead LGBTQ elders
to avoid accessing care altogether.

LGBTQ elders may hint towards a partner(s)
in their life in subtle ways, such as signaling a
"friend" with whom they spend much time.
Providers should be sensitive to these cues and
use sensitive language to encourage patients. The
providers should consider non-presumptive questions such as, "Do you live with anyone?" "Who
is your support system?" "Who do you spend the
most time with?" and "Who do you enjoy spending time with the most?"

Research has shown that among LG elder
populations, better adjustment to aging occurs in
those who accept their gay or lesbian identities or
who live with a partner. Being "out" leads to
higher levels of life satisfaction and support in
adjusting to the aging process. For these reasons,
PCPs should be available to support their patients
in coming out, keeping in mind that it may start at
any age. By providing patients with supportive
literature, practitioners can help support this transition to help their patients reap the benefits of
coming out.

While the benefits of coming out improve the
lives of LGB patients in many ways, certain risks
should be discussed. While anti-gay sentiment

has decreased significantly over the past few decades, coming out may still lead to ostracism from family or friends. Particularly in rural areas, gay men fear that coming out would lead to ridicule, hostility, and violence. They also fear for their job security. Among LGBTQ elders, the positive effects of a family of choice are believed to outweigh the possible loss of family of origin. Providers should consider and alert their patients to these risks, keeping in mind that staying in the closet often leads to further psychological distress and negative health outcomes. Overall, despite the potential negative consequences, coming out appears to have favorable outcomes.

Health Care Issues

LGBTQ elders face the same disparities already discussed in this textbook. A brief review of salient points is given in Table 7.1. First, health professionals must empathize with LGBTQ elders and try to understand prior discrimination they may have faced within the health care system. Given the horrors of the past, they may be unwilling to discuss their issues openly. As a result of systematic discrimination, LGB elders

Table 7.1 Health concerns for LGBT elder populations

Gay and bisexual men	Lesbian and bisexual women	Transgender
Psychosocial issues	Psychosocial issues	Psychosocial issues
Mental health	Mental health	Mental health
Substance use	Substance use	Substance use
Sexual health including STIs and HIV/AIDS	Sexual health including STIs	Hormone therapy
Cardiovascular disease	Breast and gynecologic cancer	Sexual health including STIs and HIV/AIDS
Anal cancer screening	Cardiovascular disease	Cardiovascular disease
		Cancer screening based on appropriate anatomy

For all: Self-defined identity, social support systems, housing, access to care, preventive care, confidentiality concerns, and end of life wishes

Adapted from Simone-Skidmore M

have higher likelihood of psychological distress and associated physical disability, substance use, and overall poor self-rated health compared to heterosexuals. While data conflict, the California Health Interview Surveys suggest higher prevalence of diabetes, hypertension, and mental health issues. While researchers have investigated the sexual health of younger LGBTQ adults thoroughly, little is known about the sexuality of LGBTQ elders, leading them to be called the "twice hidden" population. Lastly, LGB elders more often lack adequate health insurance compared to the general population despite comparable income and higher educational attainment.

Sexual Health

Providers should remain cognizant that LGBTQ elders frequently are sexually active rather than inactive. LGBTQ elders may be involved in monogamous relationships, may have several partners over their lifetime, and may have multiple partners at one time. These issues should be clarified with patients in a sensitive manner. Recommended language for taking a sexual history is reviewed in Chap. 8. Health concerns related to sexual behaviors do not disappear for LGBTQ elders. These may include STIs, HIV/AIDS, cervical cancer, and anal cancer. Appropriate screening for these should not be overlooked in this population. Further study of LGBTQ elders and sexual health is needed to improve understanding of this population's needs.

End of Life Care

LGBTQ health disparities extend to end of life conditions such as cancer and HIV/AIDS. There are few studies on end of life and palliative care experiences and needs for LGBQ patients, and existing studies are susceptible to selection bias. There are even fewer on transgender people, published only in the last few years.

In ideal circumstances, (1) end of life issues are discussed with the patient in the outpatient setting far before end of life problems are immi-nent, (2) these discussions include pertinent fam-ily and friends, (3) end of life discussions include medical proxy or power of attorney, visitation rights, living will and/or do-not-resuscitate orders, and (4) anticipated facilities, such as extended care facilities, are reviewed in advance. These ideal circumstances are rarely achieved. Therefore, primary care providers should make special efforts to review end of life care issues with their patients, anticipating both ideal and unideal circumstances.

LGBTQ patients face a few specific chal-lenges during end of life: even higher reluctance to come out to primary care provider due to wan-ing independence; lack of assured access to family of choice; and unclear availability of orga-nizations and facilities that are non-discriminatory and non-abusive.

Providers should involve relevant family and friends, as requested by the patient. If desired by the patient, partners should be involved in decision-making. Providers should be aware of legal issues related to non-legally defined part-nership, such as insurance coverage and visita-tion rights. Providers should also understand state laws regarding surrogate decision makers if none are defined and ascertain whether there are legal relatives the patient does *not* want to have in their care.

LGBTQ patients may seek religious support, support groups, and medical facilities during end-of-life. Palliative care services may be religiously-based. Providers should clarify spiri-tual and religious beliefs of patients and ensure that future services do not fundamentally conflict with the patient's beliefs. If patients or caregivers seek support groups, ideally these support groups are accepting and validating of sexual and gender minorities and their experiences. For example, breast cancer support groups are overwhelmingly heterosexual females; moreover, their concerns, particularly attractiveness to male partners, differ from the experience of lesbians with breast can-cer. Extended care facilities are yet another set-ting in which LGBTQ patients and their families may experience discrimination, violence, or refusal of care.

Housing

Older patients often identify housing as a signifi-cant part of their quality of life. It can be a matter of pride or resilience but can also have a signifi-cant effect on their health if they require a higher level of care. The ground-breaking documentary *Gen Silent* tells the story of six LGBT seniors who struggle with the health care system, with a focus on their housing issues and concerns with being out. Couples that have been together for years are now faced with the prospect of moving into assisted living facilities. As their health care needs increase and they require greater assis-tance, they feel the need to go back in the closet for their own safety. Residential institutions have reacted poorly to affection between gay couples, and loss of independence threatens the livelihood of LGBTQ elders. Nearly three-quarters of LGBT elders perceive discrimination in retire-ment facilities. Not surprisingly, nearly 100% would appreciate gay-friendly communities. LGBT elders are also less likely to have family support as they have few or no children or they end up estranged from their families. Over 35% of transgender elders say there would be no one to take care of them as they grow older. Some progress has been made. SAGE (Services and Advocacy for Gay, Lesbian, Bisexual and Transgender Elders) is a helpful resource for LGBTQ elders.

External Resource 7.6

Gen Silent is a critically acclaimed docu-mentary about LGBT older people going back into the closet to survive. http://bit.ly/TECe1ch07_04

SAGE is the country's largest and oldest organization dedicated to improving the lives of LGBT older people. Founded in 1978 and headquartered in New York City, SAGE is a national organization that offers supportive services and consumer resources to LGBT older people and their caregivers. https://www.sageusa.org

Sense of Community

Over a lifetime, LGBTQ elders have faced varying degrees of social isolation and rejection. The elder with few close friends and no connection to legal family may have essentially no social support. Social isolation may lead to adverse mental health and substance use problems. Similar to their younger counterparts, a sense of belonging in LGBTQ communities improves quality of life for elders. Especially as they age, LGBTQ people find solace in groups of friends. Their adjustment to aging then relies on family of choice and remaining social engaged.

Despite the health disparities and long-standing discrimination, LGBTQ elders demonstrate resilience, often stemming from deep involvement and solidarity with LGBTQ community centers and activities. Even elders in rural communities, who may connect only via the internet or extended personal networks, demonstrate this resilience.

Intimate Partner Violence

Intimate partner violence (IPV) was previously discussed in Section "Counseling, Patient Education and Health Concerns with Emphasis on Prevention" of this chapter. See Chap. 5 for an in-depth discussion of IPV. LGBTQ elders are still susceptible to IPV. Providers of LGBTQ elders should understand the patient's intimate relationships and maintain a realistic index of suspicion for IPV.

Key Points
- LGBTQ elders face specific challenges beyond those of their younger counterparts, including greater housing discrimination and fear of being out.
- Many LGBTQ elders find strength and resilience by accepting their sexual orientation or gender identity and by being active in their community.
- PCPs can provide helpful advice to LGBTQ patients at any stage in the coming out process. PCPs should discuss the benefits but also advise of potential consequences.
- End of life and housing require special attention in LGBTQ elders, largely because of issues relating to family choice and their concerns of discrimination and abuse.

Case 7.2

This is a follow-up care visit at a nursing home with a 78-year-old male with a past medical history significant for mild chronic obstructive pulmonary disease and coronary artery disease status-post coronary artery bypass graft (CABG). Previously, he was living at home with his wife, recuperating from his CABG, until she unexpectedly passed three months ago. After reviewing his medications, he begins to cry and says that he has started a relationship with another male resident at the nursing home. He says that he has always known he is gay but was always scared to tell his family and friends for fear of losing their trust. He asks for advice on what to do. He says he wants to tell his children so he can be open with his new partner.

- **What is the PCPs priority for this patient?**
- **How can the PCP facilitate "coming out"?**
- **What relationship dynamics should be considered?**
- **What other health concerns should be discussed?**

This man is ready to "come out," and his PCP should provide adequate support. Choice of wording is incredibly important during this sensitive period. Providing empathetic support and addressing potential consequences of coming out will facilitate growth and possible external support for the patient. The PCP should allow the patient to define himself in terms of sexual orientation. It is therapeutic for the patient to discuss sexual orientation, past and current relationships, as well as fears or concerns.

The patient wants to maintain a relationship with his new partner as well as his family and friends. The process of coming out may take time and the PCP should encourage the patient to come out at his own pace and facilitate conversations amongst persons in the patient's life, either in the office or by referral to counseling.

The provider should note mental health concerns, such as depression or anxiety, and sexual health concerns, in addition to the patient's other medical problems (COPD and CAD).

Cardiovascular Disease

Cardiovascular risks in LGBTQ people are related to four major risk factors: smoking, obesity, HIV and antiretroviral therapy, and hormone therapy.

Smoking

While there is some controversy over methods of estimation, overall prevalence of smoking among LGBT communities is significantly higher compared to other populations. Most studies estimate odds of current smoking to be 2–3 times higher and former smoking to be 1.5–2 times higher in sexual and gender minorities compared to the general population. These disparities are even worse in younger and more urban LGBT populations. However, middle-aged and older lesbians are more likely to be daily smokers compared to younger counterparts. In addition, there is also a lack of targeted interventions focusing on smoking cessation for LGBTQ people. Despite some increased focus, stronger public health campaigns on LGBTQ smoking are needed.

It is important to note that many of the surveys that have been used in past studies utilized convenience sampling in LGBT bars, and therefore numbers may be falsely elevated. More recent studies, however, have avoided this sampling bias and continue to show high prevalence. A recent study showed elevated prevalence among gay men and lesbians and even higher prevalence among bisexual men and women. The well-known consequences of long-term tobacco use include elevated risks of cardiovascular disease (CVD), chronic obstructive pulmonary disease, cognitive decline, and certain cancers. Tobacco use likely accounts for a significant number of health disparities within LGBTQ populations.

Obesity

Although researchers are still investigating the mechanisms of and exact relationship between obesity and CVD, the positive correlation has created a public health spotlight on preventing and decreasing rates of obesity. While gay and bisexual men are less likely to be overweight as compared to their heterosexual peers, lesbians and bisexual women are more likely to be obese than heterosexual women. While most studies are based solely on BMI, a less than ideal measure for obesity, other studies show elevated waist circumference and waist-to-hip ratios among lesbians as well, which have a positive correlation with CVD. In addition, a diet lacking in fruits and vegetables likely plays a large role, particularly among older lesbians. Lastly, specific surveys regarding lesbian views on obesity have shown that they are less likely to view obesity as a health problem or culturally unacceptable. While the frequency and magnitude of CVD in lesbians and its consequences, such as myocardial infarction and stroke, are debated, a focus on weight loss and exercise among lesbians remains a specific focus for health care professionals.

Fortunately, this issue is relatively well studied. Notably, a focus on physical health (as opposed to external aesthetics) among a predominantly lesbian group has led to positive behavior changes related to food choices and exercise frequency. Experts theorize that cultural connectivity helps women to overcome past failures in losing weight and to maintain successes. Further investigation into lesbian-specific weight loss programs is warranted.

HIV and Highly Active Anti-retroviral Therapy

While Chap. 11 addresses the bulk of HIV issues in this text, evaluation of all persons with HIV should include risk for CVD. With improving survival and longevity in people living with HIV, the focus on other causes of morbidity and mortality has increased. Research suggests that increased risk for CVD may come from the virus itself via endothelial dysfunction and inflammation or from its treatment with Highly Active Anti-Retroviral Therapy (HAART) via fat redistribution and metabolic derangements. Interactions between the virus and HAART (particularly protease inhibitors) may play a unique role. Whether the effects are more significant on the vasculature or the myocardium, HIV and its treatment predispose patients to CVD.

Prevention and treatment of CVD in persons with HIV includes medication changes (drug switching among HAART regimens), typical treatments of lipid and glucose abnormalities, and any other therapies that would be indicated based on risk stratification and comorbidities. While lifestyle modifications (dietary changes, smoking cessation, and increased exercise) are first line, pharmacologic treatment should not be too long delayed. Dyslipidemia should prompt initiation of a statin, while insulin resistance may require metformin or another insulin sensitizer. Overall, further studies in HIV-positive patients would be needed to formulate specific guidelines. Virologic suppression should never be deprioritized due to the disastrous long-term effects of immune system compromise.

Hormone Therapies

Aside from the risks already mentioned (obesity, tobacco use), hormone use by transgender individuals may also contribute to an increased risk of cardiovascular disease. While increased risk of embolism formulation from estrogens is known, testosterone's impact on CVD is not. The risks and benefits associated with hormone therapy should always be discussed at length with transgender patients. It is important that patients make truly informed decisions about their care and, according to their own preferences, believe that the benefits of hormone therapy outweigh risks of increased cardiovascular morbidity and mortality before beginning treatment.

Conclusion

Adult primary care has extraordinary breadth and depth. Primary care providers are positioned to ensure high-quality, equitable care by advocating for their patients; assisting to navigate the health care system; and coordinating care with specialists. For LGBTQ patients, an empathic and informed primary care provider should be skilled at discussing sensitive issues, developing care goals based on the patient's values and preferences, anticipating obstacles, and accessing special resources as needed.

Boards-Style Application Questions

Question 1. Kyle is a 34-year-old gay male presenting to your office for the first time to establish care. He has never been hospitalized, has no significant past medical or surgical history, and is up to date on all of his immunizations. He has no known allergies and is not taking any medication. He is a computer technician and says that he enjoys his job. He has a good relationship with his family and feels as though he has a strong support system. His family history is significant for hypertension (father) and breast cancer (mother). He does not smoke cigarettes and has never used any illicit drugs. He drinks alcohol occasionally. He is currently single. He has no current complaints. As you begin to ask more questions pertaining to his sexual history, Kyle becomes very defensive and accuses you of asking him questions regarding STIs and HIV/AIDS solely because he is gay. How should you respond?

A. Apologize to Kyle and move on to another topic.
B. Encourage Kyle to see another PCP who would be more understanding of his sexuality.
C. Explain to Kyle that all gay men have unprotected sex with multiple male partners and are at increased risk for STIs and HIV therefore it is important to take a thorough sexual history.
D. Tell Kyle that you ask all patients about their risks for STIs and HIV/AIDS

Question 2. A 34-year-old woman presents for evaluation of generalized fatigue, muscle aches, and abdominal pain. She notes that for the past six weeks she has had trouble finishing tasks at work and has felt too tired and achy to go to the gym. She thinks most of it is because of poor sleep over this period. Her physical exam is unremarkable except for a dysthymic and restricted affect. She has no history of mood or anxiety disorders. What is the best next step?

A. Diagnose chronic fatigue syndrome and advise exercise
B. Order CBC, TSH, ANA; call patient with results
C. Prescribe an SSRI and follow-up in six weeks
D. Prescribe sleep aid and have her call back with response
E. Screen patient for IPV

Question 3. A 33-year-old male presents for a routine health screening for a new job. He does not have any acute complaints except for recent urethritis that was treated with ceftriaxone and azithromycin a month ago. His family history is positive for colorectal cancer in his father at age 68. He is sexually active with men and women and identifies as bisexual. With women he practices penetrative vaginal and anal sex and with men practices receptive anal sex. He denies any current dysuria or penile discharge. He has consistently had undetectable viral load on HAART. His vital signs are within normal limits, his BMI is 23, and a full physical examination

(including rectal) is benign. Which of the following screening tests is indicated for this patient?

A. Anal Pap smear
B. Colonoscopy
C. HbA1C or fasting blood sugar
D. Lipid panel
E. Urine testing for Chlamydia/gonorrhea

Question 4. You are meeting a new patient for the first time. She is a 58-year-old lesbian female with a past medical history of hypertension and type II diabetes. She takes her medications (aspirin 81 mg daily, lisinopril 20 mg daily, metformin 500 mg twice daily, and atorvastatin 40 mg daily) regularly. She had a normal mammogram two months ago, and a Pap smear a year ago was normal (she has never had an abnormal one). She denies blurry vision and denies tingling and numbness in her feet. Physical examination is notable for a BMI of 34, BP 135/80. What is the *most important* thing to discuss with this patient?

A. Diet and exercise discussion
B. Increase lisinopril
C. Pap smear today
D. Podiatry referral
E. Start insulin

Question 5. Kate is a 31-year-old female presenting to your clinic for the first time to establish care. Kate is a healthy female with no current concerns or complaints. She had a Pap smear 4 years ago that was normal. She has no history of abnormal Pap smears. She has no abnormal discharge or vaginal bleeding. She is sexually active with one female partner. She has never had sex with a male partner and has been with her current female partner for the last 5 years. Kate and her partner do not use any form of barrier methods for protection. She does not smoke, consume alcohol, or use illicit drugs. She is physically fit and eats a balanced diet. You and Kate begin a discussion on preventive medicine. Which is most important for Kate at this time?

A. Routine CBC
B. Pap smear
C. Lipid panel and HbA1
D. Kate does not need any testing at this time

Question 6. Ryan is a 26-year-old male that you are seeing in your office for the first time today. Ryan is presenting today with a 10-day history of sore throat, fever, and decreased appetite. He denies cough, rash, rhinorrhea, nausea/vomiting, and diarrhea. He is otherwise healthy and has no chronic medical conditions. He is not taking any medication. You learn that Ryan is currently single and has sex with male partners only. He is routinely tested for STIs and HIV and his last tests (which were done one month ago) were all negative. What other information is important to elicit before moving on to the physical examination?

A. Recent travel
B. Sick contacts
C. Treatments tried
D. Recent sexual partners
E. All of the above

Question 7. You are taking over the care of a 56-year-old male with HIV who was admitted for hypoxic respiratory failure secondary to Pneumocystis pneumonia. He required endotracheal intubation to help his oxygenation and ventilatory status. His male partner has been at the bedside for much of the hospitalization; he called the patient's daughter, who has arrived quickly from another city. She expresses concern about her father's relationship and asks that the partner be removed from the hospital so she can attend to him. What is the most appropriate response?

A. "Go ask the nurse."
B. "I need to consult our Ethics Committee."
C. "Of course, we will have him removed right away."
D. "You should be more tolerant of your father's choices."
E. "Your father requested that his partner accompany him while in the hospital. What exactly is your concern?"

Question 8. You are visited by a patient well known to you, an 84-year-old female. She identifies as a lesbian and is single. She was previously married but divorced over 40 years ago. She has four adult children and seven grandchildren. She lives alone in an apartment building but has many close friends there. She spends her free time volunteering at the local LGBT Community Center. You have noted some mild cognitive decline recently, and she wants to discuss goals of care and decision-making processes in case her dementia progresses. What is the most important thing to do while considering this patient's advance directives?

A. Ask the patient who she wants to be her power of attorney
B. Call the eldest child
C. Send a letter to her ex-husband eliciting his feedback
D. Take a secret trip to the Community Center and ask around

Question 9. Alan is a 31-year-old male presenting to your office for the first time today to discuss immunizations. He fell on a metal fence yesterday playing basketball and sustained a puncture wound on his right hand. The wound today is not erythematous; there is no discharge, edema or tenderness to palpation of the wound. Alan cannot recall his last tetanus shot. The patient has no relevant past medical or surgical history. He has no history of depression or anxiety. All of his family members are healthy. He does not smoke, drink or abuse alcohol. He has had four different sexual partners in the last six months; three of his partners were male and one was female. The patient uses condoms consistently. He has no known history of any STIs and is routinely tested for HIV/STIs. You discuss the need for a tetanus shot with Alan and he asks about other immunizations he should receive. Given Alan's history, what immunizations are most important to discuss with Alan at this time?

A. Tdap
B. Tdap, Hepatitis B
C. Tdap, MMR
D. Tdap, Pneumovax

Question 10. Greg and Nick are both your patients. They are in a monogamous intimate relationship and usually present to your office together. Nick has HIV, which was reported to the health department when he was diagnosed. Nick presents alone today. He has been feeling well and is on HAART therapy. He takes his medications as prescribed and his CD4 count has been stable. He has not had any opportunistic infections and has no complaints today. He mentions to you today that Greg does not know about his HIV status. Nick says he has been very careful and that he is sure to always practice safer sex, but Greg is beginning to question why Nick consistently wants to use condoms during sexual activity. Nick is feeling guilty for keeping his HIV status from Greg for this long and is afraid of what may happen once he tells Greg he is HIV positive. He asks you for your advice. What is the best next step?

A. Offer to see Nick and Greg together and facilitate a conversation about Nick's HIV status
B. Tell Nick that it is wrong for him to have kept his status from Greg and that he should tell him as soon as he leaves the office
C. Tell Nick that, since Greg is your patient too, you have to call him and tell him that Nick is HIV positive
D. Tell Nick you understand the kind of situation he is in and to only tell Greg once he feels ready to do so

---

Boards-Style Application Questions Answer Key

Question 1. (D) is the correct answer. Apologizing to Kyle and moving on without obtaining a sexual history (A) is inappropriate as you may miss out on valuable information that may affect Kyle's care. It is also important to initiate a discussion on safe sexual practices and one way of ensuring Kyle is protecting himself and others is by taking a sexual history. Answer (C) is incorrect because it is imperative to always complete a thorough sexual history regardless of sexual orientation; STIs and the risk of HIV/AIDS

should be discussed with all patients who are at risk of contracting or transmitting these diseases. It is also inappropriate to make assumptions and to stereotype patients' sexual practices. Your personal discomfort with a patient's sexual orientation (B) should not interfere with your ability to provide them with comprehensive effective health care.

Question 2. (E) is the correct answer. This patient is presenting with many signs of depression, including poor sleep, fatigue and somatic complaints. While all of the answers represent possible treatments for this patient's issue, you have not yet fully evaluated this patient. The patient should undergo a full evaluation, including specific and direct yet sensitive questioning and a full physical, looking for bruising, burns or other marks of IPV. While (D) may help her sleep, it does not address her larger problem. (B) is important when evaluating someone with fatigue; however, her clinical picture points toward a more uniform diagnosis. (C) may very well be an appropriate action; however, this patient's safety comes first and she may need more immediate action. (A) is incorrect as the diagnosis of chronic fatigue syndrome has yet not been satisfied.

Question 3. (A) is the correct answer. Together with his HIV status, his sexual behavior puts him at risk for anal HPV and therefore anal intraepithelial neoplasia (AIN). While underutilized, anal Pap smears have been shown to pick up early lesions and can prevent progression to anal cancer. (C) and (D) could be helpful if he had risk factors, which he does not. Asymptomatic men should not receive urine testing for Chlamydia or gonorrhea (E). (B) is incorrect as a colonoscopy should occur at 50, as per USPSTF guidelines, based on his family history.

Question 4. (A) is the best answer. She had a normal Pap smear so is not due for one; (C) is therefore incorrect. Her blood pressure is well-controlled according to current JNC guidelines; (B) is unnecessary at this point. (D) is not right as she denies any problems with her feet; she should, however, have yearly dilated retinal examinations with an Ophthalmologist. If her diabetes were uncontrolled, she may need insulin. (E) would be correct if presented with an elevated A1C. Most importantly, however, the patient should be counseled regarding weight loss via diet and exercise. She may benefit from lesbian-specific weight-loss programs.

Question 5. (B) is the correct answer. Women who have sex with women do have a tendency towards obesity when compared to women who have sex with men, but some studies have reported that lesbians tend to be more physically active and this may be cardio-protective. Given that the clinical vignette says that this patient is physically fit and eats a well-balanced diet, there is no real clinical indication for performing the tests in answer (C). Given that Kate is a menstruating female it is very likely that she is slightly anemic; she is not complaining of any symptoms of anemia therefore a routine CBC (A) would not be indicated at this time. Aside from a Pap smear, this would be a good opportunity to facilitate a discussion on safe sexual practices amongst lesbians; Kate should also be counseled regarding STI testing for her and her partner.

Question 6. (E) is the correct answer. All of the answer choices presented are important for the establishment of an appropriate differential diagnosis. In this type of presentation, a thorough history of presenting illness should be done before proceeding to other aspects of the oral history/physical examination. Since this is the first time you are seeing Ryan you should inquire about his family and social histories; a discussion should be had regarding his social support system and current living situation. In reference to answer (D), it is unlikely that the patient has HIV with a negative test 1 month ago, but it is still possible.

Question 7. (E) is the best response. All patients reserve the right to request the visitors they desire to have with them. While this is a difficult situation, it is important to remember what the patient would want. Immediate removal of the partner would be unethical; (C) is incorrect. (B) is unnecessary, as the provider can make this decision

without utilizing outside consultation. (D) places the burden on the daughter and may exacerbate the situation. (A) puts the burden on nursing staff and shows a lack of leadership and empathy from the provider. (D) allows the daughter to describe her issues and conveys her father's expressed wishes.

Question 8. (A) is the correct answer. All elderly patients should be asked about who they want to help make decisions for them if they were to be incapacitated. Given her involvement in the LGBTQ community, she may have close friends in her family of choice that she wants involved in these decisions. While the eldest child can be consulted in an emergency, discussion prior to this can help find the best person; (B) is not the best answer. (C) is incorrect as the relationship between the patient and her ex-husband is unclear; it is a HIPAA violation to elicit his feedback without the patient's approval. While (D) would be a great way to get to know the patient, it is inappropriate for a practitioner to pry; asking the patient is easier and within the realm of the PCP's role.

Question 9. (B) is the correct answer. This would be a good opportunity to discuss the importance of hepatitis screening and immunization with Alan. Men who have sex with men are at an increased risk of contracting hepatitis which may lead to liver failure and liver cancer. The only way to protect against hepatitis C is by practicing safe sex. All men who have sex with men and have not received a complete hepatitis B vaccination series should be vaccinated against hepatitis B.

Question 10. (A) is the correct answer. This is a difficult situation for all persons involved and often times may create an ethical dilemma for a PCP who is caring for both patients (one of whom is HIV-positive and a second who may be at risk). It is important to be understanding and empathetic to the layers of emotion that may be associated with disclosing HIV status to an intimate partner. Facilitating a discussion will not only provide Nick with a safe space to disclose his HIV status but will also provide Greg with an opportunity to ask questions and to be tested.

Sources

42 CFR 482.13- Condition of Participation: Patient's Rights. US Government Printing Office Website. http://www.gpo.gov/fdsys/pkg/CFR-2011-title42-vol5/pdf/CFR-2011-title42-vol5-sec482-13.pdf. Accessed 22 Aug 2014.

Addis S, Davies M, Greene G, MacBridge-Stewart S, Shepherd M. The health, social care and housing needs of lesbian, gay, bisexual and transgender older people: a review of the literature. Health Soc Care Community. 2009;17(6):647–58.

American Medical Association. Health care needs of gay men and lesbians in the United States. JAMA. 1996;275(17):1354–9.

Ard KL, Makadon HJ. Addressing intimate partner violence in lesbian, gay, bisexual and transgender patients. J Gen Intern Med. 2011;26(8):930–3.

Boehmer U, Miao X, Maxwell NI, et al. Sexual minority population density and incidence of lung, colorectal and female breast cancer in California. BMJ Open. 2014;4:e004461. https://doi.org/10.1136/bmjopen-2013-00461.

Boehmer U, Ozonoff A, Miao X. An ecological analysis of colorectal cancer incidence and mortality: differences by sexual orientation. BMC Cancer. 2011;11:400.

Cahill S, Makadon H. Sexual orientation and gender identity data collection in clinical setting and in electronic health records: a key to ending LGBT health disparities. LGBT Health. 2014;1(1):34–41.

Calza L, Manfredi R, Pocaterra D, Chiodo F. Risk of premature atherosclerosis and ischemic heart disease associated with HIV infection and antiretroviral therapy. J Infection. 2008;57:16–32.

HPV Vaccine recommendations. Centers for Disease Control and Prevention. https://www.cdc.gov/vaccines/vpd/hpv/hcp/recommendations.html. Accessed 23 Jan 2019.

Cochran SD, Mays VM, Bowen D, et al. Cancer related risk indicators and preventative screening behaviors among lesbian and bisexual women. Am J Public Health. 2001;91(4):591–7.

Cochran SD, Mays VM. Physical health complaints among lesbians, gay men, and bisexual and homosexually experienced heterosexual individuals: results from the California quality of life survey. Am J Public Health. 2007;97(11):2048–55.

Conron KJ, Mimiaga MJ, Landers SJ. A population-based study of sexual orientation identity and gender differences in adult health. Am J Public Health. 2010;100(10):1953–60.

Davy Z. To be or not to be LGBT in primary health care: health care for lesbian, gay, bisexual, and transgender people. Br J Gen Pract. 2012;62(602):491–2.

De Vries B. LG(BT) persons in the second half of life: the intersectional influences of stigma and cohort. LGBT Health. 2014;1(1):18–23.

Dibble SL, Roberts SA. Improving cancer screening among lesbians over 50: results of a pilot study. Oncol Nurs Forum. 2003;30(4):71–9. https://doi.org/10.1188/03.ONF.E71-E79.

Ensign J. Health care for the homeless: a vision of health for all. National Healthcare for the Homeless Council. https://www.nhchc.org/wp-content/uploads/2016/12/pioneers-session-report-finalized.pdf Published 2016. Accessed 23 Jan 2019. Feldman MB, Meyer IH. Eating disorders in diverse lesbian, gay, and bisexual populations. Int J Eat Disord 2007; 40(3): 218–226.

Ferri RS. Issues in gay men's health. Nurs Clin N Am. 2004;39(39):403–10.

Fogel S, Young L, McPheron JB. The experience of group weight loss efforts among lesbians. Women Health. 2009;49(6–7):540–54.

Fogel S, Young L, Dietrich M, Blakemore D. Weight loss and related behavior changes among lesbians. J Homosex. 2012;59(5):689–702.

Fredriksen-Goldsen KI, Muraco A. Aging and sexual orientation: a 25-year review of the literature. Res Aging. 2010;32(3):372–413.

Friedman HB, Saah AJ, Sherman ME, et al. Human papillomavirus, anal squamous intraepithelial lesions, and human immunodeficiency virus in a cohort of gay men. J Infect Dis. 1998;178:45–52.

Gates GJ. Same-sex couples in US census 2010: race and ethnicity. The Williams Institute. https://williamsinstitute.law.ucla.edu/wp-content/uploads/Gates-CouplesRaceEthnicity-April-2012.pdf. Published 2012. Accessed 23 Jan 2019.

Gee R. Primary care health issues among men who have sex with men. J Am Ac Nurse Prac. 2006;18:144–53.

Gen Silent. https://www.theclowdergroup.com/gensilent. Accessed 22 Aug 2014.

Harding R, Epiphaniou E, Chidgey-clark J. Needs, experiences, and preferences of sexual minorities for end-of-life care and palliative care: a systematic review. J Palliat Med. 2012;15(5):602–11.

Health Equity Index. Human rights campaign. https://www.hrc.org/hei. Accessed 23 Jan 2019.

Jabson JM, Blosnich JR. Representation of lesbian, gay and bisexual people in clinical cancer trials. Ann Epidem. 2012;22:821–3.

Johnson CV, Mimiaga MJ, Bradford J. Health care issues among lesbian, gay, bisexual, transgender and intersex (LGBTI) populations in the United States: introduction. J Homosex. 2008;54(3):213–24.

Kerker BD, Mostashari F, Thorpe L. Health care access and utilization among women who have sex with women: sexual behavior and identity. J Urban Health. 2006;83(5):970–9.

Keuroghlian AS, Shtasel D, Bassuk EL. Out on the street: a public health and policy agenda on lesbian, gay, bisexual and transgender youth who are homeless. Am J Orthopsych. 2014;84(1):66–72.

Lastdrag.org. http://www.lastdrag.org/. Accessed 22 Aug 2014.

Lipshultz SE, Mas CM, Henkel JM, Franco VI, Fisher SD, Miller TL. HAART to heart: highly active antiretroviral therapy and the risk of cardiovascular disease in HIV-infected or exposed children and adults. Expert Rev Anti-Infect Ther. 2012;10(6):661–74.

Machalek DA, Poynten M, Jin F, et al. Anal human papillomavirus infection and associated neoplastic lesions in men who have sex with men: a systematic review and meta-analysis. Lancet Oncol. 2012;12:487–500. https://doi.org/10.1016/S1470-2045(12)70080-3.

Machalek DA, Grulich AE, Hillman RJ, et al. The study of the prevention of anal cancer (SPANC): design and methods of a three-year prospective cohort study. BMC Public Health. 2013;13:946–58. https://doi.org/10.1186/1471-2458-13-946.

Makadon HJ. Ending LGBT invisibility in health care: the first step in ensuring equitable care. Cleve Clin J Med. 2011 Apr;78(4):220–4.

Mayer KH, Bradford JB, Makadon HJ, Stall R, Goldhammer H, Landers S. Sexual and gender minority health: what we know and what needs to be done. Am J Public Health. 2008;98(6):989–95.

McNair RP, Hegarty K. Guidelines for the primary care of lesbian, gay, and bisexual people: a systematic review. Ann Fam Med. 2010;8:533–41.

Meads C, Moore D. Breast cancer in lesbians and bisexual women: systematic review of incidence, prevalence and risk studies. BMC Public Health. 2013;13:1127–37.

Mravcak SA. Primary care for lesbians and bisexual women. Am Fam Physician. 2006;74(2):279–86.

National LGBT Cancer Network. http://www.cancer-network.org/. Accessed 22 Aug 2014.

Obedin-Malliver J, Goldsmith ES, Stewart L, et al. Lesbian, gay, bisexual and transgender-related content in undergraduate medical education. JAMA. 2011;306(9):971–7. https://doi.org/10.1001/jama.2011.1255.

Recommended Adult Immunization Schedule, by Vaccine and Age Group. CDC Web site http://www.cdc.gov/vaccines/schedules/hcp/imz/adult.html. Accessed 20 Aug 2014.

Roberts SJ, Stuart-Shor EM, Oppenheimer RA. Lesbians' attitudes and beliefs regarding overweight and weight reduction. J Clin Nursing. 2010;10:1986–94.

Rosenfeld D, Bartlam B, Smith RD. Out of the closet and into the trenches: gay male Baby Boomers, aging, and HIV/AIDS. Gerontologist. 2012;52(2):255–64.

Rotondi KN, et al. Nonprescribed hormone use and self-performed surgeries: "Do-It-Yourself" transitions in transgender communities in Ontario, Canada. Am J Public Health. 2013;103(10):1830–6.

SAGE website. http://sageusa.org/. Accessed 22 Aug 2014.

Sanchez NF, Rabatin J, Sanchez JP, Hubbard S, Kalet A. Medical students ability to care for lesbian, gay, bisexual, and transgendered patients. Fam Med. 2006;38(1):21–7.

Simone-Skidmore M. LGBT Aging: addressing disparities and healthcare needs. The National LGBT Health Education Center. http://www.lgbthealtheducation.

org/wp-content/uploads/LGBT-Aging-Addressing-Disparities-and-Health-Care-Needs.pdf. Accessed 22 Jan 2019.

Steele LS, Tinmouth JM, Lu A. Regular health care use by lesbians: a path analysis of predictive factors. Fam Pract. 2006;23:631–6.

Stroumsa D. The state of transgender health care. Am J Public Health. 2014;104(3):e31–8.

Top Ten Issues to Discuss with your Health care Provider. GLMA Web site http://www.glma.org/index.cfm?fuseaction=Page.viewPage&pageId=947&grandparentID=534&parentID=938&nodeID=1. Accessed 1 Aug 2014.

United States Preventive Services Task Force Website. http://www.uspreventiveservicestaskforce.org/. Accessed 22 Aug 2014.

US Preventive Services Task Force. Screening for ovarian cancer: US Preventive Services Task Force recommendation statement. JAMA. 2018;319(6):588–94. https://doi.org/10.1001/jama.2017.21926.

Van Wagenen A, Driskell J, Bradford J. "I'm still raring to go": successful aging among lesbian, gay, bisexual, and transgender older adults. J Aging Stud. 2013;27(1):1–14.

Wallace SP, Cochran SD, Durazo EM, Ford CL. The health of aging lesbian, gay and bisexual adults in California. Policy Brief UCLA Cent Health Policy Res. 2011;1:1–8.

Wandrey RL, Qualls WD, Mosack KE. Rejection of breast reconstruction among lesbian cancer patients. LGBT Health 2015;3(1):74–8.

Ward BW, Dahlhamer JM, Galinsky AM, Joestl SS. Sexual orientation and health among U.S. adults: National Health Interview Survey, 2013. In: National health statistics reports; no. 77. Hyattsville: National Center for Health Statistics; 2014.

Wight RG, LeBlanc AJ, Detels R. Stress and mental health among midlife and older gay-identified men. Am J Public Health. 2012;102(3):503–10.

Williams ML, Bowen AM, Horvath KJ. The social/sexual environment of gay men residing in a rural frontier state: implications for the development of HIV prevention programs. J Rural Health. 2005 Winter;21(1):48–55.

Witten TM. It's not all darkness: robustness, resilience, and successful transgender aging. LGBT Health. 2014;1(1):24–33.

Women's Health Initiative. http://www.nhlbi.nih.gov/whi/. Accessed 22 Aug 2014.

Zwarenstein M, Goldman J, Reeves S. Interprofessional collaboration: effects of practice-based interventions on professional practice and health care outcomes. Cochrane.

Sexual Health

8

Carl G. Streed Jr., Ivy H. Gardner, Kara Malone,
and Brent C. Monseur

The Sexual Health History

External Resource 8.1
This short video called **"Let's Talk About Sexual Health"** covers the importance of an open dialogue between youth and providers regarding sexual health, featuring Elizabeth Torrone, PhD, MSPH, of the Centers for Disease Control and Prevention.
http://bit.ly/TECe1ch08_01

The first listed author is the chapter's associate editor from The Equal Curriculum Project. The chapter authors are otherwise ordered according to their preference.

C. G. StreedJr. (✉)
Boston University School of Medicine, Center for Transgender Medicine & Surgery, Boston Medical Center, Boston, MA, USA
e-mail: carl.streed@bmc.org

I. H. Gardner
Oregon Health & Science University, Portland, OR, USA

K. Malone
The Ohio State University College of Medicine, Columbus, OH, USA
e-mail: malone.364@osu.edu

B. C. Monseur
Thomas Jefferson University Hospital, Philadelphia, PA, USA

The World Health Organization defines sexual health as "a state of physical, emotional, mental and social well-being in relation to sexuality; it is not merely the absence of disease, dysfunction or infirmity. Sexual health requires a positive and respectful approach to sexuality and sexual relationships, as well as the possibility of having pleasurable and safe sexual experiences, free of coercion, discrimination and violence." To advocate for their patients' sexual health, health care providers must first be able to obtain detailed, respectful, and assumption-free sexual health histories from all of their patients. Unfortunately, most health care providers do not routinely take complete sexual histories.

A health care provider may avoid taking a complete sexual history because of embarrassment, lack of knowledge, time constraints, or the misperception that this information is not relevant to the patient's health. The main barriers to taking sexual histories from LGBTQ individuals are personal discomfort on the part of the health care provider and a lack of training and knowledge. Some discomfort stems from not knowing what questions to ask LGBTQ individuals because of the provider's lack of familiarity with specific sexual practices and the sexual terminology patients may use. Rarely is this discomfort a result of blatant prejudice or disgust with non-heterosexual sex.

Exposure to and education about LGBTQ individuals can mitigate the discomfort providers feel about taking a sexual history from LGBTQ individuals. Health professional students with clinical exposure to LGBTQ individuals have a more positive attitude toward LGBTQ patients and better knowledge of LGBTQ health issues and are more likely to consistently take adequate sexual histories from patients.

Another way for health care providers to feel more comfortable about taking sexual histories from LGBTQ patients is to have a systematic way of asking assumption-free questions that are sensitive and respectful of all patients regardless of their sexual orientation or gender identity. Like the general medical history, the sexual history should start with open-ended questions to make the person feel comfortable and allow them to express any concerns. Some open-ended starting questions: "What are your concerns or questions about your sexuality, sexual orientation, or sexual desires?" "What sexual concerns do you have?" "Tell me about your sexual health." Another way to start the conversation is to emphasize the importance of sexual health and ask the individual's permission to ask about their sexual health before diving into the specific questions. If the health care provider is not completely comfortable asking about sexual health or feels that the patient is uncomfortable, it may help to tell the patient these questions are routinely asked of all patients.

It is imperative that the health care provider taking a sexual history avoid making assumptions about the patient. Such assumptions may dictate which questions are asked and prevent the provider from acquiring pertinent information. Assumptions can also lead to surprise and discomfort when what the patient says does not match what the health care provider assumed, which may make the patient uncomfortable and limit their disclosure of important information. This is especially true when a sexual history is taken from an LGBTQ patient. Nothing should be assumed about an individual's sexual orientation or experiences beyond what the patient specifically discloses. An easy way to convey a lack of assumptions about a patient's sexual orientation and experiences is to use gender-neutral language and pronouns when asking about relationships and sexual partners. It is better to ask the patient whether they have a partner or significant other than to inquire about a girlfriend, boyfriend, wife, or husband. If the patient provides the gender of their partner(s),

follow that lead; if the patient does not, continue using gender-neutral language.

In addition to refraining from assumptions about a patient's sexual orientation, the health care provider should not assume how many partners the patient has or the type of relationship the patient is in. It is more respectful and informative to ask how many sexual partners the patient has than to ask about marriage or monogamy. If a provider is corrected by the patient after making an incorrect assumption, it is acceptable for the provider to briefly apologize and ask for clarification. Another way to demonstrate respect for the patient is to use the same terms the patient uses to describe their sexual orientation, gender identity, and body. It is disrespectful to use a different term to describe a patient's identity or body when the patient has already indicated their term, even when using a more medical one. For example, if a transgender woman calls her penis a clitoris, it would be disrespectful to later ask about penile discharge; simply say "discharge." Similarly, it also disrespectful to refer to a patient as homosexual when the patient has identified as queer. It is permissible to ask in a respectful manner for clarification of the terminology that the patient uses to avoid misunderstandings.

The sexuality and sexual behaviors of older adults are frequently neglected by clinicians and researchers. Negative stereotypes regarding the sex lives of older adults are abundant. Unmindful clinicians may assume that sexuality is not important to an older patient's quality of life, that the patient does not have or want any sexual contact (and therefore has negligible sexual risk), that an older patient will be unwilling to discuss sexuality and sexual health, or that an older adult will not be able to participate in discussions about sexual orientation or gender identity. These assumptions lead to missed opportunities to treat sexual dysfunctions (e.g., erectile dysfunction, vaginal atrophy), mitigate effects of illness states on sexual desire and enjoyment (e.g., urogenital cancers), identify psychosexual challenges, offer appropriate screenings and medical tests, and provide counseling on safer sex.

After the sexual history is started with an open-ended question, more direct questions are needed to obtain specific information. Clinicians should avoid using medical jargon and define terms and abbreviations such as *STI* for *sexually transmitted infection* as they come up. Table 8.1 provides examples of ways to frame questions that address components of the sexual history, categorized by the "5 P's of sexual health" recommended by the CDC—Partners, Practices, Protection from STIs,

Table 8.1 The fives P's of STI prevention (extended)

Partners
Who do you have sex with?
In the past 2 months, how many partners have you had sex with?
In the past 12 months, how many partners have you had sex with?
Prevention of pregnancy
Do you have any sexual contact that could result in pregnancy?
Are you or your partner trying to get pregnant?
If not: What are you (or your partner) doing to prevent pregnancy?
Protection from STIs
What do you do to protect yourself from STIs and HIV?
How often do you use condoms? Always? Sometimes? Never?
If never: Why don't you use condoms?
If sometimes: In what situations or with whom do you not use condoms?
When was the last time you were tested for STIs or HIV?
Are you interested in being tested for STIs or HIV?
Do you take any medication to prevent HIV?
Are there any other forms of protection that you're interested in discussing?
Practices
To understand your risk for STIs, I need to understand what kind of sex you've had recently. It's important for me to know what sexually transmitted infections you may be at risk for, so I'm going to ask what kinds of sexual activities you've engaged in in the past year.
Have you had vaginal sex, meaning "penis in vagina"?
If yes: Do you use condoms never, sometimes, or always?
Have you had anal sex, meaning "penis in rectum or anus sex"?
If yes: Do you use condoms never, sometimes, or always?
Have you had oral sex, meaning "mouth on penis or vagina"?
Do you ever have pain or discomfort during sex?
Do you or your partner(s) use any devices, toys, or substances to enhance your sexual pleasure?
Have you noticed any changes in sexual function?
Is there anything else about your sexual practices that I need to know about?

Table 8.1 (continued)

Past history of STIs
Have you ever had an STI?
Have you ever been treated for an STI? Any symptoms since?
Have any of your partners been tested for an STI? Treated?
Have you, or any of your partners, ever injected drugs?
Have you, or any of your partners, exchanged money or drugs for sex?

Past history of sexually transmitted infections, and Prevention of pregnancy.

The examples in these tables are better used as a framework than as a memorized script. This allows for adapting as needed, depending on the patient's experiences, level of disclosure, and comfort. Patients may not always feel comfortable answering all of these questions. Respecting the patient's right to disclosure is an important part of taking a sensitive sexual history. In addition, every patient should be screened for physical and sexual abuse, either during the sexual history or at some point during the encounter.

If time is limited or the patient's chief complaint is unrelated to sexual health, it is acceptable to ask just a couple of screening questions instead of getting a detailed sexual history. A screening sexual health history may include these questions:

- Have you been sexually involved with anyone in the last 6 months?
- Do you have sex with men, women, both, or neither?
- What sexual concerns do you, or your partner(s), have?

Key Points
- The best approach to taking a sexual history from any patient, including LGBTQ patients, is to employ a systematic way of asking assumption-free questions that are sensitive and respectful, regardless of the patient's sexual orientation or gender identity.

- Use gender-neutral language and pronouns when asking about relationships and sexual partners.
- Demonstrate respect by using the same terms the patient uses to describe their sexual orientation, gender identity, and body.
- Start the sexual history with open-ended questions or begin the conversation by emphasizing the importance of sexual health and asking the individual's permission to talk about their sexual health before diving into specifics.
- A detailed sexual history should include gender identity and number of partners, the sexual activities the patient engages in and their frequency, what the patient does for protection against sexual transmitted infections (STIs) and contraception (if applicable), how often and in what situations the patient uses protection, history of STIs, pain with sex or other issues, sexual satisfaction, and an opportunity for the patient to identify additional questions or concerns.

Case 8.1

A 30-year-old woman comes to the primary care clinic to establish care after moving to the area. She identifies as a cisgender queer and reports that she has been in a relationship with a woman for three years but occasionally has sex with other people. In the past six months she has had sex with two women, a genderqueer person, and a man. The patient occasionally uses condoms and dental dams but never when she has been drinking. She had Chlamydia several years ago and was adequately treated. She also often gets yeast infections that she treats with over-the-counter medications. The patient does not

remember when she was last tested for STIs. She had an elective abortion one year ago, and an IUD was placed at that time. She is generally satisfied with her sex life but has noticed recently that anal and vaginal penetration is sometimes uncomfortable.

The provider, unaware of the above, asks whether she is in a relationship now, and she replies, "Yes, my girlfriend and I have been together for three years." The provider assumes that the patient is a lesbian and monogamous and stops the sexual history at this point.

How might the health care provider have better approached the sexual health history?
Why was his sexual history so brief?
What are some questions that could have revealed her specific sexual behaviors?

The provider in this case missed a wealth of important information by cutting the sexual history short. He did not know what to ask next because he made some assumptions about the patient and, based on those assumptions, incorrectly thought that there were no more questions to ask. He may have also felt uncomfortable with his lack of knowledge and familiarity with LGBTQ health issues refrained from asking more questions to avoid offending the patient or making her uncomfortable. Without knowing this patient's sexual history, however, the provider is missing out on much vital medical information about this patient and cannot counsel her on STI prevention or clarify her pain during penetrative sex. It is to be hoped that this inadequate sexual history and his assumptions about her sexual orientation and activities will not prevent the provider from taking a more accurate sexual history in the future.

Sexual Activities

Sexual orientation does not dictate sexual behavior, and vice versa. Health care providers cannot assume what particular sexual activities patients engage in or what they find pleasurable. There is no way of knowing any of this without asking. The conflation of sex with sexual intercourse (if narrowly defined as a man's penis in a woman's vagina) is harmful not only to LGBTQ individuals but all individuals because it excludes the vast possibilities of sexual activities that people may do during intimate encounters. It is important for health care providers not to assume that they have the same definition of sex, especially when interviewing young people. Sex is any act that gives someone erotic physical pleasure, and no sexual act is better or more "normal" than others. There is no difference in sexual satisfaction or sexual dysfunction between LGBTQ and cisgender heterosexual people. It is also important to realize that knowing a patient's sexual orientation or the gender of the patient's partner(s) does not necessarily give the health care provider insight into the patient's or partner's body or either person's relationship with their body. The patient or partner(s) may be transgender or intersex and may have a different configuration of genitals than what is generally assumed from someone's gender identity. A patient may have a history of abuse or body image issues or may not feel connected with certain body parts and therefore not include them in sexual activities.

Health care providers must be knowledgeable of their patients' sexual practices to be able to educate them on their risk of STIs and how to reduce these risks. The best framework with which to appreciate and assess the STI risk of a wide array of sexual activities is to understand what body parts are involved. The STI risk involved in penetrative sex depends on the orifice being penetrated and what is used for penetration. Orifices that may be used for penetration are the vagina, anus, and mouth. (Less common are ostomies.) Objects used for penetration include the penis, fingers/hands, toes, dildos, household objects, foods, and other sex toys/devices. Anus-penis penetrative sex is associated with a high incidence of self-reported STIs in men and women of all sexual orientations. Vagina-penis and anus-penis penetrative sex carries a higher risk of STIs than do other forms of penetrative sex. This has led to the misconception that other types of penetrative sex carry no risk. The limited data on the risks associated with penetrative sex with fingers/hands or sex toys demonstrate that transmission of STIs is possible. Vagina–sex toy penetrative sex with toys that are not regularly cleaned and are shared between individuals is associated with bacterial vaginosis. Penetrative sex with fingers/hands carries a risk of transmission of herpes simplex and human papilloma virus (HPV). All forms of penetrative and nonpenetrative sex carry an increased risk of STIs when open wounds, cuts, sores, or abrasions are present on the skin or mucosa. Objects that can break can cause tears, and more aggressive or unlubricated penetration can cause fissures in the vagina or anus (uncommon with oral penetration).

Oral sex includes contact between the mouth and the vulva, penis, anus, dildos, and other sex toys. Anus-mouth, penis-mouth, and vagina-mouth sex all carry a risk of STIs and hepatitis. Other sexual activities include manual stimulation of the genitals and genital-on-genital rubbing. Research on the STIs risk associated with these sexual activities is limited, but it has been shown that recent genital-on-genital contact between women is associated with a higher rate of bacterial vaginosis. Although the evidence elucidating the STI risk of many nonpenetrative and nonpenile forms of sex is likewise limited, patients should be advised to use basic precautions—washing their hands before manual sex or finger/hand penetrative sex, cleaning sex toys before sex, using barriers such as condoms and dental dams as often as possible—to prevent the spread of infection.

Commercial over-the-counter lubricants have a significant role in sexual health. Use of lubricants can enhance pleasure while preventing pain, abrasions (small tears that increase risk of STIs), and larger tears (e.g., fissures). Commercial sex toys are typically safer than other objects that may be used for penetrative sex because they are made with designs and materials that unlikely to injure epithelia, break, or become trapped.

Some infections may be transmitted during sexual activity that are not sexually transmitted infections in the classical sense. There have been outbreaks of meningococcal meningitis due to Neisseria meningitidis serogroup C in MSM in New York City, Los Angeles, and cities in Europe. Immunization was recommended for MSM with sexual contacts in those urban centers. There have also been methicillin-resistant *Staphylococcus aureus* (MRSA) outbreaks in urban MSM in some cities, but subsequent studies of urban MSM has not found elevated MRSA colonization.

Key Points

- Sexual orientation does not dictate sexual behavior. Sex is any act that gives someone physical pleasure, and no particular sexual act is better or more "normal" than another.
- Health care providers must be knowledgeable of their patients' sexual practices to educate them on their risk of STIs and how to reduce these risks.
- Vagina-penis and anus-penis penetrative sex carry a higher risk of STIs than do other forms of penetrative sex.
- Although evidence elucidating the STI risk of many nonpenetrative and nonpenile forms of sex is limited, patients should be advised to use basic precautions (e.g., washing hands before manual sex or finger/hand penetrative sex, cleaning sex toys before sex, using condoms and dental dams as often as possible) to help prevent the spread of infection.

Case 8.2

A 27-year-old man goes to his primary care provider for his yearly physical. He identifies as gay and says that he has been in a relationship with a trans man for the past seven months. The patient says that he and his partner are monogamous and always use condoms for anal and vaginal penetrative sex. He wants to be tested for STIs today because he and his boyfriend want to be fluid-bonded and to stop using condoms. He also wants to ask about non-barrier contraceptive methods that he and his partner might use because his partner does not have a health care provider with whom he feels comfortable discussing contraception. The patient is not sure how to bring this up during the visit and feels nervous about having to explain that he and his partner have penis-vagina penetrative sex.

- **What sexual activities could this PCP have predicted from the patient's sexual orientation?**
- **Without asking about the patient's partner, what might the provider miss?**

Again, a provider knows nothing about an individual's sexual activities just from that person's sexual orientation. Even if the provider knew that this individual had a boyfriend, the provider still does not know what body parts the partner has or what sexual activities they are engaging in together. The provider in this case would probably assume that the patient's partner is cisgender, that the only high-risk sexual activity is penis-anus penetrative sex, and that the only thing the provider needs to ask about is condom use. It is often uncomfortable for patients to volunteer this kind of information, and they may not ask the provider questions or voice their concerns if the provider does not take a full sexual history.

Sexually Transmitted Infections

Although all people who are sexually active are at risk for sexually transmitted infections (STIs), men who have sex with men (MSM) and women who have sex with women (WSW) have some increased risks, regardless of self-identified sexual orientation. The following sections will describe the epidemiology, transmission, safer sex options, prophylaxis, and treatment for these STIs: bacterial vaginosis, Chlamydia, gonorrhea, hepatitis A virus, hepatitis B virus, hepatitis C virus, human papillomavirus, herpes virus, infectious proctitis, lymphogranuloma venereum, and syphilis. Human immunodeficiency virus infection (HIV) is covered in detail in Chap. 11.

Treatment for these clinical entities may change. For the most up-to-date treatment recommendations, please see the Centers for Disease Control and Prevention's most recent guidelines. As of 2018, the most current guidelines are the *2015 Sexually Transmitted Diseases Treatment Guidelines*. A dense summary of evaluation and management based on presenting signs and symptoms is available in Tables 10.4 and 10.5. *Trichomonas vaginalis* and *Haemophilus ducreyi* (chancroid), which are not covered in this chapter, are also included in those tables. In the following section, *men* refers to natal males, and *women* refers to natal females unless otherwise described.

Bacterial Vaginosis

Although most cases of bacterial vaginosis (BV) are asymptomatic, BV is the most common cause of vaginal discharge and malodor. Unlike the other infections discussed, BV is a clinical syndrome that results in changes in the normal vaginal bacterial flora. Typically, *Lactobacillus* species are replaced with high concentrations of anaerobic bacteria. Significantly, studies have shown that lesbians and individuals who have *never* been sexually active can contract BV. Still, treatment of BV has been shown to reduce the risk of Chlamydia, gonorrhea, HIV, and other viral STIs.

Signs and Symptoms. The most common symptom of BV is an abnormal homogeneous off-white vaginal discharge (especially after vaginal intercourse) that may be accompanied by an unpleasant fishy odor.

Diagnosis. Either clinical criteria or microscopic visualization of "clue cells" may be used to make the diagnosis.

Treatment. BV is treated with one week of oral 500 mg metronidazole twice daily or 0.75% gel. Alternatively, a clindamycin cream (2%) may be used for one week intravaginally at bedtime. Neither douching nor treatment of male partners has been shown to decrease the incidence of BV.

Chlamydia

Chlamydia trachomatis (CT) infection spreads through anal, oral, or vaginal sex, affects both men and women, and is the most commonly reported STI. Sexually active young people, as well as gay, bisexual, other MSM, and possibly WSW, are at increased risk for CT infection. Among MSM, urethral Chlamydia transmission is uncommon when anal sex is not practiced. However, 53–85% of CT cases among MSM may go underreported as a result of extragenital infections unless nucleic acid amplification tests of rectal and oral samples are performed in addition to urine/urethral samples. Although data specific to rectal infection in women who engage in anal intercourse is limited, one study revealed that urine-based screening would have failed to identify as many as 13.4% of rectal Chlamydia infections. See the discussion of infectious proctitis, later in this chapter, for gastrointestinal manifestations of CT.

Signs & Symptoms. Affected individuals may complain of genital discharge, dysuria, or both. Men may also complain of pain/swelling in the testes. Anal infection is often asymptomatic.

Diagnosis. Often diagnosed clinically, CT is confirmed with the use of polymerase chain reaction (PCR) of urine, urethral discharge, vaginal discharge, or throat swabs.

Treatment. CT is easily treated. Patients should be instructed to finish the prescribed regimen plus seven days before engaging in sexual activity. Among MSM sexual partners who do not come into the clinic, patient-delivered partner therapy (PDPT) increases the likelihood of partner treatment. Treatment consists of a single dose of 1 g oral azithromycin or one week of 100 mg oral doxycycline twice daily.

Prevention. CDC screening guidelines recommend annual screening for CT for sexually active cisgender gays, bisexuals, and other MSM. USPSTF recommends annual screening in all sexually active women under 24 and women over 25 with risk factors (new or multiple sex partners). The CDC recommends that MSM with more than one partner, anonymous partners, and those who use or are sexually active with those who use illicit drugs should increase their frequency of screening. MSM must be screened for both CT and gonorrhea; otherwise, more than 70% of cases may be missed. For transgender people, the decision to test is entirely individualized, based on anatomic inventory and sexual behaviors.

Health care providers have cited various barriers, such as time constraints, lack of staff, and cultural/language barriers, to maintaining these screening standards. For this reason, self-testing, self-collected rectal/pharyngeal swabs, and Internet-based testing may be suitable alternatives. Condom use with anal sex has been shown to be protective against CT infection.

Complications. Without treatment, CT can cause pelvic inflammatory disease in women (natal females) or sterility in men (natal males). HIV-positive men who engage in receptive anal intercourse have been shown to have a higher prevalence of rectal CT but not of rectal gonorrhea. Finally, untreated genital CT and rectal Chlamydia (as well as rectal gonorrhea) may increase the risk of acquiring or transmitting HIV.

Gonorrhea

Neisseria gonorrhea is a frequently reported STI that affects the rectum, throat, and genitals in both men and women. Sexually active young people are at increased risk, as are MSM, particularly HIV-positive ones. CDC reports in 2014 also establish that gonorrhea in MSM accounted for 37.1% of all the cases in the Gonococcal Isolate Surveillance Project. Incidence continues to rise, with the greatest share of cases reported from the west coast of the US. Incidence is likely to be underestimated because often the only samples that are collected are urethral swabs and urine. Unlike urethral Chlamydia, the risk of urethral gonorrhea is similar in MSM who do and do not have anal sex. More than 70% of gonorrhea infections go unreported because they are extragenital and will not be diagnosed unless nucleic acid amplification testing of rectal and oral samples is performed in addition to assays of urine and urethral samples. Although the data are specific to rectal infection in women who engage in anal intercourse, one study found that urine-based screening would have failed to identify 35% of rectal Chlamydia infections.

Signs and Symptoms. Although many cases are asymptomatic, both men and women may complain of dysuria, genital or anal discharge (white, yellow, or green), anal itching or soreness, bleeding, or painful bowel movements.

Diagnosis. Often diagnosed clinically, gonorrhea is confirmed by means of PCR of urine, urethral discharge, vaginal discharge, or throat swabs.

Treatment. Gonorrhea is easily treated, and patients should be instructed to finish the prescribed regimen plus seven days before engaging in further sexual activity. The recommended regimen is ceftriaxone 250 mg intramuscular once and azithromycin 1 g by mouth. Azithromycin treats gonorrhea by a different mechanism from cephalosporins and also treats CT, which is a very common coinfection. Cefixime 400 mg once by mouth may replace ceftriaxone. Drug-resistant strains of gonorrhea are on the rise, particularly among MSM. Patients should be instructed to return for follow-up if symptoms do not abate after a few days of treatment. Among sexual partners of MSM who do not come into the clinic, patient-delivered partner therapy (PDPT) may increase the likelihood of treatment. Treatment failures should be anticipated because MSM are particularly susceptible to antimicrobial-resistant strains. (See the discussion of Chlamydia above.)

Prevention. Prevention strategies for gonorrhea are like those for Chlamydia. The USPSTF recommends annual screening in all sexually active women under 24 and women over 25 with risk factors: "a previous gonococcal infection, other STIs, or new or multiple sex partners, as well as inconsistent condom use, commercial sex work, or illicit drug use." A study in Madrid showed that of the 89% of HIV-positive men with asymptomatic pharyngeal gonorrhea, 86% engaged in unprotected oral sex. Considering the finding that most men who used condoms only did so when engaging in anal intercourse, patients should be counseled on the importance of condom use when participating in other sexual practices. For transgender people, the decision to test is entirely individualized, based on anatomic inventory and sexual behaviors.

Complications. Gonorrhea can have complications similar to CT, including PID in women (natal females) and sterility in men (natal males). Additionally, though rare, gonorrhea can be life threatening if it spreads to the blood or joints.

Hepatitis A

Hepatitis A virus (HAV) infection is self-limited infection that infects the liver and sheds viral load in the feces. Acute liver failure is rare, and HAV infection does not become chronic. In addition to contact with contaminated foods, person-to-person sexual contact can cause transmission by way of the fecal-oral route. Approximately 10% of all new HAV cases involve MSM. All MSM should receive the HAV vaccine.

Signs and Symptoms. Often presenting with flu-like symptoms of fatigue, fever, and myalgias, HAV infection can progress to cause abdominal pain, loss of appetite, jaundice, diarrhea, and light clay–colored stools.

Diagnosis. Serologic testing is required for diagnosis.

Treatment. Treatment of HAV infection is supportive.

Prevention. HAV infection is a vaccine-preventable STI. Condoms have not been demonstrated to be protective against in HAV prevention. HIV infection may dampen immune response to HAV infection.

Hepatitis B

Unlike HAV, hepatitis B virus (HBV) is spread in bodily fluids such as blood and semen. Its incidence is high in MSM. The highest concentrations of viral load are found in the blood. HBV infection may be acute or chronic, with the risk of chronicity changing inversely with age. There is an associated increase in risk for hepatocellular carcinoma. MSM are at increased risk for HBV infection, accounting for 20% of new cases, and vaccination is strongly encouraged.

Signs and Symptoms. Early HBV may present like the flu, with malaise, fever, loss of appetite, nausea, vomiting, and body aches, progressing to include dark urine and jaundice.

Transmission. HBV can be spread through both unprotected anal sex and receptive oral sex.

Diagnosis. Serologic testing is required for diagnosis.

Treatment. As of 2008, seven medications are licensed for the treatment of hepatitis B infection in the United States: the antiviral drugs lamivudine, adefovir, tenofovir, telbivudine, and entecavir and a pair of immune modulators, interferon α_{2a} and PEGylated interferon α_{2a}.

Prevention. HBV infection is vaccine-preventable. HIV infection can dampen the immune response to vaccine. Patients with HIV should be closely followed, and the vaccination regimen may need to be modified.

Complications. Untreated, HBV infection can lead to liver cirrhosis, liver failure, and hepatocellular carcinoma.

Hepatitis C

Similar to HAV and HBV infections, HCV infection has a higher incidence in MSM, but unlike the other two hepatitis strains, it is not vaccine-preventable. As the most common chronic blood-borne infection in the US, hepatitis C is not classically categorized as an STI; however, reports of sexual transmission continue, particularly among MSM, especially HIV-infected ones. Considering this and the reported high frequency of reinfection after treatment, HIV-infected individuals should undergo HCV screening and have their liver function monitored.

Signs and Symptoms. Like HBV infection, HCV infection can present like the flu, with malaise, fever, loss of appetite, nausea, vomiting, and body aches, progressing to include dark urine and jaundice.

Treatment. Affected patients should be referred to a specialist for consultation on therapy options, including PEGylated interferon, ribavirin, and newer agents.

Prevention. Sexual transmission in people who engage exclusively in penis-vagina sex is a rare event that may not even warrant condom use; however, condom use is important for HIV-infected men, regardless of sexual practices. No effective vaccine or post-exposure follow-up is currently available. The USPSTF recommends screening for hepatitis C virus (HCV) infection in persons at high risk for infection, such as intravenous drug users. The USPSTF also recommends offering one-time screening for HCV infection to adults born between 1945 and 1965.

Complications. Prior syphilis infection, engaging in unprotected sex, and HIV infection have all been positively associated with hepatitis C. The incidence of hepatitis C infection continues to increase among HIV-positive MSM. Untreated, HCV infection can lead to liver cirrhosis, liver failure, and hepatocellular carcinoma.

Herpes

Herpes strains are often classified as oral or genital, but both herpes simplex virus (HSV)-1 and HSV-2 have been documented to cause genital herpes, a chronic viral infection. Although most genital herpes cases are in fact caused by HSV-2 (~50 million in the US), the incidence of anal infections resulting from HSV-1 infection is on the rise. HSV and syphilis are the pathogens most commonly transmitted anorectally. Approximately 18.4% of MSM were found to have HSV-2 infection in the National Health and Nutrition Examination Survey. One US-based study showed that the prevalence of HSV-2 differed for WSW by self-identified sexual orientation: 45.6% of heterosexuals, 35.9% of bisexuals, and 8.2% of homosexuals/lesbians, compared with women who do not have sex with women, who had a prevalence of 23.8%.

Signs and Symptoms. Painful blisters are widely believed to be the standard presentation, but people are often unaware that they have HSV, and their infections go undiagnosed. This presents challenges in preventing the spread of this infection.

Diagnosis. Although HSV infection is often diagnosed clinically, testing of vesicle fluid by PCR can identify HSV.

Treatment. Antiviral treatment should be aimed at treating both the acute and chronic aspects of the disease. It is important to remember that treatment cannot completely eradicate the virus. Topical antiviral therapy is of negligible benefit. Treatment regimens are broken down into first incidence, suppressive therapy, episodic, and severe infection. In an initial outbreak, the patient should be treated for 7–10 days (or until ulcers heal) with oral acyclovir (400 mg three times daily or 200 mg five times daily), oral famciclovir (250 mg three times daily), or oral valacyclovir (1 g twice daily). Suppressive therapy can be used to decrease the risk of transmission to susceptible partners and can also reduce recurrence by 70–80%. Oral daily treatment with acyclovir (400 mg, twice), famciclovir (250 mg, twice), or valacyclovir (500 mg or 1 g, once) is recommended. Therapy for recurrent episodes may be used if it is started within one day of the appearance of a new lesion. Various regimens consist of daily oral acyclovir, famciclovir, or valacyclovir. Patients should be provided the prescription in advance so they can begin treatment as soon as possible after the appearance of a lesion.

Prevention. Routine serologic screening is not recommended for genital herpes simplex virus (HSV) infection in asymptomatic adolescents and adults, including those who are pregnant. Circumcision was not observed to have a significant impact on acquisition in MSM. Barrier methods help prevent transmission.

Human Papilloma Virus

Human papilloma virus (HPV) is the most common STI worldwide. Although many HPV infections are asymptomatic (~50% of sexually active persons), certain strains are associated with genital warts (HPV-6, HPV-11) or malignancies of the cervix, anal canal, and oropharynx (HPV-16, HPV-18). HIV-infected MSM populations have a high incidence of anal cancer, exceeding that of cervical cancer in women, a finding that may support cytological screening in MSM. At this time evidence is limited, but some studies have called for an increase in HPV vaccine coverage and cancer surveillance in MSM. WSW are less likely to

undergo regular cervical screening. HPV can be transmitted during finger-genital contact. Although more studies are needed to determine the incidence of HPV among WSW, this population should be encouraged to undergo regular screening.

Signs and Symptoms. Genital warts on visual inspection are a hallmark of HPV infection.

Diagnosis. Cervical and anal Papanicolaou testing to visualize any cellular metaplasia are used to make the diagnosis. Additional testing may be used to detect HPV DNA.

Treatment. Treatment is typically aimed at genital warts or other lesions when present. Patient-applied treatments include podofilox (0.5% solution or gel), imiquimod (5% cream), and sinecatechins (15% ointment). Provider-administered treatments include multiple cryotherapy applications, podophyllin resin (10–20%, compound tincture of benzoin), trichloroacetic acid (TCA; 80–90%), bichloroacetic acid (BCA; 80–90%), and surgical removal.

Prevention. HPV infection is a vaccine-preventable illness. Three vaccines are used in the US at the time of this writing. Although all cover strands associated with malignancies, only the quadrivalent and 9-valent protect against genital wart papilloma virus types.

Complications. Left untreated, infection with high-risk HPV can result in cervical, anal, or pharyngeal cancer.

Infectious Proctitis and Enteritis

Proctitis, inflammation of the rectum, is particularly common among people who have receptive anal sex compared with the general population. Various organisms have been associated with proctitis, most commonly *Campylobacter* species, *Entamoeba histolytica*, and lymphogranuloma venereum strains of *Chlamydia trachomatis*. Immunocompromised patients (e.g., HIV-infected patients) may have proctitis as a result of other opportunistic infections. *Helicobacter* species (*H. cinaedi* and *H. fennelliae*) may also play a role as cofactors to *C. trachomatis* proctitis.

Signs and Symptoms. Affected individuals may present with abdominal cramping, diarrhea, itching, tenesmus, or anal discharge.

Transmission. Although transmission pathways depend on the causative organism, the route is typically oral or oral-anal. Cases resulting from transmission during mutual masturbation have also been reported. People who participate in anus-mouth sexual practices are at increased risk for enteritis (often due to *Giardia lamblia*), which may or may not present concurrently with proctitis.

Diagnosis. Health care providers should be cognizant that gastrointestinal outbreaks in MSM may be the result of sexually transmitted infections, HIV infection, or both. Infection with HSV, *Neisseria gonorrhoeae*, *C. trachomatis*, and *Treponema pallidum* should be considered. If enteritis is suspected, stool samples are required for definitive diagnosis of *Giardia* infection.

Treatment. Proctitis is treated with ceftriaxone 250 mg IM and one week of doxycycline 100 mg twice daily unless lymphogranuloma venereum infection is present, in which case doxycycline is administered for three weeks. Infections resulting from herpes virus can be treated like genital herpes infections.

Complications. Complications of chronic proctocolitis include colorectal fistulas and strictures, making early treatment imperative.

Lymphogranuloma Venereum

Lymphogranuloma venereum (LGV) is an STI caused by *Chlamydia trachomatis* serovars L1, L2, and L3 that has been associated with outbreaks of anorectal infections among MSM.

Signs and Symptoms. In heterosexual men and women, LGV typically presents as tender inguinal or femoral lymphadenopathy with or without genital ulcers. In people with rectal exposure as a result of anal intercourse, symptoms also include proctocolitis, mucoid/hemorrhagic rectal discharge, anal pain, constipation, tenesmus, and fever.

Diagnosis. Health care providers should consider that LGV can mimic inflammatory bowel disease, both endoscopically and histologically. When available, genetic testing for specific *C. trachomatis* strains can confirm the diagnosis. Significantly, there have been reports that specific strains exist among some subpopulations of MSM. LGV-inducing strains are often associated with HIV coinfection; genotype L infections require longer treatment protocols with antibiotics. Even if LGV-specific genital and lymph node testing for *C. trachomatis* is not available, a clinical picture consistent with LGV should be treated when other causes have been excluded.

Treatment. The treatment regimen is doxycycline 100 mg orally twice a day for 21 days. Sex partners of patients with LGV should be treated with a single 1-g dose of azithromycin or a week of doxycycline 100 mg twice daily.

Complications. Complications of chronic proctocolitis include colorectal fistula and strictures, making early treatment imperative.

Syphilis

According to recent estimates of the CDC, MSM account for approximately three out of four syphilis cases. Furthermore, MSM continue to account for a large percentage of syphilis incidence and prevalence, and cases are often associated with HIV coinfection. Black, Hispanic, and young MSM are at increased risk for primary and secondary syphilis.

Syphilis spreads by way of direct contact with sores on the penis, vagina, anus, or lips or in the rectum or mouth. Untreated syphilis has long-term consequences. Infection is classified in four stages: primary, secondary, latent, and late. Even MSM who do not practice anal sex may have a risk of urethral primary syphilis similar to that of MSM who do: receptive unprotected oral sex and use of anal sex toys have been positively correlated with syphilis despite a low risk of HIV transmission.

Signs and Symptoms. Syphilis can have vague symptoms, making it difficult to distinguish from other diseases. In the primary stage, a patient may complain of what they assume to be an ingrown hair or nick from a zipper. There may be one or more sores that last anywhere from three to six weeks. In second stage, the patient may note a nonpruritic rash on the palms and soles. The rash, like the sores, will resolve without treatment. Latent syphilis, the next phase, is not associated with any symptoms. If the disease goes untreated, late-stage syphilis may develop 10–30 years after the initial infection and often involves the nervous system (neurosyphilis). It can cause uncoordinated movement, paralysis, numbness, blindness, or even death as a result of damage to internal organs. Asymptomatic syphilis is also possible, as is nervous system involvement in early stages.

Diagnosis. The use of PCR to diagnose primary syphilis may be useful when a serological response is not yet present.

Treatment. Early syphilis is easy to cure, with penicillin G being the preferred agent. Preparation, dosage, and duration of treatment all depend on the stage of disease.

Prevention. CDC screening guidelines call for annual screening for syphilis in sexually active gay and bisexual men and in other MSM. Persons with HIV are also at high risk. MSM with more than one partner, anonymous partners, and those who use or are sexually active with users of illicit drugs should increase their frequency of screening. Discussing syphilis screening recommendations, as well as the risk factors of syphilis, with patients may improve compliance with screen-

ing. For transgender people, the decision to test is entirely individualized, based on anatomic inventory and sexual behaviors. Regional prevalence and membership in a high-prevalence demographic also guide the decision to test.

Complications. Unsafe sex practices are reemerging in part because of the availability of anti-retroviral drugs for HIV. For this reason, health care providers should be sure to counsel patients on the risk of reinfection and repeat infection if they do not comply with medical recommendations and encourage them to seek follow-up testing. Syphilis infection increases the risk of both acquiring and transmitting HIV. HIV-positive syphilis patients should undergo neurologic, ophthalmic, and otologic examinations to catch cases of early neurosyphilis. Although ocular manifestations of syphilis are rare, they are more likely in MSM. An acute febrile reaction known as the Jarisch-Herxheimer reaction is possible with treatment. It is typically managed with antipyretics.

External Resource 8.2
The CDC continually updates epidemiologic data on **Special Populations**, including MSM and WSW. http://bit.ly/TECe1ch08_02

Additional training **Tools & Materials** addressing STIs are hosted by the CDC. http://bit.ly/TECe1ch08_03

Key Points
- Health care providers should counsel patients on the risk of reinfection and repeat infection if they do not comply with medical recommendations and encourage them to seek follow-up testing.
- Because almost 10% of all new hepatitis A cases involve MSM, this population should receive the HAV vaccination in

addition to the strongly encouraged routine HBV vaccination.

- WSW are an at-risk population whose members are less likely to undergo cervical screening. This population should obtain regular Pap smears and the HPV vaccine.
- Many STIs go undiagnosed because of their extragenital presentations. Health care providers should consider obtaining rectal and pharyngeal samples in addition to the standard urine and urethral samples to rule out infection.

Case 8.3

A 21-year-old woman comes to her primary care physician for the physical she must have to try out for her college basketball team. During her visit, she reports that she does not regularly see an obstetrician-gynecologist because she is not currently sexually active with men and has no desire to take birth control pills. She adds that she is in a monogamous relationship with her girlfriend of two years and says that her girlfriend's health care provider informed her that she would not need regular cervical cancer screening because she is "low-risk."

How should the health care provider advise this patient?

What modes of transmission of STIs should be considered?

What prevention counseling can be offered?

Many health care providers and LGBTQ people are unaware that WSW need regular cancer screenings (Pap smears). Although many WSW have had or will have sex with a man, regardless of sexual orientation, studies have shown that cervical neoplasia occurs whether or not these individuals have had male sexual partners. HPV, which can cause cervical cancer, is the most common STI and has been shown to be transmitted during oral sex, genital-to-genital contact, and finger-to-genital contact. Every individual with a cervix requires Pap smears, starting at the age of 21, regardless of sexual orientation or sexual activity.

WSW should be counseled to use barrier methods when engaging in sexual activity: condom use with sex toys, dental dams during oral sex, and gloves during penetrative sex that carries an increased risk of bleeding.

Although the HPV vaccine is most effective when given at an earlier age because it induces a higher immune response when administered before the first sexual encounter (i.e., 11–12 years), this individual should be also be offered vaccination. Currently the vaccine is approved for male and female patients ages nine through 45. See the HPV section of this chapter and Chap. 5 for more details.

Boards-Style Application Questions

Question 1. A 17-year-old youth comes to get the results of a prior STI screen that was performed with urethral swabs. According to his chart, he has been sexually active with men and has had multiple partners, and some of whom he met through online dating sites were anonymous. He also notes that he always uses protection during anal intercourse. The result of his gonococcal urethral swab is negative. What is the most appropriate next step in the management of this individual?

A. Prescribing antibiotic prophylaxis
B. Counseling him to limit his sexual partners
C. Recommending that he avoid anal intercourse with men
D. Performing an STI screen with pharyngeal and rectal swabs
E. Educating him on consistent condom use during anal intercourse

Question 2. A 23-year-old college student comes into your office complaining of general malaise and fatigue for the past couple of days. He is up to date on his routine vaccinations and has not traveled abroad. The patient reports that he has recently become sexually active with his boyfriend but says that he has never participated in anal sex. A rapid HIV test performed on a buccal swab sample is negative. What is the most appropriate next step in this individual's care?

A. Administering a viral vaccine
B. Prescribing a course of acyclovir treatment
C. Referring him to an infectious disease specialist
D. Running nucleic acid testing on a blood specimen
E. Performing a rectal swab to rule out bacterial infection

Question 3. A 50-year-old woman presents with a chief complaint of a six-month history of hot flashes and night sweats. Her vital signs are normal and abdominal examination findings are normal; pelvic examination reveals pale, thin, dry vaginal mucosa. At the end of the visit, the patient seems embarrassed as she asks whether she may discuss one more thing. She states that she is having problems with vaginal dryness and pain during sex. You suggest a vaginal lubricant during sexual activity and discuss more comfortable sexual positions to alleviate discomfort. How could the patient's anxiety about her sexual dysfunction have been minimized?

A. By asking her what impact this was having on her partner
B. By reassuring her that these are common symptoms among women
C. By providing adequate counseling and specific suggestions for management
D. By discussing her pelvic exam findings during the exam and asking whether she had any questions

Question 4. A 27-year-old woman with a history of migraines presents to your clinic complaining of two weeks of lower back pain. She rates the pain as 8 on a 1-to-10 scale and says that it is dull in quality, with occasional episodes of stabbing pain brought on by prolonged sitting. The patient does not recall what she was doing when it started. She can alleviate the pain by lying flat on her back. It is aggravated by sitting. She has also noticed that it is worse in the morning. The woman's boyfriend was recently found to have ankylosing spondylitis, and she is concerned that she may have it as well. During the sexual history you learn that over the last six months she has been sexually active with her wife and boyfriend only. The most appropriate question to ask next is:

A. Do you use any form of birth control?
B. What do you use for protection against STIs?
C. Would you like to be tested for HIV and other STIs?
D. In the past six months, what kinds of sexual activities have you engaged in?

Question 5. A 41-year-old nonbinary transgender person with a history of systemic lupus erythematosus (SLE) and hypertension presents with a two-day history of dysuria and suprapubic pain. SLE was diagnosed 12 years ago, and the patient is taking hydroxychloroquine. The patient reports having similar episodes of pain over the last two years but denies any urinary frequency, fever, flank pain, nausea or vomiting. What is usually the greatest barrier faced by the provider in taking a complete sexual history with LGBTQ patients?

A. Limited time during a patient encounter
B. Not wanting to make the patient uncomfortable
C. Limited knowledge of LGBTQ patients' health concerns
D. Disgust with queer sex or prejudice against LGBTQ people

Question 6. A 53-year-old transgender woman with no significant past medical history presents to you, worried that she has an STI. She is concerned because she has just learned that her current sexual partner has Chlamydia and herpes.

Although she generally uses protection, she recalls two occasions on which she and her partner did not use a condom. You are familiar with this patient and know that she calls her penis a clitoris. You notice a more blunted affect than normal, as well as several 1.5-cm bruises on the patient's upper arms. The patient denies fever or burning with urination. What question is the most appropriate?

A. "Do you feel safe with your boyfriend?"
B. "Have you noticed any penile discharge?"
C. "Have you noticed any sores on your clitoris?"
D. "Does your boyfriend ever hurt or threaten you?"

Boards-Style Application Question Answer Key

Question 1. As many as 85% of cases of gonorrhea are missed when only urethral swabs are obtained. Because the individual has only had urethral swabs collected, performing an STI screen with pharyngeal and rectal swabs is the most appropriate next step in managing the individual (option D). Gonorrhea is not prevented by antibiotic prophylaxis (option A). Counseling the patient to limit his sexual partners (option B) and recommending that he avoid anal sex (option C) are neither feasible nor evidence-based. Option E does not apply because the patient already uses condoms during anal sex.

Question 2. MSM should be vaccinated against hepatitis A (option A, the correct answer), but this is not part of a routine vaccination schedule. Hepatitis A is transmitted by the fecal-oral route, and its presentation is consistent with the patient's history of fatigue and general malaise. Although MSM have increased prevalence of herpes, the clinical picture is not consistent with herpes infection (option B). A referral is not appropriate at this time (option C). The individual has already had a negative HIV test in the office (option D). Blood samples (option E) are drawn to confirm positive test results, not after a negative finding.

Question 3. A new complaint should be explored thoroughly and in a sensitive manner. In this case, this would include reassurance that the patient's symptoms are common among perimenopausal women (option B), plus an explanation that the symptoms should still be further explored to exclude other causes of dyspareunia. Option C may be helpful, but jumping immediately to recommendations may not allay the patient's anxiety. Option D is poor timing for counseling. Option A is perhaps outside the scope of the acute complaint.

Question 4. Although all these questions are appropriate during a sexual history, the next question should be which sexual activities the patient engages in (option D). Knowing this information helps you determine which STIs they are at risk for, what kinds of protection they can use, and whether you need to ask and provide counsel about contraception. From the information given it is not clear whether the patient's partners are transgender or intersex, and there is no information about the kinds of sex they have. Going straight to asking about contraception (option A) or STIs (option B) after a patient discloses the number and genders of sexual partners may make the patient think that you are making assumptions of high-risk sexual behavior and may cause the patient to be hesitant to disclose information in the future. Option C is not objectively poor, but for an acute complaint, gathering more information for differential diagnosis would be prudent.

Question 5. The greatest barrier providers face in taking a complete sexual history from an LGBTQ patient specifically is discomfort due to a lack of training and knowledge about LGBTQ patients (option D). In this case, it may not be immediately apparent that an anatomic inventory needs to be performed. A small minority of providers may be uncomfortable or disgusted with the idea of queer sex or are prejudiced against LGBTQ people (option C), but this is not a barrier in the majority of providers. Health care providers may avoid taking a full sexual history in general due to limited time (option A) or to avoid making the patient or themselves uncomfortable (option B).

Question 6. There are several things going on in this question. The patient is concerned about STIs, but the change in affect and her bruises raise the possibility of abuse. Both issues must be addressed during this visit. Because this patient uses the term *clitoris* to describe her penis, that is the term you should use as well, so option C, in which the provider mentions the patient's clitoris, is more appropriate than referring to the patient's penis (option B). Options A and D are both incorrect because you do not know the gender of the patient's sexual partner or their relationship status, and you want to avoid making any assumptions about a patient's sexual or social history.

Sources

Ahdoot A, Kotler DP, Suh JS, Kutler C, Flamholz R. Lymphogranuloma venereum in human immunodeficiency virus-infected individuals in New York City. J Clin Gastroenterol. 2006;40(5):385–90.

American College of Obstetricians and Gynecologists. Addressing health risks of noncoital sexual activity. Obstet Gynecol. 2013;122(6):1378–83.

Anderson JS, Hoy J, Hillman R, Barnden M, Fu B, McKenzie A, Gittleson C. A randomized, placebo-controlled dose-escalation study to determine the safety, tolerability, and immunogenicity of an HPV-16 therapeutic vaccine in HIV-positive participants with oncogenic HPV infection of the anus. J Acquir Immune Defic Syndr. 2009;52(3):371–81.

Bevier PJ, Chiasson MA, Heffernan RT, Castro KG. Women at a sexually transmitted disease clinic who reported same-sex contact: their HIV seroprevalence and risk behaviors. Am J Public Health. 1995;85(10):1366–71.

Blackwell CW. Men who have sex with men and recruit bareback sex partners on the Internet: implications for STI and HIV prevention and client education. Am J Mens Health. 2008;2(4):306–13.

Blaxhult A, Samuelson A, Ask R, Hökeberg I. Limited spread of hepatitis C among HIV-negative men who have sex with men in Stockholm, Sweden. Int J STD AIDS. 2014;25(7):493–5.

Borg ML, Modi A, Tostmann A, Gobin M, Cartwright J, Quigley C, et al. Ongoing outbreak of *Shigella flexneri* serotype 3a in men who have sex with men in England and Wales, data from 2009-2011. Euro Surveill. 2012;17(13):20137.

Bradshaw D, Matthews G, Danta M. Sexually transmitted hepatitis C infection: the new epidemic in MSM? Curr Opin Infect Dis. 2013;26(1):66–72.

Brown B, Davtyan M, Galea J, Chow E, Leon S, Klausner JD. The role of human papillomavirus in human immunodeficiency virus acquisition in men who have sex with men: a review of the literature. Viruses. 2012;4(12):3851–8.

Caceres CF, Konda K, Segura ER, Lyerla R. Epidemiology of male same-sex behaviour and associated sexual health indicators in low- and middle-income countries: 2003-2007 estimates. Sex Transm Infect. 2008;84(Suppl 1):i49–56.

Carter JW Jr, Hart-Cooper GD, Butler MO, Workowski KA, Hoover KW. Provider barriers prevent recommended sexually transmitted disease screening of HIV-infected men who have sex with men. Sex Transm Dis. 2014;41(2):137–42.

Centers for Disease Control and Prevention. Sexually transmitted disease surveillance 2010. Atlanta: US Department of Health and Human Services; 2011.

Centers for Disease Control and Prevention. Sexually transmitted disease surveillance 2012. Atlanta: US Department of Health and Human Services; 2013.

Chin-Hong PV, Husnik M, Cranston RD, Colfax G, Buchbinder S, Da Costa M, et al. Anal human papillomavirus infection is associated with HIV acquisition in men who have sex with men. AIDS. 2009;23(9):1135–42.

Ciesielski CA. Sexually transmitted diseases in men who have sex with men: an epidemiologic review. Curr Infect Dis Rep. 2003;5(2):145–52.

Cohen J, Lo YR, Caceres CF, Klausner JD. WHO guidelines for HIV/STI prevention and care among MSM and transgender people: implications for policy and practice. Sex Transm Infect. 2013;89(7):536–8.

Coleman E. What is sexual health? Articulating a sexual health approach to HIV prevention for men who have sex with men. AIDS Behav. 2011;15(Suppl 1):S18–24.

Council on Scientific Affairs, American Medical Association. Health care needs of gay men and lesbians in the United States. JAMA. 1996;275(17):1354–9.

Cox P, McNair R. Risk reduction as an accepted framework for safer-sex promotion among women who have sex with women. Sex Health. 2009;6(1):15–8.

Cranston RD, Murphy R, Weiss RE, Da Costa M, Palefsky J, Shoptaw S, Gorbach PM. Anal human papillomavirus infection in a street-based sample of drug-using HIV-positive men. Int J STD AIDS. 2012;23(3):195–200.

Dahlberg M, Nordberg M, Pieniowski E, Boström L, Sandblom G, Hallqvist-Everhov Å. Retained sex toys: an increasing and possibly preventable medical condition. Int J Color Dis. 2018;34(1):181–3. https://doi.org/10.1007/s00384-018-3125-4.

Davis TW, Goldstone SE. Sexually transmitted infections as a cause of proctitis in men who have sex with men. Dis Colon Rectum. 2009;52(3):507–12.

de Vries HJ. Sexually transmitted infections in men who have sex with men. Clin Dermatol. 2014;32(2):181–8.

de Vries H, Zingoni A, White J, Ross J, Kreuter A. 2013 European Guideline on the management of proctitis, proctocolitis and enteritis caused by sexually transmissible pathogens. Int J STD AIDS. 2013;25(7):465–74. https://doi.org/10.1177/0956462413516100.

Dietz CA, Nyberg CR. Genital, oral, and anal human papillomavirus infection in men who have sex with men. J Am Osteopath Assoc. 2011;111(3 Suppl 2):S19–25.

Douglas JM Jr, Peterman TA, Fenton KA. Syphilis among men who have sex with men: challenges to syphilis elimination in the United States. Sex Transm Dis. 2005;32(10 Suppl):S80–3.

Edwards A, Thin RN. Sexually transmitted diseases in lesbians. Int J STD AIDS. 1990;1(3):178–81.

Einhorn L, Polgar M. HIV-risk behavior among lesbians and bisexual women. AIDS Educ Prev. 1994;6(6):514–23.

El-Bassel N, Gilbert L, Witte S, Wu E, Hunt T, Remien RH. Couple-based HIV prevention in the United States: advantages, gaps, and future directions. J Acquir Immune Defic Syndr. 2010;55(Suppl 2):S98–S101.

Everett BG. Sexual orientation disparities in sexually transmitted infections: examining the intersection between sexual identity and sexual behavior. Arch Sex Behav. 2013;42(2):225–36. https://doi.org/10.1007/s10508-012-9902-1.

Fenton KA. Time for change: rethinking and reframing sexual health in the United States. J Sex Med. 2012;7(Suppl 5):250–2.

Fethers K, Marks C, Mindel A, Estcourt CS. Sexually transmitted infections and risk behaviours in women who have sex with women. Sex Transm Infect. 2000;76(5):345–9.

Gao L, Zhou F, Li X, Yang Y, Ruan Y, Jin Q. Anal HPV infection in HIV-positive men who have sex with men from China. PLoS One. 2012;5(12):e15256.

Ghosh I, Ghosh P, Bharti AC, Mandal R, Biswas J, Basu P. Prevalence of human papillomavirus and co-existent sexually transmitted infections among female sex workers, men having sex with men and injectable drug abusers from eastern India. Asian Pac J Cancer Prev. 2012;13(3):799–802.

Gilbert M, Kwag M, Mei W, Rank C, Kropp R, Severini A, et al. Feasibility of incorporating self-collected rectal swabs into a community venue-based survey to measure the prevalence of HPV infection in men who have sex with men. Sex Transm Dis. 2011;38(10):964–9.

Gilbert M, Hottes TS, Kerr T, Taylor D, Fairley CK, Lester R, et al. Factors associated with intention to use Internet-based testing for sexually transmitted infections among men who have sex with men. J Med Internet Res. 2013;15(11):e254.

Goldstone SE, Kawalek AZ, Goldstone RN, Goldstone AB. Hybrid capture II detection of oncogenic human papillomavirus: a useful tool when evaluating men who have sex with men with atypical squamous cells of undetermined significance on anal cytology. Dis Colon Rectum. 2008;51(7):1130–6.

Grace D, Chown S, Jollimore J, Parry R, Kwag M, Steinberg M, et al. HIV-negative gay men's accounts of using context-dependent sero-adaptive strategies. Cult Health Sex. 2014;16(3):316–30. https://doi.org/10.1080/13691058.2014.883644.

Grov C, Rendina HJ, Breslow AS, Ventuneac A, Adelson S, Parsons JT. Characteristics of men who have sex with men (MSM) who attend sex parties: results from a national online sample in the USA. Sex Transm Infect. 2014;90(1):26–32.

Gunn RA, O'Brien CJ, Lee MA, Gilchick RA. Gonorrhea screening among men who have sex with men: value of multiple anatomic site testing, San Diego, California, 1997-2003. Sex Transm Dis. 2008;35(10):845–8.

Halioua B, Bohbot JM, Monfort L, Nassar N, de Barbeyrac B, Monsonego J, Sednaoui P. Ano-rectal lymphogranuloma venereum: 22 cases reported in a sexually transmitted infections center in Paris. Eur J Dermatol. 2006;16(2):177–80.

Henderson HJ. Why lesbians should be encouraged to have regular cervical screening. J Fam Plann Reprod Health Care. 2009;35(1):49–52.

Hinchliff S, Gott M, Galena E. "I daresay I might find it embarrassing": general practitioners' perspectives on discussing sexual health issues with lesbian and gay patients correspondence. Health Soc Care Community. 2001;13(4):345–53.

Hospers HJ, Kok G. Determinants of safe and risk-taking sexual behavior among gay men: a review. AIDS Educ Prev. 1995;7(1):74–96.

Institute of Medicine. The health of lesbian, gay, bisexual, and transgender people: building a foundation for better understanding. Washington, DC: The National Academies Press; 2011.

Kent CK, Chaw JK, Wong W, Liska S, Gibson S, Hubbard G, Klausner JD. Prevalence of rectal, urethral, and pharyngeal Chlamydia and gonorrhea detected in 2 clinical settings among men who have sex with men: San Francisco, California, 2003. Clin Infect Dis. 2005;41(1):67–74.

Kirkcaldy RD, Zaidi A, Hook EW 3rd, Holmes KK, Soge O, del Rio C, et al. *Neisseria gonorrhoeae* antimicrobial resistance among men who have sex with men and men who have sex exclusively with women: the Gonococcal Isolate Surveillance Project, 2005-2010. Ann Intern Med. 2013;158(5 Pt 1):321–8.

Kirkcaldy R, Harvey A, Papp J, Del Rio C, Soge OO, Holmes KK, et al. *Neisseria gonorrhoeae* antimicrobial susceptibility surveillance—the Gonococcal Isolate Surveillance Project, 27 sites, United States, 2014. MMWR Surveill Summ. 2016;65(7):1–19. https://doi.org/10.15585/mmwr.ss6507a1.

Koblin BA, Husnik MJ, Colfax G, Huang Y, Madison M, Mayer K, et al. Risk factors for HIV infection among men who have sex with men. AIDS. 2006;20(5):731–9.

Kratz M, Weiss D, Ridpath A, Zucker JR, Geevarughese A, Rakeman J, Varma JK. Community-based outbreak of *Neisseria meningitidis* serogroup C infection in men who have sex with men, New York City, New York, USA, 2010–2013. Emerg Infect Dis. 2015;21(8):1379–86. https://doi.org/10.3201/eid2108.141837.

Kreuter A, Skrygan M, Gambichler T, Brockmeyer NH, Stücker M, Herzler C, et al. Human papillomavirus–associated induction of human beta-defensins in anal intraepithelial neoplasia. Br J Dermatol. 2009;160(6):1197–205.

Kropp RY, Wong T, The Canadian LGV Working Group. Emergence of lymphogranuloma venereum in Canada. CMAJ. 2005;172(13):1674–6.

Kuyper L, Vanwesenbeeck I. Examining sexual health differences between lesbian, gay, bisexual, and heterosexual adults: the role of sociodemographics, sexual behavior characteristics, and minority stress. J Sex Res. 2011;48(2–3):263–74. https://doi.org/10.1080/00224491003654473.

Lambers FA, Prins M, Thomas X, Molenkamp R, Kwa D, Brinkman K, et al. Alarming incidence of hepatitis C virus re-infection after treatment of sexually acquired acute hepatitis C virus infection in HIV-infected MSM. AIDS. 2011;25(17):F21–7.

Lehmiller JJ, Ioerger M. Social networking smartphone applications and sexual health outcomes among men who have sex with men. PLoS One. 2014;9(1):e86603.

Lemp GF, et al. HIV seroprevalence and risk behaviors among lesbians and bisexual women in San Francisco and Berkeley, California. Am J Public Health. 1995;85(11):1549–52.

Leung N, Vidoni M, Robinson D, Padgett P, Brown E. A community-based study of Staphylococcus aureus nasal colonization and molecular characterization among men who have sex with men. LGBT Health. 2017;4(5):345–51. https://doi.org/10.1089/lgbt.2017.0016.

Lewnard J, Berrang-Ford L. Internet-based partner selection and risk for unprotected anal intercourse in sexual encounters among men who have sex with men: a meta-analysis of observational studies. Sex Transm Infect. 2014;90(4):290–6. https://doi.org/10.1136/sextrans-2013-051332.

Makadon HJ. Ending LGBT invisibility in health care: the first step in ensuring equitable care. Cleve Clin J Med. 2011;78(4):220–4. https://doi.org/10.3949/ccjm.78gr.10006.

Marrazzo JM, Stine K, Koutsky LA. Genital human papillomavirus infection in women who have sex with women: a review. Am J Obstet Gynecol. 2000;183(3):770–4.

Marrazzo JM, Koutsky LA, Eschenbach DA, Agnew K, Stine K, Hillier SL. Characterization of vaginal flora and bacterial vaginosis in women who have sex with women. J Infect Dis. 2002;185(9):1307–13. https://doi.org/10.1086/339884.

Marrazzo JM, Coffey P, Bingham A. Sexual practices, risk perception and knowledge of sexual transmitted disease risk among lesbian and bisexual women. Perspect Sex Reprod Health. 2005;37(1):6–12.

Mathews WC, Booth MW, Turner JD, Kessler L. Physicians' attitudes toward homosexuality: survey of a California county medical society. West J Med. 1986;144(1):106–10.

McMillan A, van Voorst Vader PC, de Vries HJ. The 2007 European Guideline (International Union Against Sexually Transmitted Infections/World Health Organization) on the management of proctitis, proctocolitis and enteritis caused by sexually transmissible pathogens. Int J STD AIDS. 2007;18(8):514–20.

McNair R. Risks and prevention of sexually transmissible infections among women who have sex with women. Sex Health. 2005;2(4):209–17.

Mimiaga MJ, Noonan E, Donnell D, Safren SA, Koenen KC, Gortmaker S, et al. Childhood sexual abuse is highly associated with HIV risk-taking behavior and infection among MSM in the EXPLORE study. J Acquir Immune Defic Syndr. 2009;51(3):340–8.

Morton L. Sexuality in the older adult. Prim Care. 2017;44(3):429–38. https://doi.org/10.1016/j.pop.2017.04.004.

Muzny CA, Harbison HS, Pembleton ES, Hook EW, Austin EL. Misperceptions regarding protective barrier method use for safer sex among African-American women who have sex with women. Sex Health. 2013a;10(2):138–41.

Muzny CA, Harbison HS, Pembleton ES, Austin EL. Sexual behaviors, perception of sexually transmitted infection risk, and practice of safe sex among Southern African American women who have sex with women. Sex Transm Dis. 2013b;40(5):395–400.

Nieuwenhuis RF, Ossewaarde JM, Götz HM, Dees J, Thio HB, Thomeer MG, et al. Resurgence of lymphogranuloma venereum in western Europe: an outbreak of Chlamydia trachomatis serovar l2 proctitis in the Netherlands among men who have sex with men. Clin Infect Dis. 2004;39(7):996–1003.

Noor S, Rosser B. Enema use among men who have sex with men: a behavioral epidemiologic study with implications for HIV/STI prevention. Arch Sex Behav. 2013;43(4):755–69. https://doi.org/10.1007/s10508-013-0203-0.

Nusbaum MRH, Hamilton CD. The proactive sexual health history. Am Fam Physician. 2002;66(9):1705–12.

Pando MA, Balán IC, Marone R, Dolezal C, Leu CS, Squiquera L, et al. HIV and other sexually transmitted infections among men who have sex with men recruited by RDS in Buenos Aires, Argentina: high HIV and HPV infection. PLoS One. 2012;7(6):e39834.

Price JH, Easton AN, Telljohann SK, Wallace PB. Perceptions of cervical cancer and Pap smear screening behavior by women's sexual orientation. J Community Health. 1996;21(2):89–105.

Quint K, Bom R, Quint W, Bruisten SM, van der Loeff MF, Morré SA, de Vries HJ. Anal infections with concomitant Chlamydia trachomatisgenotypes among men who have sex with men in Amsterdam, the Netherlands. BMC Infect Dis. 2011;11(1):63. https://doi.org/10.1186/1471-2334-11-63.

Rankow EJ, Tessaro I. Cervical cancer risk and Papanicolaou screening in a sample of lesbian and bisexual women. J Fam Pract. 1998;47(2):139–43.

Reinton N, Moi H, Olsen AO, Zarabyan N, Bjerner J, Tønseth TM, Moghaddam A. Anatomic distribution of *Neisseria gonorrhoeae, Chlamydia trachomatis* and *Mycoplasma genitalium* infections in men who have sex with men. Sex Health. 2013;10(3):199–203.

Richardson D, Goldmeier D. Lymphogranuloma venereum: an emerging cause of proctitis in men who have sex with men. Int J STD AIDS. 2007;18(1):11–4; quiz 15.

Robertson P, Schachter J. Failure to identify venereal disease in a lesbian population. Sex Transm Dis. 1981;8(2):75–6.

Sanchez NF, Rabatin J, Sanchez JP, Hubbard S, Kalet A. Medical students' ability to care for lesbian, gay, bisexual, and transgendered patients. Fam Med. 2006;38(1):21–7. Available at: http://www.ncbi.nlm.nih.gov/pubmed/16378255.

Sinković M, Towler L. Sexual aging: a systematic review of qualitative research on the sexuality and sexual health of older adults. Qual Health Res. 2019;29(9):1239–54. https://doi.org/10.1177/1049732318819834.

Skinner CJ, Stokes J, Kirlew Y, Kavanagh J, Forster GE. A case-controlled study of the sexual health needs of lesbians. Genitourin Med. 1996;72(4):277–80.

Smith EM, Johnson SR, Guenther SM. Health care attitudes and experiences during gynecologic care among lesbians and bisexuals. Am J Public Health. 1985;75(9):1085–7.

Sonnex C, Strauss S, Gray JJ. Detection of human papillomavirus DNA on the fingers of patients with genital warts. Sex Transm Infect. 1999;75(5):317–9.

Stall R, Mills TC, Williamson J, Hart T, Greenwood G, Paul J, et al. Association of co-occurring psychosocial health problems and increased vulnerability to HIV/AIDS among urban men who have sex with men. Am J Public Health. 2003;93(6):939–42.

Stark D, van Hal S, Hillman R, Harkness J, Marriott D. Lymphogranuloma venereum in Australia: anorectal *Chlamydia trachomatis* serovar L2b in men who have sex with men. J Clin Microbiol. 2007;45(3):1029–31.

Stevens PE. Lesbian health care research: a review of the literature from 1970 to 1990. Health Care Women Int. 1992;13(2):91–120.

Stevens PE, Hall JM. Stigma, health beliefs and experiences with health care in lesbian women. J Nurs Scholarsh. 1988;20(2):69–73.

Sullivan PS, Hamouda O, Delpech V, Geduld JE, Prejean J, Semaille C, et al. Reemergence of the HIV epidemic among men who have sex with men in North America, Western Europe, and Australia, 1996-2005. Ann Epidemiol. 2009;19(6):423–31.

Sullivan PS, Peterson J, Rosenberg ES, Kelley CF, Cooper H, Vaughan A, et al. Understanding racial HIV/STI disparities in black and white men who have sex with men: a multilevel approach. PLoS One. 2014;9(3):e90514.

Tian LH, Peterman TA, Tao G, Brooks LC, Metcalf C, Malotte CK, et al. Heterosexual anal sex activity in the year after an STD clinic visit. Sex Transm Dis. 2008;35(11):905–9.

Tinmouth J, Rachlis A, Wesson T, Hsieh E. Lymphogranuloma venereum in North America: case reports and an update for gastroenterologists. Clin Gastroenterol Hepatol. 2006;4(4):469–73.

van de Laar TJ, van der Bij AK, Prins M, Bruisten SM, Brinkman K, Ruys TA, et al. Increase in HCV incidence among men who have sex with men in Amsterdam most likely caused by sexual transmission. J Infect Dis. 2007;196(2):230–8.

van de Laar T, et al. Evidence of a large, international network of HCV transmission in HIV-positive men who have sex with men. Gastroenterology. 2009;136(5):1609–17.

Van der Bij AK, Pybus O, Bruisten S, Brown D, Nelson M, Bhagani S, et al. Diagnostic and clinical implications of anorectal lymphogranuloma venereum in men who have sex with men: a retrospective case-control study. Clin Infect Dis. 2006;42(2):186–94.

van Griensven F, de Lind van Wijngaarden JW, Baral S, Grulich A. The global epidemic of HIV infection among men who have sex with men. Curr Opin HIV AIDS. 2009;4(4):300–7.

van Krosigk A, Meyer T, Jordan S, Graefe K, Plettenberg A, Stoehr A. Dramatic increase in lymphogranuloma venereum among homosexual men in Hamburg. J Dtsch Dermatol Ges. 2004;2(8):676–80.

van Rijckevorsel G, Whelan J, Kretzschmar M, Siedenburg E, Sonder G, Geskus R, et al. Targeted vaccination programme successful in reducing acute hepatitis B in men having sex with men in Amsterdam, the Netherlands. J Hepatol. 2013;59(6):1177–83.

White JC, Dull VT. Health risk factors and health-seeking behavior in lesbians. J Womens Health. 1997;6(1):103–12.

WHO. Defining sexual health: report of a technical consultation on sexual health. Geneva: World Health Organization; 2002.

Wolitski RJ, Fenton KA. Sexual health, HIV, and sexually transmitted infections among gay, bisexual, and other m en who have sex with men in the United States. AIDS Behav. 2011;15(Suppl 1):S9–S17.

Xia Q, Osmond DH, Tholandi M, Pollack LM, Zhou W, Ruiz JD, Catania JA. HIV prevalence and sexual risk behaviors among men who have sex with men: results from a statewide population-based survey in California. J Acquir Immune Defic Syndr. 2006;41(2):238–45.

Xu F, Sternberg MR, Markowitz LE. Men who have sex with men in the United States: demographic and behavioral characteristics and prevalence of HIV and HSV-2 infection: results from National Health and Nutrition Examination Survey 2001-2006. Sex Transm Dis. 2010;37(6):399–405.

Ye S, Yin L, Amico R, Simoni J, Vermund S, Ruan Y, et al. Efficacy of peer-led interventions to reduce unprotected anal intercourse among men who have sex with men: a meta-analysis. PLoS One. 2014;9(3):e90788.

Zheng B, Yin Y, Han Y, Shi MQ, Jiang N, Xiang Z, et al. The prevalence of urethral and rectal Mycoplasma genitalium among men who have sex with men in China, a cross-sectional study. BMC Public Health. 2014;14(1):195. https://doi.org/10.1186/1471-2458-14-195.

Transgender Health

James R. Lehman, Lydia A. Fein, Elan L. Horesh,
Marina Petsalis, Erryn E. Tappy, Christopher Estes,
and Christopher J. Salgado

Introduction

Both for transition and for other medical care, transgender individuals need competent, longitudinal management that integrates primary and specialty care. Primary care and preventive health recommendations are often the same for transgender persons as they are for the general popula-

The first listed author is the chapter's associate editor from The Equal Curriculum Project. The chapter authors are otherwise ordered according to their preference.

J. R. Lehman (✉)
Department of Psychiatry, University of Wisconsin–Madison, Madison, WI, USA
e-mail: james.lehman@uwalumni.com

L. A. Fein
University of Miami Miller School of Medicine, Miami, FL, USA
e-mail: lafein@med.miami.edu

E. L. Horesh
Mount Sinai Hospital, New York, NY, USA
e-mail: elan.horesh@mountsinai.org

M. Petsalis
University of Texas Health Science Center at Houston, Houston, TX, USA
e-mail: marina.e.petsalis@uth.tmc.edu

E. E. Tappy
George Washington University Hospital, Washington, DC, USA

C. Estes · C. J. Salgado
University of Miami, Miami, FL, USA
e-mail: cestes@med.miami.edu;
ChristopherSalgado@med.miami.edu

tion. Most preventive screening needs can be rationally predicted on the basis of a patient's anatomic inventory. However, some recommendations change if a transgender patient has undergone hormone therapy or certain surgical procedures. Refer to Chaps. 5 and 7 for a more complete discussion of preventive and primary care for transgender patients.

> **External Resource 9.1**
> In "**Transgender Health: Simon's Story**," a transgender man discusses sensitive issues relevant to the patient-provider relationship, addressing both positive and negative experiences. Total time 6:36. http://bit.ly/TECe1ch09_01

Gender Dysphoria and Gender Identity

In the *Diagnostic and Statistical Manual of Medical Disorders*, fifth edition (*DSM-5*), the condition *gender dysphoria* is defined as clinically significant distress or impairment in social, occupational, or other areas of function that occurs when the gender with which a person identifies does not match the sex that was assigned at birth. It is diagnosed when the gender discrepancy and associated distress affect functional capacities in the person's daily life for at least six months.

Gender dysphoria has replaced the diagnosis of gender identity disorder, which appeared in *DSM-IV*. The decision to favor the term *dysphoria* over *disorder* in the *DSM-5* provides a more appropriate label for this condition, removing the connotation that the patient is "disordered" while protecting patients' access to care by maintaining a diagnosable condition. Often a diagnosable psychiatric condition is required to gain access to insurance coverage for medically necessary treatment or to garner legal and social protections.

Recall that **gender identity** is a person's internal sense of gender. It does not always align with the sex assigned to the person at birth, which is most commonly based on the appearance of external genitalia. **Gender nonconformity** occurs when a person's gender identity differs from the societal norms of gender expression for a particular sex. Gender has evolved from the historically accepted binary of man/woman or male/female and is now thought to exist on a spectrum. *Nonbinary* refers to someone who does not identify exclusively as male or female. *Gender fluid* refers to someone whose gender identity changes over time across the spectrum. People who identify as **genderqueer** usually do so in reaction to the gender binary system. They consider themselves neither male nor female but rather between, beyond, or some combination of genders. It is important to note that gender-nonconforming persons are not inherently gender dysphoric. The diagnosis of gender dysphoria can only be applied if the gender nonconformity causes significant distress to the person.

As discussed in previous chapters, *transgender* is an extremely broad term that simply means having a gender identity that does not match one's sex assigned at birth. In the medical literature, this differentiation is often signified with the terms *male-to-female (MtF)* or *female-to-male (FtM)* to clarify natal sex and gender identity. *Transgender woman (TGW)* and *transgender man (TGM)* are used interchangeably for MtF and FtM, respectively. Persons whose gender identity is congruent with their natal sex are referred to as *cisgender*.

Transsexual is sometimes used interchangeably with *transgender* but more specifically refers to a person who has undergone or who is undergoing medical or surgical therapy to align physical sex characteristics with the gender identity. **Cross-dressers** are people who dress as members of the opposite gender, occasionally or all the time. Unlike transgender and transsexual persons, cross-dressers' gender identity is not misaligned with their assigned gender, and they do not generally experience gender dysphoria.

The sexual orientation of gender variant people encompasses a wide range of sexualities. Although some transgender persons report a strictly heterosexual or homosexual orientation, others will identify with broader identities such as bisexual, pansexual, or queer. *Pansexuality*, also known as *omnisexuality*, refers to attraction toward someone of any gender identity, rejecting the binary system of attraction that is the societal norm. Refer to Chap. 1 for a more complete discussion of terminology used for the sexual and gender minorities.

The prevalence of gender nonconformity is difficult to quantify primarily because no national studies have included gender identity among their measured variables. In many societies, stigmatization of gender variance makes the identification of transgender persons challenging. It is estimated that approximately 0.6% of the US population identifies as transgender. There appears to be approximately twice as many TGW as TGM. Most epidemiologic studies of gender dysphoria primarily include people seeking treatment and therefore do not capture gender incongruent persons who have undiagnosed gender dysphoria or who are not undergoing treatment.

Key Points
- Gender dysphoria may be diagnosed only if gender discrepancy causes a clinical level of distress or impairment in function. It is not inherent in all gender-nonconforming persons.

- Because gender variant persons encompass a variety of sexual orientations and gender identities, it is essential that health care providers understand the unique feelings, perspectives, and needs of their gender variant patients.
- Stigmatization and lack of epidemiologic studies make it difficult to quantify the prevalence of gender nonconforming or transgender persons.

Case 9.1

A 20-year-old natal male named Paul has made an appointment with a psychiatrist to discuss his worsening anxiety regarding his appearance. Since adolescence Paul has felt increasingly uncomfortable with the appearance of his body. He does not like his male genitalia and started making efforts to conceal them several years ago. Paul also dislikes his body and facial hair and spends an extra 30 minutes in the bathroom each morning to ensure that it is all removed. He has grown his hair long and started wearing women's clothes. Despite these changes, he still suffers significant anxiety in social settings and has had difficulty holding a job because of his reluctance to leave home for the past several years. When asked by the psychiatrist about gender identity, Paul states that he wishes he had been born female.

May the psychiatrist apply a diagnosis of gender dysphoria to Paul? Why or why not?

If Paul simply preferred to take on a more feminine appearance but was content with his natal gender, into what gender classification might he fit? Why?

Paul meets the criteria for gender dysphoria as set forth in the DSM-5. *He has clinically significant distress because of the gender incongruence that has affected his*

daily function. His natal gender does not match the gender with which he identifies. His distress is evidenced by his social anxiety and related inability to maintain a job. Paul would also be considered transgender because his gender identity that does not match his genetic sex.

If Paul preferred to adopt a more feminine appearance without actually suffering distress or possessing the desire to be female rather than male, he would fall into the classification of gender nonconforming. He would not meet diagnostic criteria for gender dysphoria.

Health Disparities and Barriers to Health Care in the Trans Population

It is well established that numerous health disparities exist between transgender and cisgender persons. In the United States, HIV prevalence in the transgender population is much higher than the national average. In a survey conducted by the National Center for Transgender Equality, 2.64% of transgender persons were HIV positive, compared with 0.6% in the general population. The prevalence in transgender women was 3.76%. Compared with cisgender individuals, transgender persons encounter increased social stigmatization, more threats of violence, and greater socioeconomic challenges such as unemployment. These factors heighten their risk for mental health problems such as depression, anxiety, post-traumatic stress disorder, substance use disorder, and suicide attempts. In the United States, 41% of transgender persons have attempted suicide, compared with less than 2% of the general population.

Transgender persons face enormous barriers to receiving appropriate general health care and specialized gender-affirming care. These barriers can be classified in four main categories: reluctance to disclose, systemic barriers, lack of provider experience and resources, and financial barriers.

Reluctance to Disclose

The National Transgender Discrimination Survey revealed that nearly 20% of respondents had been refused care because of their gender identity and that nearly 30% had been verbally assaulted while attempting to seek care. Negative interactions in a health care setting, from inappropriate or belittling comments to refusal or inability to address relevant issues by any member of the health care team or health care facility, can deter transgender individuals from seeking medical care and drive them to obtain treatment in nontraditional and potentially dangerous settings. The prevalence of unsupervised hormone therapy has been estimated to be as high as 63% in some urban transgender populations.

Systemic Barriers

It is important for the health care system and its associated structural components to be sensitive to the needs of transgender patients. Unisex or non-gendered public restrooms, private hospital rooms or arrangement of a roommate of the same gender identity for trans patients, and use of the patient's preferred name and correct pronouns are all factors that contribute to a transgender-affirming environment. Having a support staff whose members are sensitive to the specific needs of transgender patients is also crucial to eliminating systemic barriers. Oftentimes, institutional or insurance-based billing policies can be problematic. Some procedures and tests that are gender specific cannot be performed unless they are congruent with the gender identification on the insurance card. Additionally, hospitals may lack policies and electronic health records that accommodate transgender identities.

Financial Barriers

As many as 48% of transgender persons have reported not seeking medical care when they were sick or injured because they could not afford it. The cost of transition-related medical care can also be prohibitive. Hormone therapy can cost several hundred dollars per month, and surgical procedures frequently cost more than $10,000. Contributing to the financial burden is the high rate of unemployment among transgender persons. Approximately 14% are unemployed—twice the national average. The Patient Protection and Affordable Care Act eliminated discrimination based on gender identity, making it so gender identity can no longer be considered a preexisting condition for insurance coverage. However, because of the high unemployment rate, the number of transgender persons able to use employment-based coverage remains small. Fortunately, more insurance providers are expanding coverage of transgender health services. In 2014, Medicare changed its policy to no longer universally deny coverage of gender confirmation surgery, deferring the question to local Medicare agencies.

Provider Barriers

Transgender care, particularly hormonal and surgical treatments, can be extremely difficult to find. Even communities with a large number of transgender individuals may not have physicians who are experienced with transgender care. It is challenging for transgender persons seeking basic health care to find a provider who has been educated in transgender health. Health care providers acknowledge that they face barriers in treating transgender patients. Providers often approach transgender patients with uncertainty, and trans patients frequently report having to educate their doctors about their own care. Provider-identified barriers to providing health care to transgender patients include discomfort about influencing decision-making in light of the importance of decisions about the medical transition process, not knowing appropriate care strategies or resources for trans patients, not knowing which colleagues might be "trans friendly," knowledge deficits stemming from a lack of formal education about trans health care, and difficulty predicting realistic treatment outcomes and managing patients who expect unrealistic outcomes.

Overcoming barriers to health care for transgender patients is crucial to reduce health disparities for the transgender population. Lessening the stigma, improving the health care system to become more trans-accepting, easing financial barriers, and increasing provider knowledge and training are all critical ways in which health care as a whole can become more responsive to the needs of transgender patients.

Key Points

- Transgender persons have a significantly higher prevalence of HIV infection than the general population.
- Transgender persons face a disproportionately high amount of social stigma, violence, and socioeconomic challenges, heightening risks for such mental health problems as depression, anxiety, and posttraumatic stress disorder, substance use disorder, and suicide attempts.
- Transgender individuals encounter barriers to care that can be classified in four main categories: reluctance to disclose, systemic barriers, lack of provider experience and resources, and financial barriers.

Case 9.2

Maria is a transgender woman. She began identifying as female during adolescence and subsequently made changes to her clothes and grooming habits to appear more feminine. After high school, Maria became very depressed because she was still unhappy with the way she looked, and she attempted suicide. Soon after her suicide attempt, a friend told her to try taking hormones to appear more feminine. Maria wanted to start hormone therapy but was unemployed and did not have insurance to pay for a visit to a doctor. She bought hormones and needles from a neighbor and began injecting herself at the dosage her neighbor recommended. Recently Maria noticed an infection at the site where she injects her hormones. She was reluctant to go to the doctor because she was still unemployed and uninsured. She had heard from a transgender friend recently that his experience at the doctor had been very unpleasant.

What are some of the reasons that transgender persons such as Maria might experience depression?

In addition to infection, what else might Maria be at risk of contracting from using hormones purchased without medical prescription and supervision?

What are some other barriers that Maria might face as a transgender person?

What are some ways in which a health care setting might be more conducive to and health care providers might be more responsive to the needs of a transgender patient population?

Transgender individuals are at increased risk for many mental health problems because they face social stigma, increased threats of violence, and socioeconomic challenges such as a high likelihood of unemployment. They are also at increased risk of substance use disorder and attempting suicide.

Transgender persons are at an increased risk of HIV infection compared with the general population. Maria's use of street-purchased hormones gives her a higher risk of contracting HIV because she may be injecting herself with used needles.

Transgender individuals report a reluctance to disclose because many have been denied care or even been verbally assaulted after revealing their gender identity. Systemic barriers to care include gender-specific bathrooms and facilities, insensi-

tive support staff, and institutional policies that are insensitive to the needs of transgender patients. Provider barriers are generally related to a deficit of transgender health–knowledgeable clinicians. Gender-neutral facilities, a staff that calls patients by the correct name and pronouns, and billing policies that do not restrict certain laboratory tests on the basis of gender are all ways in which a health care setting can be made more attractive to the transgender population.

The Transition: Mental Health, Gender-Affirming Hormones, Surgery, and Additional Treatments

The transition process is highly individualized and often takes years, depending on a patient's specific needs and desires, in addition to the person's insurance coverage or financial situation. Health care professionals play a role in transition by assisting gender dysphoric individuals in affirming their gender identities through mental health, medical, and surgical interventions. Health professionals from multiple specialties and disciplines must work together in an interdisciplinary and interprofessional capacity to provide optimal care for every transgender patient. The World Professional Association for Transgender Health (WPATH) has developed standards of care (SOC) to provide clinical guidance for health care professionals when treating transgender patients.

External Resource 9.2
The **World Professional Association for Transgender Health**, formerly known as the Harry Benjamin International Gender Dysphoria Association, is an interdisciplinary professional and educational organization devoted to transgender health. https://www.wpath.org

External Resource 9.3
Jazz, a transgender adolescent girl, discusses the challenges and decisions she now faces as she nears puberty. Total time 5:28. http://bit.ly/TECe1ch09_02

Mental Health

Mental health is a crucial aspect of the transition, and transgender persons may seek psychotherapy from a mental health professional to cope with gender dysphoria and, as necessary, to acquire the letters of referral necessary for them to pursue the medical and surgical aspects of transition. The primary responsibilities of a mental health professional in treating a person with gender dysphoria are:

- Assessing gender dysphoria
- Providing information regarding options for gender identity and expression and possible medical interventions
- Assessing, diagnosing, and discussing treatment options for coexisting mental health disorders, which are common in patients with gender dysphoria
- Assessing the patient's eligibility, then preparing and referring the patient for hormone or surgical therapy if it is needed
- Supporting the psychological and emotional needs of an individual as they move through transition

Although psychotherapy is not a requirement for a patient with gender dysphoria, it is highly recommended. The goal of psychotherapy is to maximize a person's well-being and quality of life by finding ways to alleviate gender dysphoria and achieve comfort in long-term gender expression.

Hormone Therapy

Hormone therapy is a medically necessary component of the transition process for many transgender individuals. It is also associated with improved self-esteem, reduction of depression symptoms, and improved quality of life. Some people seek to achieve maximum feminization or masculinization; others find relief in hormonally minimizing existing secondary sex characteristics and maintaining an androgynous presentation.

Hormone therapy must be tailored to the patient's goals, the risk/benefit ratio of medications, the presence of other medical conditions, and any applicable social and economic issues. According to the WPATH SOC, hormone therapy may be initiated after the patient meets the following criteria:

- Persistent, well-documented gender dysphoria
- The capacity to make a fully informed decision and consent to treatment
- Being of the age of majority in the country in question (if younger, a protocol set forth in the SOC is followed)
- Reasonably good control of any significant medical or mental health concerns

The goals of hormone therapy are to reduce endogenous hormone levels, thereby minimizing the secondary sex characteristics of the patient's assigned or natal sex, and to replace endogenous sex hormones with those of the identified gender. The Endocrine Society has published clinical practice guidelines for the administration of **gender-affirming hormone therapy**. Some of the core recommendations are (1) that gender dysphoria be diagnosed by a qualified health professional, (2) that medical conditions that can be exacerbated by hormone depletion and gender-affirming hormone therapy be evaluated and addressed before the start of treatment, and (3) that hormone levels be maintained in the normal physiological range for the identified gender.

Hormone therapy is generally lifelong and requires close monitoring, typically every two or three months in the first year and annual or biannual checks thereafter. If a patient undergoes gonadectomy, hormone therapy is continued but at lower dosages. Cardiovascular risk factors should be monitored and assayed regularly in patients on hormone therapy. Prior to initiation of hormone therapy, all individuals should be asked about desire for fertility and counseled on options for fertility preservation.

MtF Hormone Therapy

The hormone regimen for MtF persons generally consists of estrogen and anti-androgen therapies (Table 9.1), with the goal of achieving estrogen levels of 100–200 pg/mL and testosterone levels <50 ng/dl. The effects of feminizing hormones include:

- Body fat redistribution
- Breast growth
- Decreased muscle mass/strength
- Decreased testicular volume
- Decreased libido
- Male-pattern baldness
- Decreased incidence of spontaneous erections
- Decreased sperm production
- Softening of skin/decreased oiliness
- Thinning and slowed growth of body and facial hair

Most effects are noticeable after three to six months of therapy. The expected maximal effects are achieved in two to three years. The administration of estrogen may exacerbate venous thromboembolism (VTE), thrombophilia, prolactinoma, severe liver dysfunction, breast cancer, coronary artery disease, cerebrovascular disease, or severe migraines in patients with these pre-existing conditions. Oral ethinyl estradiol is associated with a significantly increased risk of VTE and cardiovascular mortality, so its use should be avoided. Therefore 17β-estradiol is recommended in an oral, transdermal, or parenteral preparation. The transdermal preparation is especially recommend in the aging patient. Although long-term exposure to feminizing hormones is associated with an increased risk of breast cancer, it is not known whether this risk is different in a transgender woman from that of person born genetically female. The benefit of progestin in feminizing hormone therapy has not been determined. Some clinicians add progestin

Table 9.1 Male-to-female hormone therapy

Therapy	Mechanism	Effects	Risks/Adverse Events	Monitoring
Estrogen	Steroid hormone interacts with cytoplasmic cell receptor; hormone-receptor complex enters nucleus to regulate gene transcription	Induction of feminine secondary sex characteristics	VTE, hypertriglyceridemia, cardiovascular disease, hypertension, type 2 diabetes (greater risk with oral therapy), breast cancer (inconclusive evidence)	Goal serum estradiol: 100–200 pg/mL Check every 2 to 3 months in the first year and once or twice per year thereafter
Anti-androgens	*Spironolactone* Inhibition of enzymes in androgen biosynthesis pathway; direct blockade of androgen receptor; acceleration of rate of metabolism of testosterone, enhancing rate of peripheral conversion to estrogen *Cyproterone acetate* Progestational compound competitively antagonizes androgen receptor and blocks enzymes in androgen biosynthesis pathway *GnRH agonists* Neurohormones block GnRH to inhibit release of FSH and LH, suppressing testosterone production *5α-Reductase inhibitors* Block conversion of testosterone to more active 5α-dihydrotestosterone	Decrease masculine characteristics; minimize testosterone level to that of a natal female 5α-Reductase inhibitors reduce male pattern baldness and body hair growth; improve skin consistency	*Spironolactone* Hyperkalemia, dizziness, GI upset *Cyproterone acetate* Not available in US because of hepatic toxicity	Goal total serum testosterone: <55 ng/dL *Spironolactone* Check potassium every 2 to 3 months in first year; check blood pressure regularly *Cyproterone acetate* Monitor liver function
Progestin	Steroid hormone interacts with cytoplasmic cell receptor; hormone-receptor complex enters nucleus to regulate gene transcription	Potentially enhances growth breast tissue, decreases irritability and breast sensitivity	Depression, weight gain, hyperlipidemia, coronary vascular disease (oral therapy), increased risk of breast cancer	

GI gastrointestinal, *GnRH* gonadotropin-releasing hormone, *FSH* follicle-stimulating hormone, *LH* luteinizing hormone

to the regimen to enhance breast development because it is known to be integral to mammary development, but a clinical benefit has yet to be established.

Side effects of feminizing hormones include impairment of fertility, fewer nocturnal and sexually stimulated erections, and diminished libido. Even though MtF persons may desire these side effects, it is important to make patients aware of all the potential outcomes before starting therapy, particularly because many transgender patients want to preserve fertility and sexual function. If these side effects are in fact unwanted, steps can be taken to deal with them—for example, cryopreservation of sperm can be undertaken if fertility is desired. However, it should be noted that fertility could return if hormone therapy is discontinued.

FtM Hormone Therapy

Testosterone is the primary component of masculinizing hormone therapy. Testosterone is

Table 9.2 Female-to-male hormone therapy

Therapy	Mechanism	Effects	Risks/adverse events	Monitoring
Testosterone	Steroid hormone interacts with cytoplasmic cell receptor; hormone-receptor complex enters nucleus to regulate gene transcription	Development of masculine secondary sex characteristics	Breast or uterine cancer, erythrocytosis, dyslipidemia, liver dysfunction	Goal total serum testosterone: 320–1000 ng/dL Check testosterone every 2 to 3 months in the first year and once or twice per year thereafter
Progestin	Steroid hormone interacts with cytoplasmic cell receptor; hormone-receptor complex enters nucleus to regulate gene transcription	Menstrual cessation at start of therapy Reduction of estrogen to level seen in natal males	Depression, weight gain, dyslipidemia, coronary artery disease, increased risk of breast cancer	Goal serum estradiol: <50 pg/mL Check during first 6 months of therapy or until menstrual bleeding ceases

present in serum as free testosterone, albumin-bound, and bound to sex hormone-binding globulin. It is generally administered parenterally or transdermally with the goal of maintaining the total serum testosterone level within the normal male range (320–1000 ng/dL). A supraphysiologic concentration increases the risk of adverse reactions, and excess testosterone can be converted to estrogen, counteracting the desired effects of therapy. Conversely, if the testosterone level is too low, the patient is at risk for decreased bone density and maximal masculinizing effects may not be achieved. The effects of masculinizing hormones typically become noticeable within twelve months of the initiation of therapy; maximal effects are achieved in one to five years. The effects of masculinizing therapy include:

- Body fat redistribution
- Cessation of menses
- Clitoral enlargement
- Deepened voice
- Facial/body hair growth
- Increased muscle mass/strength
- Scalp hair loss
- Skin oiliness/acne
- Vaginal atrophy

Absolute contraindications to testosterone therapy include pregnancy, unstable coronary artery disease, and untreated polycythemia.

Patients with underlying cardiovascular or cerebrovascular disease or history of estrogen-dependent cancers such as breast cancer should consult a cardiologist or oncologist before initiating testosterone therapy.

Masculinizing therapy can limit fertility. It is recommended that health care providers discuss reproductive options and desires before starting therapy. If fertility is desired, cryopreservation of oocytes, ovarian tissue, or embryos is possible. Health care providers must also discuss the limitations of hormonal therapy with patients. However, fertility could return with cessation of hormone therapy. Though variable across persons, certain characteristics of the natal sex—including the relatively lower height, broader hip configuration, and greater percentage of subcutaneous fat of FtM adults—will not change with androgen treatment. Progestin can be used at the beginning of hormone therapy to stop menstruation more rapidly. A description of FtM hormone therapies is provided in Table 9.2.

Gender Affirming Surgery

Any surgical procedure performed for the treatment of gender dysphoria is considered a gender affirming surgery. Typically surgery performed to convert the genitalia to those of the desired gender is known as **gender affirmation surgery**. It is also called *sex reassignment surgery, gender con-*

Fig. 9.1 Example of phalloplasty. (**a**) FtM patient before phalloplasty with hypertrophic clitoris, a result of long-term testosterone therapy; (**b**) Same FtM patient one year after phalloplasty

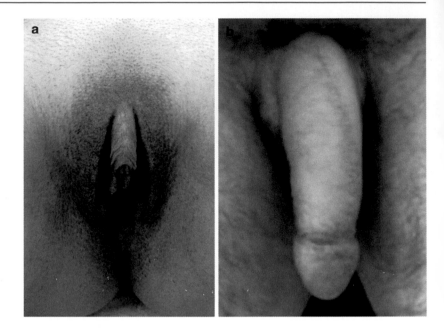

firmation surgery, or *gender reassignment surgery.* Genital and non-genital surgeries exist as integral components in the management of gender dysphoria alongside psychotherapy and hormonal therapy. Although many transsexual, transgender, and gender-nonconforming individuals do not need gender affirming surgery to alleviate gender dysphoria, a majority require one or more of these procedures. For such individuals, these procedures are essential to improving quality of life and to establishing a greater congruence with their gender identity, role, and expression.

WPATH publishes and reviews guidelines and SOC, including surgical options and eligibility criteria for surgery, based on expert clinical consensus and available evidence. The common cases FtM and MtF will be discussed, but the guidelines and SOC can also be applied more broadly to nonbinary and gender nonconforming patients. **Subsequently, this chapter will follow WPATH guidelines and SOC closely**.

General criteria for genital and non-genital surgeries in both FtM and MtF patients are the same as listed above for hormone therapy. Gender affirmation surgery should not take place unless the surgeon has received referrals from separate mental health professionals. Under the SOC, one letter is required for breast/chest surgery, com-

monly referred to as "top surgery," and two letters are required for sex reassignment surgery, commonly referred to as "bottom surgery" (conversion of penis to vagina or vagina to penis). Figures 9.1 and 9.2 are presurgical and postsurgical images of FtM patients. Figure 9.3 shows pre- and postoperative images of a transgender women who underwent vaginoplasty.

FtM patients seeking hysterectomy and salpingo-oophorectomy—or, in MtF patients, orchiectomy or vaginoplasty—are required to undergo 12–24 continuous months of hormone therapy and to be under the care of a mental health professional. A FtM patient desiring metoidioplasty or phalloplasty or MtF patient desiring vaginoplasty is also required to live in the desired gender for 12 months. These experiences are expected to provide ample opportunities for the patient to adjust to the desired gender role before undergoing irreversible surgical procedures. The health care provider should document the patient's experience in the medical record. By following this procedure, mental health professionals, physicians, and patients collaborate in the decision-making process required to make irreversible changes to the body. A variety of surgical options, with their benefits and limitations, are outlined in Tables 9.3 and 9.4.

Fig. 9.2 Example of chest reconstruction. (**a**) FtM patient before chest reconstruction; (**b**) Same FtM patient one year after chest reconstruction (right)

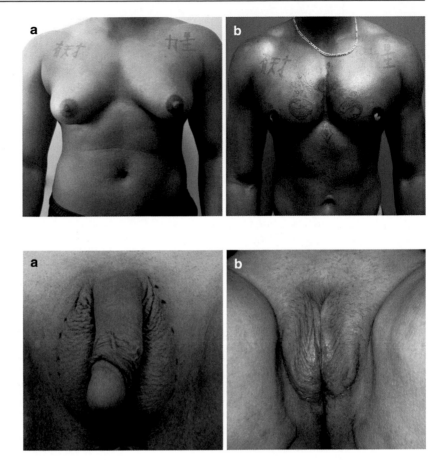

Fig. 9.3 Example of vaginoplasty. (**a**) MtF patient before and (**b**) after vaginoplasty

Table 9.3 Male-to-female surgical procedures

Procedure	Description	Limitations/considerations
Genital		
Orchiectomy	Removal of the testes; often permits lower dosages of estrogen therapy and eliminates need for testosterone blockers	
Penectomy	Removal of penis, usually performed in conjunction with vaginoplasty	
Vaginoplasty	Creates a functional and cosmetically acceptable vagina; sexual sensation preserved with clitoral reconstruction; may involve use of grafts from penis, colon, or other tissue	Neovagina may be too small or short for coitus; skin conduit may require lubrication for sex; colon grafts must be screened for cancer and monitored for the development of inflammatory bowel disease; complications include vaginal stenosis and rectovaginal fistula
Clitoroplasty	Utilizes the glans penis to create a clitoris with preserved erotic sensation	
Labioplasty	Construction of labia majora from scrotal tissue; construction of labia minora from penile skin, if available	Construction of labia minora and aesthetic outcome depend on the tissues that have been used for vaginoplasty

(continued)

Table 9.3 (continued)

Procedure	Description	Limitations/considerations
Non-genital		
Breast augmentation	Construction of breasts appearing and feeling similar to those of natal females	Outcomes vary with shape of the thorax, position of nipple-areola complex, size of pectoral muscles and, usually, presence of a minimal amount or an absence of breast tissue
Reduction thyroid chondroplasty	Removes the protruding part of the thyroid cartilage ("Adam's apple")	
Voice modification surgery	Raises the pitch of the voice; often combined with reduction thyroid chondroplasty	Speech therapy before surgical intervention is recommended; often required to achieve a satisfactory postoperative result
Liposculpture for gluteal augmentation	Body contouring provides more feminine features	
Rhinoplasty (nose job), forehead reduction, malar and mandibular contouring	Assists in facial feminization; considered medically necessary by patient	

Table 9.4 Female-to-male surgical procedures

Procedure	Description	Limitations/considerations
Genital		
Hysterectomy Salpingo-oophorectomy	Eliminates most endogenous estrogen production and permanently ends menstruation	Should be done in patients with family history of gynecological malignancies, especially with the risk of endometrial cancer posed by testosterone therapy Usually laparoscopic to avoid lower abdominal scar
Vaginectomy	Removal vagina, required if the vaginal opening is to be closed	Typically anterior vaginal tissue is used for urethral lengthening; the posterior vagina is discarded
Metoidioplasty	Creates male-appearing genitalia with hypertrophic clitoris (from testosterone therapy) as the phallus; erectile tissue and erotic sensation is preserved	Less invasive than phalloplasty May permit standing urination; small phallus cannot be used in vaginal or anal penetration
Scrotoplasty with placement of testicular prosthesis	Scrotum may be constructed with labia majora tissue and placement of saline or silicone testicular implants, often when a penile implant is placed	May be delayed in many urethroplasty/phalloplasty procedures until sensation is achieved Testicular prostheses may be extruded if too large
Urethroplasty	Creation of a urethral canal through the neophallus	Permits standing urination Great potential for complications, including strictures and fistulas; usually done with phalloplasty
Phalloplasty	Tissue from another part of the patient's body (abdominal, radial forearm, latissimus dorsi, fibula), as a free tissue transfer, is used Nerves may be connected to the pudendal nerve to provide erotic sensation; erectile capability with semirigid or inflatable penile prosthesis, autogenous bone, or cadaver-derived bone	Phallus is closer to the size a natal male's Pedicled abdominal flaps and anterolateral thigh flaps may not provide sensation, and prelaminated flaps for neourethra will require another surgery Incidence of complications such as urethral cutaneous fistulas and stenosis are as high as 50% to 60%
Non-genital		
Chest reconstruction/bilateral mastectomy	Specific technique depends on the amount of breast tissue available; often done at the time of hysterectomy and oophorectomy	Scarring may result Nipples may be large, small, or grafted
Voice surgery	May help deepen the voice	Should be used only when hormone or speech therapy fails to deepen the voice

It is important to note that WPATH is currently developing a newer version of their SOC, so certain criteria may change.

Surgery Outcomes

It is crucial that the health care team make an appropriate diagnosis, select eligible surgical candidates, and decide on the appropriate timing and type of procedures with the patient that optimize the benefits and minimize the risks for the patient. These steps may reduce dissatisfaction or regret resulting from complications or results that differ from expectations. That said, follow-up studies have demonstrated an undeniable beneficial effect on such postoperative outcomes as subjective well-being, cosmesis, and sexual function in most individuals. Even patients who experience severe surgical complications rarely regret having undergone surgery. Therefore the importance of the surgery and surgical outcomes to the patient should be appreciated as one of the best predictors of the overall outcome of gender affirmation surgery.

Non-hormonal and Non-surgical Transition Options

In addition to psychological, medical, and surgical treatment options for treating gender dysphoria, other options can be incorporated into the transition process. These include:

- Voice and communication therapy to help develop the verbal and nonverbal communication skills associated with the identified gender
- Peer and personal resources for social support and advocacy for the gender dysphoric person and friends and family, including community organizations and online and in-person support groups
- Hair removal by means of electrolysis, laser treatments, or waxing
- Breast binding or padding, genital tucking or penile prosthesis, padding of hips or buttocks
- Change in name and gender marker on identity documents
- Image consulting for transgender patients

Key Points

- The management of gender dysphoria must be individualized but generally includes psychotherapy, hormonal therapy, surgery, and non-hormonal and non-surgical management and support options.
- Transitioning is a complex multistep process that is highly individualized and can often take many years, depending on the patient's specific needs and desires, in addition to insurance coverage or financial situation.
- Health professionals from various specialties and disciplines must work together in an interdisciplinary and interprofessional capacity to appropriately manage gender dysphoria and follow clinical guidelines set forth by WPATH.
- Hormone therapy consists primarily of estrogen and androgen blockers for MtF patients and testosterone for FtM patients.
- Gender affirmation surgery includes both genital and non-genital procedures, all with the goal of creating a feminine or masculine appearance that is more congruent with the desired gender identity.

Case 9.3

A 19-year-old MtF transgender woman presents to her primary care physician's office for a consultation on beginning hormone therapy. When puberty began, the patient started experiencing severe discomfort with the changes happening to her body. She did not like her body or facial hair, nor did she feel comfortable with her male genitalia and deepening voice. The patient felt some relief from this distress when she started dressing in feminine clothes, removing her unwanted hair, and tucking her genitalia to make them less noticeable. Soon after graduating from high school, she visited a psychiatrist for the first time because her discomfort persisted. The psychiatrist diagnosed gender dysphoria and referred the patient to an endocrinologist for hormone therapy. During her initial visit, the patient tells the endocrinologist that her maternal grandmother was found to have breast cancer at the age of 45. In light of her family history, she wonders whether hormone therapy will increase her risk of breast cancer. Despite this concern, the patient is eager to start treatment and wants to know the effects of the hormones and when she might start seeing changes.

What clinical guidelines should the physician follow in treating this woman?

What physician specialist is the most appropriate person to oversee hormonal transition?

What is this patient's risk for breast cancer with hormone therapy? Is the treatment contraindicated? What should the endocrinologist do before starting therapy?

What hormone regimen is likely best for this patient? Why?

What are the effects of feminizing hormones, and when do they become noticeable?

The Endocrine Society has published clinical guidelines for the administration of hormone therapy in transgender patients, discussed above. There are no strict rules about which specialty should begin or manage gender-affirming hormone therapy. Previous experience in the area or, at a minimum, professional support from knowledgeable peers, is significantly helpful. Family physicians, general internists, and endocrinologists have all demonstrated proficiency in monitoring gender-affirming hormone therapy. It is the clinician's responsibility to appraise the situation and determine their own comfort level in offering hormone therapy to a patient. Indeed, some clinicians may not feel comfortable performing the initial assessment but may feel comfortable conducting maintenance.

Breast cancer is a preexisting condition that can be exacerbated by gender-affirming hormone therapy. Long-term exposure to estrogens is associated with an increased risk of breast cancer, but it is not known whether this risk is higher than that of a natal female. Although hormone therapy is not contraindicated, the physician should ensure that the patient is properly evaluated by the appropriate physician for her family history of breast cancer before any therapy is initiated.

Because oral ethinyl estradiol is associated with an increased risk of venous thromboembolism and increased cardiovascular mortality, 17β-estradiol is recommended. Hormone therapy is generally lifelong and dosed to maintain the physiologic levels of a natal female. If a patient undergoes gonadectomy, hormone therapy is generally maintained at a lower dosage. Patients are usually also started on an anti-androgen such as spironolactone to minimize masculine characteristics. Patients taking spironolactone must be monitored for hyperkalemia and hypotension. Progestin may also be added because it is thought to enhance breast growth, but this benefit has not yet been definitively demonstrated.

The feminizing effects of MtF hormone therapy include body fat redistribution, decreased muscle mass/strength, softening of skin/decreased oiliness, diminished libido, reduced incidence of spontaneous erections, breast growth, reduced testicular volume, decreased sperm production, thinning and slowed growth of body and facial hair, and male-pattern baldness. These effects are noticeable after three to six months of therapy, and maximal effects are achieved after two to three years. Fertility intentions should be discussed before the start of therapy.

Case 9.4

A FtM transgender man presents to a plastic surgeon to inquire about "sex reassignment surgery." He has been under the care of a psychiatrist and an endocrinologist for mental health counseling and hormone therapy, respectively, for many years. His only previous surgery was a hysterectomy and bilateral salpingo-oophorectomy to remove his female reproductive organs. At this time he is interested in top surgery to remove his breasts but also asks the surgeon to discuss some options for bottom surgery in the future. He is hesitant at this time because he has heard of a high risk of complications with bottom surgery. The patient's partner is present for the consultation and confesses that she is apprehensive about surgery because, in light of the risk for complications, she is worried it might not be beneficial to the patient.

Before the plastic surgeon agrees to perform surgery, what requirements must the patient fulfill in order to adhere to the Standards of Care set forth by WPATH?

When performing top surgery (chest reconstruction), what anatomic considerations must the plastic surgeon be aware of? What complication may arise?

What are the various options for bottom surgery and their associated outcomes and complications?

What might the doctor tell this patient's partner to reassure her that surgery will likely be beneficial to the patient?

WPATH has published criteria for eligibility for sex reassignment surgery: The patient must have persistent and well-documented gender dysphoria, must be capable of making informed decisions and to consent, must be the age of majority, and must have any significant medical or mental health concerns well controlled. Documented gender dysphoria requires a letter of diagnosis from one mental health

professional for top surgery and two letters from separate mental health professionals for bottom surgery. The patient must have undergone 12–24 months of hormone therapy for top surgery and must have lived in his or her desired gender role for 12 months, in addition to undergoing hormone therapy, to be eligible for bottom surgery.

Top surgery in transgender men, referred to as chest reconstruction, is the surgery most commonly requested by transmen. There are many possible techniques; the one used depends on the amount of breast tissue present. Scarring is a common complication.

The FtM individual has multiple options for bottom surgery. This patient has already undergone hysterectomy and salpingo-oophorectomy. He may also choose to undergo metoidioplasty or phalloplasty. A metoidioplasty converts a testosterone-enlarged clitoris into a small phallus. Erotic sensation is preserved, and the patient will usually be able to urinate standing up. However, because of its small size, the patient will unlikely be able to use his phallus for penetrative sex. The patient may instead opt to undergo phalloplasty, in which tissue from another part of the patient's body is used to construct a phallus that is more comparable in size to a natal male's penis. Erectile capacity is provided by a penile prosthesis or autogenous bone. The patient will be able to have penetrative sex with his neophallus (the pudendal nerve supplies erotic sensation), and the patient will be able to urinate standing up. Phalloplasty is generally combined with vaginectomy and urethroplasty. Common complications are strictures, fistulas, and urethral stenosis.

Most transgender persons will undergo at least one surgery to alleviate gender dysphoria. Studies of patients who have undergone sex reassignment surgery have shown overwhelming benefit for well-being, cosmesis, and sexual function. Even those patients who sustain postoperative complications rarely regret having undergone surgery.

A patient considering surgery should work closely with an interdisciplinary team of health care providers, including a mental health professional, to ensure that the correct diagnosis and appropriate procedures are chosen on the basis of specific needs.

Gender Dysphoria in Children and Adolescents

Gender identity begins to develop between the ages of 18 and 24 months. Early indications include gender-typed preferences such as the selection of gender stereotyped toys and playmates of the same sex. Most children express a gender identity that is congruent with their natal sex, but as many as 6% of boys and 12% of girls express gender variant behavior in childhood.

Common features of gender dysphoria in children include a desire to be of the other sex; unhappiness with physical characteristics and functions; a preference for toys, clothes, and games commonly associated with the other sex; and a preference for playing with opposite-sex peers. These features can vary greatly from child to child, particularly in their intensity and frequency. Gender dysphoric children also tend to have psychiatric comorbidities such as anxiety or depression. For gender dysphoria to be diagnosed in a child, the desire to express the unassigned gender must be present and verbalized.

In most gender dysphoric children, these feelings do not persist into adolescence and adulthood. Persistence of gender dysphoria into adolescence and adulthood is associated with higher intensity of gender dysphoria in childhood and is more likely to persist in natal girls. In studies of prepubertal children with gender dysphoria, natal boys were more likely to identify as gay than as transgender in adulthood.

Whether gender dysphoria persists from childhood or has its onset in adolescence, the start of puberty and development of secondary sex characteristics can be particularly distressing for the gender dysphoric adolescent. Gender dysphoria presents similarly in adolescents as it does in children. However, the distress associated with puberty may result in morbidity related to hormone self-medication, self-harm, or suicide, particularly if left untreated.

Recall that physical changes in puberty (secondary sex characteristics) are a result of stimulation of production of estrogen or testosterone via the hypothalamic-pituitary-gonadal axis. In girls, puberty begins with the development of breast buds, followed by growth of pubic hair and, two to three years later, menarche. In boys the first physical change is testicular enlargement, followed by facial and axillary hair growth approximately two years later.

Treatment Options

As with the treatment of gender dysphoria in adults, it is important to individualize therapy for the child or adolescent because treatment goals are unique to each patient. Effective communication among health care professionals, the child or adolescent, and family members is crucial. Expectations of the treatment outcomes should be discussed at length with the patient and the patient's family to identify unrealistic expectations held by the patient and to reduce the risk of harm if treatment goals cannot be met.

Children
The main modalities of treatment for gender dysphoric children are psychological and social interventions. Overall the goal of these treatments is to ease the distress experienced by the child. It is important to keep in mind the likelihood that gender dysphoria in a child will desist. For this reason, any changes made to the child's gender expression should be fully reversible. Mental health practitioners play an important role in the treatment of the gender dysphoric

child, particularly for assessing the extent of gender dysphoria, providing counseling to the child and the family, identifying and treating any coexisting mental health conditions, and educating and advocating on behalf of the patient, such as when facing maltreatment at school. Another important role of the mental health professional is to assist the family with the child's gender expression, particularly in determining to what extent the child will socially transition and how to facilitate the necessary changes. Mental health providers caring for gender dysphoric children should be experienced in child psychiatry or therapy.

Adolescents

Treatment for adolescents should incorporate mental health counseling in the same way that the treatment of children does. Physical interventions may be initiated after an appropriate exploration of psychological, family, and social issues. Three types of physical interventions exist for adolescents: (1) fully reversible, (2) partially reversible, and (3) irreversible. It is generally advised that these measures be taken in a stepwise fashion, with adequate time allowed for the child to adjust to the outcomes of each stage.

Pubertal suppression is a fully reversible intervention. Pubertal suppression is effective in alleviating gender dysphoria. It prevents the development of sex characteristics that may be difficult or impossible to reverse if sex reassignment is ultimately desired. It also provides the adolescent time to explore and develop their cross-gender role before experiencing permanent pubertal changes. A positive response to pubertal suppression also has diagnostic value because it confirms the diagnosis of gender dysphoria. The WPATH criteria for initiation of puberty-suppressing therapy are:

- Demonstration by the adolescent of a long-lasting and intense pattern of gender nonconformity or gender dysphoria (whether suppressed or expressed)
- Emergence or worsening of gender dysphoria with the onset of puberty

- Handling of any coexisting psychological, medical, or social problem that could interfere with treatment (e.g., that may compromise treatment adherence) such that the adolescent's situation and function are stable for treatment to be started
- Provision of informed consent by the adolescent and, particularly when the adolescent has not reached the age of medical consent, by the parents or other caregivers or guardians, who are involved in supporting the adolescent throughout the treatment process

It is recommended that pubertal suppression be started when a girl or and boy first exhibits physical changes of puberty, typically Tanner stage 2. Pubertal suppression maintains end-organ sensitivity to sex steroids, permitting reversal of effects if therapy is stopped. In adolescents who present with gender dysphoria at later stages of puberty, suppression is still possible. However, certain pubertal changes may already be irreversible—particularly the development of breast tissue in biological females and deepening of the voice and outgrowth of the jaw and brow in biological males.

Pubertal suppression is best achieved with gonadotropin-releasing hormone (GnRH) analogues that block gonadotropins and luteinizing hormone and, consequently, testosterone and estrogen production in natal males and females, respectively. With exposure to GnRH agonists, development of secondary sex characteristics halts and atrophy ensues in breast tissue and testicles. Menstruation ceases in natal girls. One concern often raised is the possibility of interfering with bone mineral density during crucial developmental years. However, current data show that GnRH analogue therapy does not affect bone density. Although pubertal suppression has so far been shown to be both safe and effective, it should be kept in mind that data on longer-term effects are not yet available, particularly with regard to bone density and psychological development.

Regular assessment of the patient's gonadotropin and sex steroid levels guides therapy to ensure complete suppression of the gonadal axis.

Adolescents should also be monitored for negative effects of blocked puberty, such a halted growth spurt, impaired bone accretion (bone density), and dysfunction of lipid and glucose metabolism, as well as renal and liver function.

An important benefit of pubertal suppression is the reversibility of therapeutic effects. This is important for patients who may wish to stop therapy and transition back to the sex assigned at birth. Cessation of GnRH analogue therapy results in spontaneous onset of pubertal development and the resumption of reproductive capability.

Gender-affirming hormone therapy is considered partially reversible and may be initiated in adolescent patients who wish to induce pubertal development of their desired sex characteristics. The aim of this treatment is to decrease the levels of endogenous hormones responsible for the development of characteristics of the natal and to supplement hormones to reach the physiologic levels produced in the reassigned sex. It is generally recommended that gender-affirming hormone therapy be started at the age of 16. However, the decision of when to initiate hormone therapy ultimately rests with the patient when they are able to make informed, mature decisions and able to engage in the therapy. Additionally, many providers will time gender affirming hormone therapy to match normal pubertal development of the patient's peers. Before initiation of treatment, it is important to discuss the adolescent's expectations for the outcomes of treatment.

Gender-affirming hormone therapy is administered in a stepwise approach, with a gradual increase of hormone dosages over time in order to mimic the effects of increasing endogenous sex hormones in puberty. Estrogen therapy is initiated in natal males and testosterone therapy in natal females. Puberty-suppressing hormone therapy should initially be maintained to achieve full suppression of the pituitary gonadotropin level. Clinical pubertal development and laboratory markers (luteinizing hormone [LH], follicle-stimulating hormone [FSH], estradiol/testosterone) should be monitored. Liver and renal function, glycosylated hemoglobin, bone density, and bone age should all be monitored.

The adverse effects of and contraindications to gender-affirming hormone therapy in adolescents are the same as they are for adults and should be discussed as part of informed consent. Patients must be counseled about their future reproductive ability and be provided with options for maintaining fertility. However, it should be noted that patients started on pubertal blockers or gender-affirming hormones before the development of reproductive function may not have reproductive function.

Surgery is irreversible. WPATH recommends withholding genital surgery until the patient reaches the legal age required for consent to medical procedures and until the patient has lived in their desired role for at least 12 consecutive months. Breast development can be particularly distressing for FtM patients, so chest surgery may be offered earlier after the patient spends a year living in the identified gender and undergoing a year of hormone therapy. However, the ultimate decision of when to undergo surgery is based on the specific clinical situation and goals for gender identity expression of each individual patient.

> **Key Points**
> - In most gender dysphoric children, dysphoria does not persist into adulthood.
> - Pubertal development can be particularly distressing for gender dysphoric adolescents, and treatment during this time is important to reduce the risks of self-medication with hormones, self-harm, and suicide.
> - Reversible psychological and social interventions are the mainstay of treatment for gender dysphoric children.
> - Physical interventions for gender dysphoric adolescents include reversible, partially reversible, and irreversible treatment options.
> - Pubertal suppression with the use of GnRH analogues is a reversible intervention that provides the adolescent time to explore their desired cross-gender role before the development of permanent secondary sex characteristics begins.

Case 9.5

A 12-year-old trans adolescent is called into her principal's office after missing several days of school and receiving a failing grade in one of her classes. The student, a natal male, began engaging in gender variant behavior as a child but was strongly discouraged by her parents, who told her that this behavior was abnormal and that she would be laughed at in school. She promised only to dress in her sister's clothes in private and tried to stop thinking about her feelings. This was adequate until recently, when she started noticing pubertal changes. She began feeling disgusted by her body and hated looking at herself in the mirror. It became difficult for the girl to pay attention in class, and she frequently thought about hurting herself so doctors would need to "fix" her body. Fearing her parents' reaction, she took matters into her own hands and begged one of her friends to get her birth control pills from a local clinic. She had read online that estrogen is the hormone responsible for puberty in girls and thought that it would help her look more feminine. The girl started taking three pills a day, despite the headaches, nausea, and occasional vomiting that they induced; some days the side effects were so bad, she skipped school.

Does this adolescent meet the criteria for gender dysphoria? Why or why not?

What role can pubertal changes play in adolescents with gender dysphoria?

What psychological and social stressors are present here? What treatment options are available?

Which physical treatment option could be considered at this time?

The DSM-5 diagnostic criteria for gender dysphoria includes clinically significant distress associated with gender discrepancy that affects important areas of function in a person's daily life for at least six months. Gender dysphoria can manifest in many different ways, including a strong desire to be treated as of the other sex, a strong desire to be rid of one's sex characteristics, or a strong belief that the person has feelings and reactions typical of the other gender. In this case, the patient displayed gender variant behavior as a child. Though negatively affected by her family's response to her behavior, she was largely able to effectively cope with gender discrepant feelings. With the onset of puberty, however, clinically significant distress became apparent in the girl's decreased function in school, preoccupation with being rid of her sex characteristics, and self-harming ideation. Pubertal changes such as breast development, testicular growth, and growth of body hair can be particularly distressing to a gender dysphoric adolescent, as seen in this case. If the dysphoric feelings go untreated at this time, the girl has is at increased risk for hormone self-medication, self-harm, and suicide.

In this patient's case, a lack of familial support and acceptance posed a significant barrier treatment and worsened the girl's vulnerability to self-medication and self-harm. Mental health professionals play an important role by advocating for gender dysphoric adolescents, educating family members about gender dysphoria, and helping the family support the adolescent's gender expression through social transitions or physical intervention. School faculty may be included in psychological and social interventions to help reduce the stigma the child may face at school and reduce potential challenges that may occur in gender-specific settings such as bathrooms and locker rooms.

Pubertal suppression is a reversible physical intervention that should be offered at this time. GnRH analogues are provided to halt the development of secondary sex characteristics. This gives the adolescent time to explore the desired cross-gender role before permanent development of secondary sex characteristics occurs and

> *eases the stress associated with the development of secondary sex characteristics. This therapy is most effective in adolescents who have not developed beyond Tanner stage 2 or 3. More invasive procedures may be required in the future to alter the appearance of undesirable sex characteristics. In this case, pubertal suppression therapy could help alleviate the patient's distress at pubertal changes and reduce the risks of self-medication and self-harm.*

Conclusion

This chapter introduced key aspects of transgender health. It is important that health care professionals and trainees acquire the knowledge, tools, and compassion necessary to treat transgender persons. Understanding the spectrum of gender identity, the diagnostic criteria for gender dysphoria in the *DSM-5*, and the complex steps in transitioning is essential to delivering care that meets the needs of transgender people. Standards and practices continue to evolve in this area of medicine. Consulting the most recent guidelines by WPATH and the Endocrine Society is recommended.

Boards-Style Application Questions

Question 1. Jaime, a 25-year-old transgender man, presents to his psychiatrist because he would like to pursue hormone therapy and wants a referral to an endocrinologist. Jaime has identified as male since the age of eight but did not begin dressing and living as a man until the age of 18 because his parents did not allow him to live as his identified gender while still at home. This was distressing to Jaime and caused him much unhappiness throughout adolescence, particularly in social settings such as school. After graduating from high school he was able to move out, seek the care of a psychiatrist, and express himself as his identified gender. Jaime's psychiatrist diagnosed gender dysphoria after the initial

visit. What factor in Jaime's history would contribute to the psychiatrist's diagnosis?

A. Jaime had difficulty adjusting to new social situations
B. Jaime excelled in school and was a well-adjusted teenager
C. Jaime's inability to live as his identified gender caused him distress for many years
D. Jaime had a happy childhood and adolescence even though his parents would not allow him to dress as a boy

Question 2. A 22-year-old transgender woman presents to the emergency department with a two-day history of fever (T_{max} 101.5 ° F) and chills. On physical examination the physician notes a well-demarcated area of erythema, 2 cm in diameter, on each of the patient's buttocks. The patient explains that she attended a "pumping party" a week earlier, during which a friend injected the patient's and other partygoers' buttocks with silicone. Because the patient has not been able to afford to see a physician, she has been attending these parties and also getting hormone injections from a neighbor. The patient does not know where her friends obtained the silicone, hormones, or needles used in the injections. She admits that she knows that these are risky behaviors but says that her previously masculine appearance had caused her significant distress for many years. In addition to appropriate workup and treatment for her presenting symptoms, what other evaluations or screenings should be performed in the hospital?

A. HIV test, Pap smear, colonoscopy
B. Pap smear, HIV test, hepatitis C antibodies
C. Depression screen, HIV test, hepatitis C antibodies
D. Pap smear, depression screen, hepatitis C antibodies
E. Hepatitis C antibodies, depression screen, colonoscopy

Question 3. Alexandra is an 18-year-old transgender woman who presents to her psychiatrist for a one-year follow-up visit. She started identifying as female, particularly in the way she wanted to dress and wear her hair, in childhood. Her parents did not accept this and forced her to dress as a boy and keep her hair short until she reached her teenage years. Puberty caused her much distress, particularly when she started growing body and facial hair. She exhibited signs of depression and even attempted suicide during this time. Now that Alexandra has moved out of her parents' home, she wears feminine clothes, wears her hair long, and undergoes regular electrolysis to remove facial hair. She was given the diagnosis of gender dysphoria by a psychiatrist one year ago and would now like to consider irreversible therapies, particularly hormone therapy and gender confirmation surgery, to acquire a more feminine appearance. According to the WPATH Standards of Care, what should her psychiatrist advise?

A. That no further intervention may be recommended until Alexandra has changed her gender legally
B. That hormone therapy may not be started until Alexandra undergoes breast augmentation and gender confirmation surgery
C. That hormone therapy may be initiated, but Alexandra must undergo breast augmentation before considering gender confirmation surgery
D. That hormone therapy may be started, but gender confirmation surgery requires a diagnosis of gender dysphoria from a second mental health professional
E. That neither hormone therapy nor gender confirmation surgery may be initiated without a diagnosis of gender dysphoria from one additional mental health professional

Question 4. Sarah, a 24-year-old African-American transgender woman, is being seen by Dr. Smith, her family physician, for her six-month follow-up visit for gender-affirming hormone therapy. Sarah tells Dr. Smith that she is concerned because she has been feeling increasingly weak and tired. Otherwise she is happy with the results that she has noticed so far, including some breast growth and a noticeable decrease in the size of her testicles. Dr. Smith reviews Sarah's medications with her. These include transdermal 17β-estradiol, spironolactone, and progesterone. After a physical examination, Dr. Smith tells Sarah that he would like to draw some blood for laboratory studies. In light of Sarah's concerns and the laboratory results shown here, what are the most important changes that Dr. Smith should make to Sarah's medication regimen?

Basic metabolic panel results (normal range):

- Na^+: 140 mmol/L (135–145 mmol/L).
- K^+: 5.8 mmol/L (3.5–5.5 mmol/L).
- Cl^-: 102 mmol/L (95–110 mmol/L).
- CO_2: 27 mmol/L (19–34 mmol/L).
- BUN: 8 mg/dL (6–22 mg/dL).
- Cr: 0.9 (0.6–1.3 mg/dL).

Complete blood count results (normal range).

- White blood cell count: $8.0 \times 10^3/\mu L$ (3.6–$11.0 \times 10^3/\mu L$).
- Hemoglobin: 10.9 g/dL (12.0–15.6 g/dL).
- Hematocrit: 41% (36%–46%).
- Platelets: $300 \times 10^3/\mu L$ (150–$400 \times 10^3/\mu L$).

A. Add an iron supplement
B. Increase the dosage of spironolactone
C. Decrease the dosage of spironolactone
D. Switch her to oral estradiol and add iron supplements
E. Decrease the dosage of transdermal estradiol and add iron supplements

Question 5. A 25-year-old MtF transgender woman presents to her surgeon, complaining of foul-smelling vaginal discharge one month after the completion of vaginoplasty. She tells the surgeon that she recently engaged in nonpenetrative sexual activity with a new partner. Pelvic examination reveals a foul-smelling discharge at the neovaginal opening and foul-smelling pus containing feculent material in the neovaginal canal. No masses or foreign bodies are palpated in the vaginal canal. What is the most likely cause of these findings?

A. Overgrowth of normal vaginal flora
B. Rectovaginal fistula in the neovagina
C. Infection with Gram-negative diplococci
D. Infection with a parasite that shows corkscrew motility on wet mount
E. Urinary tract infection with gram negative bacilli resulting from chronic urine retention

Question 6. A 42-year-old transgender woman comes to the emergency room complaining of pain and swelling in her right leg that started one day ago and has been getting worse. She recalls tripping and falling last week on her way to work, resulting in some minor bruises on her thigh and hip. Because of the injury she has been resting in bed for most of the day and using pain relievers. She has no significant past medical or family history and reports smoking a half-pack of cigarettes daily. Cardiac and pulmonary findings are within normal limits; examination of the right leg reveals +1 edema and warmth in the calf. There is minor ecchymosis along the lateral aspect of the right thigh. Findings on examination of the left leg are within normal limits.

Complete blood count results (normal range):

- White blood cell count: $9.23 \times 10^3/\mu L$ ($3.6–11.0 \times 10^3/\mu L$).
- Hemoglobin: 14.1 g/dL (12.0–15.6 g/dL).
- Hematocrit: 45.3% (36%–46%).
- Platelets: $320 \times 10^3/\mu L$ ($150–400 \times 10^3/\mu L$).

Which medication would most significantly contribute to her clinical presentation?

A. Oral finasteride
B. Oral 17β-estradiol
C. Oral spironolactone
D. Oral ethinyl-estradiol
E. Transdermal 17β-estradiol

Question 7. Sam is a 12-year-old biologically female adolescent in whom gender dysphoria was just diagnosed by a pediatric psychiatrist. He has identified as male since the age of 4. Recently Sam's breasts have started to develop, and this has caused him more distress. His par-

ents bring him to a pediatric endocrinologist to discuss the initiation of medicine to cause pubertal suppression. The doctor discusses the risks associated with puberty-blocking therapy, such as the potential for restriction of bone development, with Sam and his parents. By what mechanism of action will the medicine have its effect?

A. Stimulating the GnRH receptor in the pituitary to increase production of FSH and LH
B. Desensitizing the GnRH receptor in the pituitary to decrease production of FSH and LH
C. Stimulating 17β-hydroxysteroid dehydrogenase to increase estradiol production in the ovary
D. Irreversibly binding to the FSH receptors on the granulosa cells to decrease production of estradiol
E. Inhibiting the conversion of estrone to estradiol by 17β-hydroxysteroid dehydrogenase in the ovary

Question 8. An 11-year-old boy is brought to a pediatric psychiatrist by his parents, who have become increasingly concerned with their son's behavior. From a young age the child has asked his parents buy him dolls, has preferred to play with girls rather than boys, and has frequently worn his sister's clothes. Despite his parents' concerns, they note that their son has always been a happy child. The psychiatrist meets with the child, a pleasant, friendly boy who is dressed in a pink T-shirt and shorts. He is wearing his hair long and in a ponytail, and the psychiatrist notices that he has pink polish on his fingernails. After their initial interview, the psychiatrist confirms that the child is indeed a well-adjusted 11-year-old boy who meets all the cognitive and developmental milestones for that age. At this point, what diagnosis can the psychiatrist give the child?

A. No diagnosis
B. Gender dysphoria
C. Gender identity disorder
D. Gender nonconforming disorder
E. Gender dysphoria, adjustment type

Boards-Style Application Questions Answer Key

Question 1. The essential component of the diagnosis of gender dysphoria is distress caused by natal and identified gender incongruence lasting longer than six months (option C). Difficulty adjusting to new social situations (option A) can be part of the diagnosis. Any functional impairment, be it social, familial, or occupational, can be attributed to gender dysphoria, but it must be specifically related to the distress caused by a person's assigned gender's differing from their identified gender. A happy, well-adjusted childhood and adolescence (option D) suggests gender variance more than it does gender dysphoria. Gender variance, or gender nonconformity, occurs when a person's gender identity differs from societal norms of gender expression, with no associated distress or disruption of functioning (options B and D).

Question 2. The patient should be screened for HIV, hepatitis C, and depression (option A). She has indicated that she is getting hormones and silicone injections from a nonmedical source. This carries risk, particularly because the source of the injected materials, and the needles, is unknown. In light of the group setting in which the silicone was injected, the needles may have been used on multiple people. Needle-sharing puts people at increased risk for HIV and hepatitis C. The prevalence of HIV is much higher in transgender populations than among the general population. Additionally, this patient has gender dysphoria. The suicide rate in the transgender population is high, as is the incidence of psychiatric comorbidities, warranting depression screening at this time. The patient, though she identifies as a woman, does not have a cervix, making a Pap smear unnecessary (options C, D, and E). The patient does not meet the age requirement for a screening colonoscopy and has no symptoms, such as bleeding from the rectum, that might warrant a colonoscopy (options B and C).

Question 3. The initiation of hormone therapy only requires a diagnosis and letter of support of one mental health professional (option D). According to the WPATH SOC, hormone therapy may be initiated after a mental health professional has documented that the patient (1) has persistent, well-documented gender dysphoria, (2) has the capacity to make a fully informed decision and to consent to treatment, (3) is of the age of majority in the country in question (in younger patients, SOC protocols are followed), and (4) has any significant medical or mental health concerns well controlled (option). A legal gender change is not one of the requirements for someone to pursue irreversible interventions for the alleviation of gender dysphoria (option A). Prior breast augmentation or sex reassignment is not required to for hormone therapy to be initiated (options B and C). In fact, hormone therapy is generally started before any surgical interventions for the alleviation of gender dysphoria. A second mental health professional is required to make a diagnosis of gender dysphoria before the patient may undergo genital sex reassignment surgery (option E).

Question 4. Sarah has hyperkalemia, one of the potential side effects of spironolactone therapy. This is likely causing her fatigue and weakness. Measuring K+ is an important component of monitoring MtF patients who take spironolactone. Her dose should be decreased (option C), not increased (option B), to achieve a normal physiologic level of potassium. Another common cause of weakness and fatigue is iron-deficiency anemia. While the patient has a mildly low hemoglobin level, a further work-up to establish the etiology of the anemia is necessary before starting iron therapy (options A, D, and E). Oral ethinyl-estradiol (option D) should not be used because of the increased risk for venous thromboembolism.

Question 5. The correct answer is B, rectovaginal fistula (RVF), an epithelium-lined tract between the rectum and vagina. Development of an RVF in the neovagina is a devastating complication of male-to-female surgery. Most patients with RVF report the passage of flatus or stool through the vagina, which is understandably distressing. The affected patient may also experience vaginitis or cystitis. At times, a foul-smelling vaginal discharge is noted, and frank stool per vagina may occur when the patient has diarrhea. The patient in question recently underwent pelvic surgery for gender confirmation and is experiencing signs and symptoms of RVF, making this the most likely diagnosis. The normal vaginal flora found in a natal female would not be expected to be present in a neovagina (option A). Although it is possible that a transgender woman might become infected with a sexually transmitted organism such as trichomonas or gonorrhea, this patient has not had penetrative sexual sex, and these infections would not cause feculent material to appear in her neovagina (options C and D). Similarly, a urinary tract infection (option E) is possible but would not likely cause a foul-smelling discharge or feculent material in the neovagina.

Question 6. This patient likely has a venous thromboembolism (VTE). Her recent bed rest, leg injury, smoking history, and physical examination findings all put this patient at a high risk for deep venous thrombosis, and, as a transgender woman, the patient is likely taking estrogen replacement therapy. Studies have shown that MtF transgender persons who are treated with oral ethinyl-estradiol (option D, the correct answer) are exposed to a higher thrombotic risk than those who are treated with transdermal preparations or formulations containing 17β-estradiol (options B and E). Oral ethinyl-estradiol has also been linked to increased cardiovascular mortality. Anti-androgen medications (e.g., option A, finasteride; option C, spironolactone), which are also used in the hormonal transition from male to female, are not linked with an increase in risk for VTE.

Question 7. The correct answer is B, desensitizing the GnRH receptor in the pituitary to decrease production of FSH and LH. GnRH agonists are puberty-blocking agents that are administered continuously to desensitize the pituitary receptors and suppress the production of LH and FSH, resulting in the inhibition of ovarian steroid

production. Endogenously secreted GnRH stimulates the pituitary in a pulsatile fashion to produce FSH and LH (option A), and agonists interfere with the normal pulsatility of this stimulus. This must be suppressed in puberty to prevent development of secondary sex characteristics. The goal of puberty blocking hormones is to decrease estradiol production by the ovary, not increase it (option C). GnRH agonists bind to GnRH receptors in the pituitary, not FSH receptors on granulosa cells, to decrease the production of estradiol (option D). They also do not function within the estrogen conversion pathway within the ovary (option E).

Question 8. The correct option is A. At this time, no diagnosis can be given to this child. Although he does exhibit preferences that are consistent with gender variant behavior, he does not display any signs of a diagnosable condition. For gender dysphoria (option B) to be diagnosed, a person must display clinically significant distress or impairment in function caused by identification with a gender differing from that which was assigned at birth. Also, for this diagnosis to be made in a child, the child must verbally express a desire to be of the other gender. The child presented in this case does not display distress or verbalize a desire to change genders. Gender identity disorder (option C) is an outdated term found in the *DSM-IV* that has been replaced by gender dysphoria in the *DSM-5*. This patient might be considered gender nonconforming, but this is not a disorder (option D). Gender dysphoria has not been subclassified into types (E).

Sources

American Psychiatric Association. Gender Dysphoria http://www.dsm5.org/Documents/Gender%20 Dysphoria%20Fact%20Sheet.pdf. Accessed June 20, 2014.

Asscheman H, Giltay EJ, Megens JA, de Ronde WP, van Trotsenburg MA, Gooren LJ. A long-term follow-up study of mortality in transsexuals receiving treatment with gender-affirming hormones. Eur J Endocrinol. 2011;164(4):635–42.

Bauer GR, Hammond R, Travers R, Kaay M, Hohenadel KM, Boyce M. "I don't think this is theoretical; this is our lives": how erasure impacts health care for transgender people. J Assoc Nurses AIDS Care. 2009;29(5):348–61.

Bazargan M, Galva F. Perceived discrimination and depression among low-income Latina male-to-female transgender women. BMC Public Health. 2012;12:663–82.

California Department of Health Services, Tobacco Control Section. California LGBT Tobacco Survey, 2004. Author analyses using machine-readable data file. Available at http://www.cdph.ca.gov/programs/tobacco/Documents/CTCP-LGBTTobaccoStudy.pdf. Accessibility verified June 20, 2014.

Cohen-Kettenis PT, Owen A, Kaijser VG, Bradley SJ, Zucker KJ. Demographic characteristics, social competence, and behavior problems in children with gender identity disorder: a cross- national, cross-clinic comparative analysis. J Abnormal Child Psychol. 2003;31(1):41–53.

Cohen-Kettenis PT, Delemarre-van de Waal HA, Gooren LJ. The treatment of adolescent transsexuals: changing insights. J Sex Med. 2008;5:1892–7.

Conron KJ, Scott G, Stowell GS, Landers SJ. Transgender health in Massachusetts: results from a household probability sample of adults. Am J Public Health. 2012;102(1):118–22.

De Cuypere G, T'Sjoen G, Beerten R, Selvaggi G, De Sutter P, Hoebeke P, et al. Sexual and physical health after sex reassignment surgery. Arch Sex Behav. 2005;34(6):679–90.

Delemarre-Van de Waal HA, Cohen-Kettenis PT. Clinical management of gender identity disorder in adolescents: a protocol on psychological and pediatric endocrinology aspects. Eur J Endocrinol. 2006;155(Suppl 1):S131–7.

Drummond KD, Bradley SJ, Peterson-Badali M, Zucker KJ. A follow-up study of girls with gender identity disorder. Dev Psychol. 2008;44:34–45.

Fagot B. Consequences of moderate cross-gender behavior in pre-school children. Child Dev. 1977;48:902–7.

Feldman J, Bockting W. Transgender health. Minn Med. 2003;86(7):25–32.

Forcier M, Johnson M. Screening, identification, and support of gender non-conforming children and families. J Pediatr Nurs. 2013;28(1):100–2.

Fraser L. Psychotherapy in the World Professional Association for Transgender Health's standards of care: background and recommendations. Int J Transgender. 2009;11(2):110–26.

Gates GJ. How many people are lesbian, gay, bisexual, and transgender? Los Angeles: The Williams Institute; 2011. http://williamsinstitute.law.ucla.edu/wp-content/uploads/Gates-How-Many-People-LGBT-Apr-2011.pdf. Accessed June 20, 2014.

Gijs L, Brewaeys A. Surgical treatment of gender dysphoria in adults and adolescents: recent developments, effectiveness, and challenges. Ann Rev Sex Res. 2007;18:178–224.

Gooren L. Hormone treatment of the adult transsexual patient. Horm Res Paediatr. 2005;64(Suppl 2):31–6.

Gooren LJ. Management of female-to-male transgender persons: medical and surgical management, life expectancy. Curr Opin Endocrinol Diabetes Obes. 2014;21(3):233–8.

Gooren LJ, Giltay EJ. Review of studies of androgen treatment of female-to-male transsexuals: effects and risks of administration of androgens to females. J Sex Med. 2008;5:765–76.

Gorin-Lazard A, Baumstarck K, Boyer L, Maquigneau A, Penochet JC, Pringuey D, et al. Hormonal therapy is associated with better self-esteem, mood, and quality of life in transsexuals. J Nerv Ment Dis. 2013;201(11):996–1000.

Grant J, Mottet L, Tanis J, Herman J, Harrison J, Keisling M. National transgender discrimination survey report on health and health care. Washington, DC: National Gay and LesbianTask Force Foundation; 2010.

Green R. The "Sissy Boy Syndrome" and the development of homosexuality. New Haven: Yale University Press; 1986.

Hage JJ, Karim RB. Ought GIDNOS get nought? Treatment options for nontranssexual gender dysphoria. Plastic Reconstr Surg. 2000;105(3):1222–7.

Hembree WC, Cohen-Kettenis PT, Gooren L, Hannema SE, Meyer WJ, Murad MH, et al. Endocrine treatment of gender-dysphoric/gender-incongruent persons: an Endocrine Society clinical practice guideline. J Clin Endocrinol Metab. 2017;102(11):3869–903.

Hewitt JK, Paul C, Kasiannan P, Grover SR, Newman LK, Warne GL. Hormone treatment of gender identity disorder in a cohort of children and adolescents. Med J Aust. 2012;196(9):578–81.

Institute of Medicine. The Health of Lesbian, Gay, Bisexual, and Transgender People: Building a Foundation for Better Understanding. Washington, DC: The National Academies Press; 2013.

Khan L. Transgender health at the crossroads: legal norms, insurance markets, and the threat of healthcare reform. Yale J Health Policy Law Ethics. 2011;11:375–418.

Klein C, Gorzalka BB. Sexual functioning in transsexuals following hormone therapy and genital surgery: a review. J Sex Med. 2009;6(11):2922–39.

Kuper LE, Nussbaum R, Mustanski B. Exploring the diversity of gender and sexual orientation identities in an online sample of transgender individuals. J Sex Res. 2012;49(2):244–54.

Lawrence AA. Patient-reported complications and functional outcomes of male-to-female sex reassignment surgery. Arch Sex Behav. 2006;35(6):717–27.

Levy A, Crown A, Reid R. Endocrine intervention for transsexuals. Clin Endocrinol. 2003;59:409–18.

Manasco PK, Pescovitz OH, Feuillan PP, Hench KD, Barnes KM, Jones J, et al. Resumption of puberty after long term luteinizing hormone–releasing hormone agonist treatment of central precocious puberty. J Clin Endocrinol Metab. 1988;67:368–72.

Menvielle E, Gomez-Lobo V. Management of children and adolescents with gender dysphoria. J Pediatr Adolesc Gynecol. 2011;24(4):183–8.

Meyer WJ, Webb A III, Stuart CA, Finkelstein JW, Lawrence B, Walker PA. Physical and hormonal evaluation of transsexual patients: a longitudinal study. Arch Sex Behav. 2001;15(2):121–38.

Michel A, Mormont C, Legros J. A psychoendocrinological overview of transsexualism. Eur J Endocrinol. 2001;145:365–76.

Mizock L, Lewis TK. Trauma in transgender populations: risk, resilience, and clinical care. J Emot Abuse. 2008;8:335–54.

Money J, Russo AJ. Homosexual outcome of discordant gender identity/role in childhood: longitudinal follow-up. J Pediatr Psychol. 1979;4(1):29–41.

Murad MH, Elamin MB, Garcia MZ, Mullan RJ, Murad A, Erwin PJ, et al. Hormonal therapy and sex reassignment: a systematic review and meta-analysis of quality of life and psychosocial outcomes. Clin Endocrinol. 2010;72(2):214–31.

Nemoto T, Bodeker B, Iwamoto M. Social support, exposure to violence and transphobia, and correlation of depression among male-to-female transgender women with a history of sex work. Am J Public Health. 2011;101(10):1980–8.

Obedin-Maliver J, Goldsmith ES, Stewart L, White W, Tran E, Brenman S, et al. Lesbian, gay, bisexual, and transgender-related content in undergraduate medical education. JAMA. 2011;306:971–7.

Oriel KA. Clinical update: medical care of trans- sexual patients. J Gay Lesbian Med Assoc. 2000;4(4):185–94.

Pfafflin F, Junge A. Sex reassignment: thirty years of international follow-up studies after sex reassignment surgery: a comprehensive review, 1961–1991. Düsseldorf: Symposium Publishing; 1998.

Poteat T, German D, Kerrigan D. Managing uncertainty: a grounded theory of stigma in transgender health encounters. Soc Sci Med. 2013;84:22–9.

Rachlin K, Green J, Lombardi E. Utilization of health care among female-to-male transgender individuals in the United States. J Homosex. 2008;54(3):243–58.

Roberts TK, Fants CR. Barriers to quality health care for the transgender population. Clin Biochem. 2014;47(10–11):983–7.

Sanchez NF, Rabatin J, Sanchez JP, Hubbard S, Kalet A. Medical students' ability to care for lesbian, gay, bisexual, and transgendered patients. Fam Med. 2006;38:21–7.

Sanchez NF, Sanchez JP, Danoff A. Health care utilization, barriers to care, and hormone usage among male-to-female transgender persons in New York City. Am J Public Health. 2009;99:713–9.

Selvaggi G, Bellringer J. Gender reassignment surgery: an overview. Nat Rev Urol. 2011;8:274–81.

Serbin LA, Poulin-Dubois D, Colburne KA, Sen MG, Eichstedt JA. Gender stereotyping in infancy: visual preferences for and knowledge of gender-stereotyped toys in the second year. Int J Behav Dev. 2001;25:7–15.

Shipherd JC, Maguen S, Skidmore WC, Abramovita SM. Potentially traumatic events in a transgender sample: frequency and associated symptoms. Traumatology. 2011;17(2):56–67.

Snelgrove JW, Jasudavisius AM, Rowe BW, Head EM, Bauer GR. "Completely out-at-sea" with "two-gender medicine": a qualitative analysis of physician-side barriers to providing healthcare for transgender patients. BMC Health Serv Res. 2012;12:110–23.

Spack NP. Management of transgenderism. JAMA. 2013;309(5):478–84.

Steensma TD, Cohen-Kettenis PT. Gender transitioning before puberty? Arch Sex Behav. 2011;40(4):649–50.

Steensma TD, McGuire JK, Kreukels BP, Beekman AJ, Cohen-Kettenis PT. Factors associated with desistence and persistence of childhood gender dysphoria: a quantitative follow-up study. J Am Acad Child Adolesc Psychiatr. 2013a;52(6):582–90.

Steensma TD, McGuire JK, Kreukels BP, Beekman AJ, Cohen-Kettenis PT. Factors associated with desistence and persistence of childhood gender dysphoria: a quantitative follow-up study. J Am Acad Child Adolesc Psychiatr. 2013b;52(6):582–90.

T'Sjoen G, Van Caenegem E, Wierckx K. Transgenderism and reproduction. Curr Opin Endocrinol Diabetes Obes. 2013;20(6):575–9.

Thole Z, Manso G, Salgueiro E, Revuelta P, Hidalgo A. Hepatotoxicity induced by an-tiandrogens: a review of the literature. Urol Int. 2004;73(4):289–95.

Toorians AW, Thomassen MC, Zweegman S, Magdeleyns EJ, Tans G, Gooren LJ, et al. Venous thrombosis and changes of hemostatic variables during gender-affirming hormone treatment in transsexual people. J Clin Endocrinol Metab. 2003;88(12):5723–9.

UCSF Center of Excellence for Transgender Health. Surgical options. Primary Care Protocol for Transgender Patient Care. Available at http://transhealth.ucsf.edu/trans?page=protocol-surgery. Accessibility verified June 21, 2014.

UCSF Center of Excellence for Transgender Health. Fertility. Primary Care Protocol for Transgender Patient Care. Available at http://transhealth.ucsf.edu/trans?page=protocol-fertility. Accessibility verified February 9, 2015.

University of California Berkeley Gender Equity Resource Center. Definition of terms. Available at http://geneq.berkeley.edu/lgbt_resources_definiton_of_terms. Accessibility verified June 20, 2014.

Van Kesteren P, Lips P, Gooren LJ, Asscheman H, Megens J. Long-term follow-up of bone mineral density and bone metabolism in transsexuals treated with cross-sex hormones. Clin Endocrinol. 1998;48:347–54.

Wierckx K, Gooren L. T'sioen G. Clinical review: breast development in trans women receiving cross-sex hormones. J Sex Med. 2014;11(5):1240–7.

World Professional Association for Transgender Health. Standards of care for the health of transsexual, transgender, and gender-nonconforming people, version 7. Available at http://admin.associationsonline.

com/uploaded_files/140/files/Standards%20of%20 Care,%20V7%20Full%20Book.pdf. Accessibility verified June 20, 2014.

Zosuls KM, Ruble DN, Tamis-LeMonda CS, Shrout PE, Bornstein MH, Greulich FK. The acquisition of gender labels in infancy: implications for gender-typed play. Dev Psychol. 2009;45:688–701.

Zucker KJ, Bradley SJ. Gender identity disorder and psychosexual problems in children and adolescents. New York: Guilford Press; 1995.

Zuger B. Early effeminate behavior in boys: outcome and significance for homosexuality. J Nerv Ment Dis. 1984;172(2):90–7.

Emergency Medicine

10

Carl G. Streed Jr., Elizabeth A. Samuels, and Joyce Rosenfeld

Introduction

Patients come to receive care in the ED not only for emergent conditions but also for primary care concerns because of limited access to primary care or a lack of health insurance. LGBTQ people often face barriers to high-quality, appropriate emergency care as a result of a combination of implicit or explicit discrimination and a lack of proper training and cultural competency among health care providers. LGBTQ people are more likely to be uninsured and to face significant disparities in access to primary or specialty care. Currently there are no accurate estimates of LGBTQ ED use and accessibility because of failures to collect data on patient sexuality orientation and gender identity and because of patients'

The first listed author is the chapter's associate editor from The Equal Curriculum Project. The chapter authors are otherwise ordered according to their preference.

C. G. Streed Jr. (✉)
Boston University School of Medicine, Center for Transgender Medicine & Surgery, Boston Medical Center, Boston, MA, USA
e-mail: carl.streed@bmc.org

E. A. Samuels
Alpert Medical School, Brown University, Providence, RI, USA
e-mail: elizabeth_samuels@brown.edu

J. Rosenfeld
Harrington Memorial Hospital, Southbridge, MA, USA

hesitancy to disclose. LGBTQ elders and adolescents have been noted to be the least likely to disclose their sexual orientation or gender identity. Some studies indicate that LGBT people may use the ED more frequently than others because they lack access to primary care and have disproportionately high rates of sexual and physical assault, psychiatric disorders, substance dependency, homelessness, HIV infection, and death by suicide and homicide.

The Approach to the Patient in the Emergency Department

The diagnostic approach for emergency medicine providers begins when the provider enters the examination room. When considering the origin of a patient's constellation of presenting symptoms, the emergency medicine provider must always focus first on the diagnosis that would be most lethal—ruling out "the big and the bad"—then move on to the most common or likely diagnosis. When an LGBTQ person presents to the ED, it will most likely be for a complaint unrelated to sexual orientation or gender identity. However, from the patient's perspective, the possibility of being insulted or abused or of not having their relationships and identity respected may be more significant than a laceration, bowel obstruction, or respiratory problem.

© Springer Nature Switzerland AG 2020
J. R. Lehman et al. (eds.), *The Equal Curriculum*, https://doi.org/10.1007/978-3-030-24025-7_10

Even though prejudice against LGBTQ individuals is diminishing among health care providers, many still do not feel comfortable taking the social and sexual histories from LGBTQ patients. In many cases this is the result of a lack of training or reliance on assumptions. The ED poses special challenges of limited time and privacy. Quickly establishing a good rapport with patients will yield more accurate histories and help providers render effective, high-quality care. Simple strategies such as sitting down when speaking to the patient, allowing the patient to speak uninterrupted, and maintaining good eye contact can all help build trust in a relatively short period. Careful consideration of past medical history, surgical history, social history, medications, allergies, and review of systems must be accomplished in a quick and considerate manner. Providers must remain mindful that LGBTQ patients— especially transgender patients who report frequent discriminatory treatment—may have had negative, discriminatory, or even traumatizing experiences in health care environments before.

Building rapport with the family and friends of the patient can be just as important as developing a good provider-patient relationship. An LGBTQ patient may not be in communication with their biological family, or the patient's significant other may not have a legal partner status. Introductions should include all individuals who are with the patient. It cannot be assumed that everyone accompanying a patient is aware of the patient's gender and sexual identity. The patient is generally allowed to decide who is present for the interview and physical exam, but other people in the room should be asked to leave when the topics of safety in interpersonal relationships, mental health, sexual health, gender and sexuality identities, and sensitive lab results such as rapid HIV testing are discussed.

Providers must be respectful and supportive of partners being present for as much of the care interaction as the patient prefers. Partners—or indeed any person(s) designated by the patient— must have all of the same visitation rights and privileges as partners with legal relationship status provided by a state sanctioned marriage even if unmarried. Depending on the policies of the institution, partners and designees may need to advocate for the patient's right to dictate who may visit, and providers may need to intervene to ensure that these rights and privileges are observed.

The physical layout of an ED can pose major obstacles to privacy. In EDs with serious overcrowding, it is not unusual for patients to wait in hall beds or be doubled up in rooms. The provider must be mindful of the volume of their voice when asking sensitive questions or reporting test results. A willing patient may write answers down if being heard is a concern. A full sexual history may not be relevant to a presenting concern such as a sprained ankle. When it *is* relevant, the physical examination and history should be taken in the most private setting possible, because being outed publicly may pose a safety risk for the patient. Similarly, it is appropriate to ask about hormone medications or **gender affirmation surgeries** when the topic is relevant to the patient's care or the chief concern.

Before the provider takes a sexual history, it is helpful to explain that the questions are asked of all patients when it is relevant to the chief complaint. The best way to take a sexual history is to ask direct, nonjudgmental, open-ended questions about sexual partners and practices. This approach to the interview should be applied universally—not only when the provider suspects that the patient is LGBTQ.

Though universal screening for intimate partner violence is controversial, providers must take care to avoid applying biases to non-heterosexual persons or relationships. Intimate partner violence can be fatal. Just under half of all women murdered by their partners had presented to the ED in the two years before death, and 93% had had a visit related to an injury. Red flags for physical or sexual abuse include injuries that are not consistent with the stated mechanism of injury, multiple ED visits for vague concerns, a much younger appearance than that of the patient's stated age, and a partner who is much older than the patient.

Unfortunately, domestic violence resources for gay men and transgender people are limited. Sources of support and information for

LGBTQ individuals experiencing intimate partner violence include:

- National Domestic Violence Hotline (24 hours a day; 800-799-SAFE)
- The Network/la Red (tnlr.org), Boston
- Communities United Against Violence (CUAV 415-333-HELP), San Francisco
- The Northwest Network (206-568-7777), Seattle
- Survivor Project (503-288-3191), Portland, OR

▶ **Discussion Questions**
- Name some strategies beyond to those already mentioned for building rapport with patients.
- Imagine a scenario in which an assumption or implicit bias interferes with building rapport with LGBTQ patients.
- Identify specific policies regarding LGBTQ patients at a health care facility in your region.
- Research whether your state is a "next of kin" or "family consent" state, i.e., whether your state identifies a relative as the surrogate decision-maker by default for an incapacitated patient who has no advance directives naming a surrogate decision-maker. How may this policy affect LGBTQ patients?

Key Points
- Patients may use the ED both for emergency treatment and because they lack access to health insurance and primary care.
- The primary constraints on patients and providers in the ED are time and privacy.
- Building trust and rapport with patients in the ED is central to providing good emergency care. Strategies include sitting down, making good eye contact, and allowing the patients to initially speak uninterrupted.
- In many EDs, privacy is limited. Speak at an appropriately low volume, ask the patient's permission to discuss sensitive topics in the presence of the people accompanying the patient, and offer other means of communicating to maintain privacy.

Emergency Medicine Case Presentations

The communication skills acquired by the trainee working under the supervision of an emergency physician depend on the situations encountered by the trainee and by the urgency of patients' presentations. Providers and trainees care for multiple patients simultaneously across a range disease severity. A patient's history and physical exam must be distilled into a relevant and brief summary. Good histories contain the seven cardinal features of a presenting illness (Table 10.1).

Presentations are focused and presented in an organized, succinct manner. The presenter may also follow one of several established formats to organize a presentation. Generally, the presenter should deliver an opening statement that characterizes the case presentation and assessment, supported by history, physical, and test findings, and follow up with a treatment plan. One frequently used format is SBAR: Situation, Background, Assessment, and Recommendations (Table 10.2).

Key Points
- Patient presentations in the ED are succinct.
- After the history and physical exam findings are summarized, the presenter should offer a differential diagnosis and plan for evaluation.

Table 10.1 Seven cardinal features of a presenting illness

1. Quality
2. Location
3. Chronology
4. Setting and onset
5. Severity
6. Modifying factors
7. Associated symptoms

Table 10.2 The SBAR system of case presentation

Situation	Patient is a 57-year-old transgender man with abdominal pain and fever.
Background	Patient started experiencing lower abdominal pain a week ago; it is associated with nausea and vomiting. No diarrhea. Fevers at home measured to 103.3 °F. Patient had a hysterectomy a week ago. On exam, the patient is tachypneic and tachycardic and appears uncomfortable. His abdomen is diffusely tender to palpation, with voluntary guarding but no rebound. The surgical incision is erythematous and without drainage.
Assessment	I am concerned that the patient has an intraabdominal infection following hysterectomy.
Recommendations	Plan to order complete blood count, chemistry panel, liver panel, lipase, lactic, and blood cultures. Will get a CT of the abdomen and pelvis to evaluate for intraabdominal abscess. I think we should give empiric antibiotics and anticipate that patient will need a surgical consultation and hospital admission.

Case 10.1

HPI: Patient is a 59-year-old woman with history of chronic obstructive pulmonary disease (COPD), hypertension, hyperlipidemia, and gout. She presented to the ED with one week of shortness of breath and chest pain. She recently flew from California to New York. She has been admitted to the hospital four times in the past six months for COPD exacerbations and pneumonia. She continues to smoke cigarettes. During the interview, the patient says she is transgender and reports taking oral estrogen daily.

Physical Exam
- Vital signs: HR 117, BP 146/82, RR 28, O$_2$ sat 92% on 4 L NC, T 98.5 °F

- GEN: Awake, alert, and oriented × 3. Appears uncomfortable, anxious, sitting upright in bed and leaning forward.
- HEENT: normocephalic, atraumatic. EOMI, PERRL, moist mucosal membranes, no oropharyngeal erythema, swelling, or exudate.
- CV: Tachycardic with regular rhythm, no m/r/g.
- PULM: Tachypneic with moderate accessory respiratory muscle use, CTAB, no wheezing.
- ABD: Soft, NTND.
- MSK: FROM of all extremities. RLE swelling with mild erythema, calf tender to palpation. 2+ DP pulses bilaterally.
- Neuro: A&O × 3, no focal neuro deficits, 5/5 strength in all extremities.

Discussion Questions
- Write or present an SBAR for this case. Alternatively, write an assessment and plan for a SOAP note or present a hand-off of this patient in your preferred format (e.g., I-PASS, IDEAL).
- What is the differential diagnosis of the cause of this patient's shortness of breath?
- How does the patient's past medical history change the differential diagnosis?
- How does the patient's gender identity change the differential diagnosis?
- What tests should be ordered next?

Sexually Transmitted Infections

Presenting Complaints of Sexually Transmitted Infections

The Centers for Disease Control and Prevention (CDC) estimate that there are 20 million new sexually transmitted infections (STIs) annually, with 110 million total STIs nationally as of 2013. LGBTQ individuals are disproportionately affected by STIs compared with their heterosexual peers. This is the result of a combination of factors, including barriers to or lack of access to care, lack of preventive measures, and sexual violence. Patients should be tested for STIs depending on their presenting concern and risk factors for disease transmission.

A thorough history will help you discern whether a patient is at risk for STIs. The history should cover sexual partners and practices, methods of preventing STIs and pregnancy, and history of STIs. Because the sex and gender of a patient or any sexual partners can never be assumed, questions about sexual activity must elicit specific practices and body parts. It is also important to consider testing lesbian and bisexual cisgender women and WSW for pregnancy if it is relevant to the presenting concern. Table 10.3 outlines *The Equal Curriculum*'s version of the CDC's recommended questions for

Table 10.3 The fives P's of STI prevention (brief)

Partners
Who do you have sex with?
In the past 12 months, how many partners have you had sex with?
Prevention of pregnancy
Are you or your partner trying to get pregnant?
If not: What are you (or your partner) doing to prevent pregnancy?
Protection from STIs
What do you do to protect yourself from STIs and HIV?
How often do you use condoms? Always? Sometimes? Never?
When was the last time you were tested for STIs or HIV?
Are you interested in being tested for STIs or HIV?
Practices
To understand your risk for STIs, I need to understand what kind of sex you've had recently. What kind of sex do you and your partner(s) have? Vaginal? Anal? Oral?
Do you ever have pain or discomfort during sex?
Do you or your partner(s) use any devices, toys, or substances to enhance your sexual pleasure?
Past history of STIs
Have you ever had an STI?
Have any of your partners been tested or treated for an STI?
Have you or any of your sex partners ever injected drugs? Exchanged money or drugs for sex?

Modified from information from the Centers for Disease Control and Prevention

STI prevention, categorized by the "5 P's of sexual health"—Partners, Practices, Protection from STIs, Past history of sexually transmitted infections, and Prevention of pregnancy. An extended version is Table 8.1.

Sexually transmitted infections can be divided into broad categories based on their presenting symptoms:

- Cervicitis, urethritis, and discharge
- Genital ulcers
- Other infections

Infections that cause cervicitis, urethritis, and discharge vary in their severity (Table 10.4). The patient should be tested not just for the suspected STI but for others as well; many infections are transmitted concurrently. In addition to undergoing the appropriate screening and treatment, any patient who does not already have a primary care provider should be referred for follow-up. Diseases marked by genital ulcers—syphilis, herpes, and chancroid—vary in their presentation and severity (Table 10.5). All have a high incidence of cotransmission with HIV, so patients should be tested if they have not been already. For an in-depth discussion of STIs, see Chap. 8.

Other Sexually Transmitted Infections

Human Papilloma Virus

Human papilloma virus (HPV), the most commonly transmitted STI, has more than 100 genotypes. Most HPV infections are cleared by the immune system, but genotypes 6 and 11 often remain and are responsible for genital warts, and genotypes 16 and 18 have been linked to cervical, anal, and oropharyngeal malignancies. Genital warts are usually painless fleshy cauliflower-like growths on external genitalia and the anus.

Contrary to common misconception, cisgender women can pass HPV on to their sexual partners. This is significant because women who have sex with women (WSW) are less likely to get Pap smears for cervical cancer screening. The incidence of HPV-related anal cancers is increasing

Table 10.4 Evaluation and management of cervicitis, urethritis, and discharge

Epidemiology	Symptoms	Testing	Treatment	Counseling	Complications if untreated
Chlamydia trachomatis					
Intracellular bacterium Most frequently reported STI; most commonly affects people <25 years; high incidence of gonorrhea coinfection	Dysuria and urethral, vaginal, or anal discharge	Urine culture; urethral, vaginal, or cervical swab and nucleic acid amplification test (NAAT)	Azithromycin 1 g PO once or doxycycline 100 mg BID for 7 days Safe in pregnancy	Inform all sexual partners in the last 60 days of need to be tested No sexual contact for 7 days after completion of antibiotic treatment	Pelvic inflammatory disease, chronic pelvic pain, infertility, ectopic pregnancy
Neisseria gonorrhoeae					
Gram-negative diplococcus Second most commonly reported STI; gonococcal cervicitis increases concentration of semen HIV-1, thereby increasing infectiousness	Lower abdominal/ pelvic pain, mucopurulent cervicitis, purulent penile or rectal discharge, testicular pain Disseminated infection: petechial or pustular skin lesions, asymmetric arthralgias, septic arthritis, fever	Urine culture; urethral, vaginal, or cervical swab and NAAT	Ceftriaxone 250 mg IM once or cefixime 400 mg PO once -----AND----- Azithromycin 1 g PO once Disseminated infection requires hospitalization for IV antibiotics; all septic joints need orthopedic washout	Inform all sexual partners of the last 60 days of need to be tested No sexual contact until 7 days after antibiotic treatment	Pelvic inflammatory disease, chronic pelvic pain, infertility, ectopic pregnancy
Trichomonas vaginalis					
Protozoal organism	Vaginal irritation, burning, pruritus, dyspareunia, malodorous watery discharge (70%), and lower abdominal pain; discomfort may increase with menstruation; urethritis in natal males is usually asymptomatic (77%)	Wet mount microscopy, NAAT	Metronidazole 2 g PO once or Tinidazole 2 g PO once -----OR----- Metronidazole 500 mg PO BID for 7 days	Treat all sexual partners in the last month No sexual contact until 7 days after antibiotic treatment	

among MSM, who are 17 times more likely to have anal cancer than are men who only have sex with women.

Everyone who has a cervix, including WSW, ages 21–29 years should undergo cervical cancer screening with cytology every three years. People 30–65 years of age who have a cervix may receive screening every three years with cytology alone, every five years with testing for high-risk HPV with or without cytology. These recommendations apply to all people who have a cervix, including transgender men.

At this time there is no evidence to suggest that anal cancer screening reduces morbidity or mortality in HIV-negative MSM or other HIV-negative people who have receptive anal sex. However, the 9-valent HPV vaccine is approved for use in all people ages 9–45. HPV screening is

Table 10.5 Evaluation and management of genital ulcers

Epidemiology	Clinical diagnosis	Pain	Inguinal adenopathy	Comment	Treatment
Syphilis					
Spirochete bacterial infection Increasing in prevalence; MSM account for three out of four cases; young, black, and Latino MSM disproportionately affected Cofactor in HIV transmission	Indurated, with a relatively clean base; heals spontaneously VDRL and RPR testing	No	Firm, rubbery, discrete nodes; nontender	Primary: chancre Secondary: rash, mucocutaneous lesions, lymphadenopathy Tertiary: cardiac, ophthalmic, auditory CNS involvement possible at any stage	Primary or secondary: penicillin G benzathine, 2.4 million units IM single dose Tertiary: penicillin G benzathine, 2.4 million units IM weekly × 3 weeks Counseling: Treat all sexual partners in past 90 days; test for HIV upon diagnosis of 1° and 2° infection, repeat in 90 days if initially negative in high-HIV prevalence areas
Herpes simplex virus					
HSV-1 or HSV-2 (most genital infections) 2–24 hours of painful prodrome at site of eruption Cofactor in HIV transmission	Multiple small, grouped vesicles coalescing and forming shallow ulcers; vulvovaginitis Culture, PCR, serologic tests	Yes	Bilateral adenopathy, tender	Cytology insensitive; culture has high false negatives	Acyclovir 400 mg PO TID daily × 7–10 days or until ulcers healed Counseling: Notify partner, use barrier methods for transmission prevention
Haemophilus ducreyi (Chancroid)					
Gram-negative bacillus Cofactor in HIV transmission	Multiple painful, irregular, purulent ulcers with exudative bases Culture, PCR	Yes	Half of affected have painful suppurative inguinal lymph nodes that may require drainage	10% are coinfected with herpes simplex virus or syphilis Culture is definitive but sensitivity is <80%	Azithromycin 1 g PO once Treat partners from last 10 days; no sex until lesions have healed Test for HIV at diagnosis and HIV and syphilis in 90 days

not routinely performed in the ED, but it is appropriate to refer individuals who have not had the necessary screening tests to a primary care provider or gynecologist.

Hepatitis

The five most common strains of viral hepatitis (A, B, C, D, and E) vary in their epidemiology and routes of transmission. MSM make up 10% of new hepatitis A cases and 15–25% of new hepatitis B cases. Hepatitis A is spread by the fecal-oral route, often in contaminated food or water. Hepatitis B, spread in semen or blood, is easily transmitted sexually. Although most cases of hepatitis A are self-limited, hepatitis B is the most common cause of liver failure worldwide. Both are preventable with vaccination, but vaccination prevalence among MSM is low.

There is no vaccine to prevent hepatitis C transmission. LGBTQ individuals are not at higher risk of contracting hepatitis C than their heterosexual peers unless they are using intravenous drugs or receiving nonsterile tattoos. The disease is rarely transmitted sexually. Currently screening is recommended for individuals born between 1945 and 1965 (the "baby boomer" generation), intravenous drug users, and people with HIV.

HIV/AIDS

In the 1980s and 1990s, human immunodeficiency virus (HIV) and acquired immune deficiency syndrome (AIDS) ravaged the gay community. The World Health Organization estimates that 35.3 million people are living with HIV/AIDs worldwide and that in 2012, 1.6 million people died of AIDS-related illnesses. The CDC estimates that just over 1.1 million people are living with HIV in the United States. Since the identification of the virus and development of antiretroviral treatments, transmission of HIV has diminished. However, MSM continue to be disproportionately affected by HIV. Although gay and bisexual men make up 2% of the total population, in 2010 they accounted for more than two-thirds (67%) of new HIV infections and currently make up more than half of people currently living with HIV. Men of color who have sex with men are at especially high risk for HIV transmission. Young African-American MSM are the most likely to be affected, accounting for 38% of new infections among MSM in 2016. From 2011 to 2015, rates of HIV infection increased 35% among Asian MSM and 13% among Latino MSM. Transgender women, and transgender women of color in particular, also have a disproportionately high prevalence of HIV infection. The CDC estimates that around one quarter (22–28%) of transgender women are currently living with HIV and more than half (56%) of black transgender women currently live with HIV.

There has been no confirmed case of female-to-female sexual transmission, but because WSW may have sex with people of any gender and can still acquire HIV through nonsexual means (e.g., intravenous drug use), they are still at risk.

Between 50% and 90% of individuals acutely infected with HIV will experience a flu-like syndrome two to four weeks after exposure that lasts about two weeks. Seroconversion, when antibodies can be detected in the serum, occurs three to eight weeks after infection. HIV viral load and CD4+ count are most predictive of disease severity. AIDS is defined as a CD4+ T-cell count less than 200 cells/mm^3 or the presence of an AIDS-defining illness (Table 10.6). More details about the diagnosis and treatment of HIV and AIDS can be found in Chap. 11.

Table 10.6 AIDS-defining illnesses

Esophageal candidiasis
Cryptococcosis
Cryptosporidiosis
Cytomegalovirus retinitis
Herpes simplex virus infection
Kaposi sarcoma
Brain lymphoma
Mycobacterium avium complex infection
Pneumocystis jiroveci (*P. carinii*) pneumonia
Progressive multifocal leukoencephalopathy
Brain toxoplasmosis

HIV testing in the ED is recommended by the CDC. Laws concerning informed consent and the process of consent vary state to state, but testing should always be discussed with the patient. Testing may be diagnostic, performed because HIV infection or AIDS is suspected, or it may be targeted screening, focused on individuals at risk for HIV, or performed as a general screening. There are many different types of tests. Many EDs use rapid serum or saliva tests. Like the traditional serum HIV test, rapid tests are antibody-based, and a positive test should be confirmed with the Western blot. In the ED, any individual with a new diagnosis of HIV should be provided supportive counseling and offered follow-up with an infectious disease specialist. The patient requires confirmatory testing in addition to measurement of serum viral load and CD4+ T-cell count.

Key Points
- Coinfection with multiple STIs is common. Test and consider treating the patient for other common STIs.
- The prevalence of syphilis is increasing and disproportionately affecting MSM. Consider testing for STIs in MSM who present with genitourinary or neurologic concerns.
- Despite advances in treatment and prevention, HIV continues to disproportionately affect MSM and transgender women. Rapid testing is available and should be used in the ED.

Case 10.2

HPI: Patient is a 16-year-old boy who has presented to the ED with a sore throat. He has had symptoms for a few days but no fever. No cough or nausea or vomiting. No trouble handling secretions, no change in voice. He says he has had strep throat in the past. He says he is bisexual and sexually active with men and women.

Physical Exam
- Vital signs: HR 105, BP 123/79, RR 21, O_2 sat 100% on RA, T 98.5 °F
- GEN: Awake, alert, and oriented ×3, NAD.
- HEENT: Normocephalic, atraumatic. EOMI, PERRL, moist mucosal membranes. Posterior pharynx is erythematous, with white exudate. No peritonsillar swelling. No anterior lymphadenopathy. No meningeal signs.
- CV: Tachycardic w/ regular rhythm, no m/r/g
- PULM: CTAB, no wheezing, rhonchi, or rales.
- ABD: Soft, NTND, no organomegaly.
- MSK: FROM of all extremities, warm and well perfused.
- Neuro: A&O × 3, no focal neuro deficits, 5/5 strength in all extremities.

A rapid strep test was sent and returned as negative.

Discussion Questions
- Write or present an SBAR for this case. Alternatively, write an assessment and plan for a SOAP note or present a hand-off of this patient in your preferred format (e.g., I-PASS, IDEAL).
- What is the differential diagnosis for the cause of this patient's sore throat?
- How does this patient's sexual history change the differential?
- What tests should be ordered?

Trauma

LGBTQ individuals are frequently targets of physical, interpersonal, and sexual violence. Compared with their heterosexual peers, LGBTQ people are at greater risk for exposure to violence, are exposed to violence at an earlier age, are more likely to have seen trauma inflicted on a close friend or relative and are more likely to have experienced the unexpected death of someone close to them. The clinician's consideration for the possibility of previous psychological traumas related to sexual or gender minority status can improve a patient's experience during a very vulnerable time.

The approach to the victim of physical trauma is different from that to other patients. All patients will first get a primary survey (Table 10.7), followed by a secondary survey, or complete physical examination. Often there are many people in the room trying to assess the extent of a trauma victim's injuries, resulting in a lack of privacy and making the patient feel exposed and vulnerable. Providers should make efforts to explain what they are doing and how each action is involved in

Table 10.7 Primary trauma survey

A	Airway	Assessment of airway with cervical spine precautions. If airway is not patent or protected, this needs to be addressed before the physician, moves to the next step.
B	Breathing	Visual inspection, palpation, and auscultation of the chest. Is the patient breathing? Are there bilateral breath sounds? Is there chest wall crepitus or some other sign of pneumothorax? If breathing is impaired, this should be addressed before the physician moves to the next step.
C	Circulation	Assessment of pulse and any sites of hemorrhage. Hemorrhagic bleeding must be stopped before the physician moves to the next step.
D	Disability	Neurologic status. Patients with impaired mental status may require intubation.
E	Exposure/ environmental	Full exposure of patient to aid assessment for injuries.

the trauma assessment. For example, a patient may feel that it is inappropriate to exert pressure over the pelvic bones or perform a rectal exam (if needed) and may benefit from a brief explanation of the importance of such assessment. It is best to help the patient understand that the provider is not simply medically curious and that the exam is medically necessary.

During the primary or secondary survey, it may become clear that the patient is transgender or gender nonconforming based on the presence or absence of some anatomy. At that time, it may be necessary to acknowledge the patient's gender identity if it had not already been disclosed. An **anatomic inventory**, or assessment of what organs the patient has or does not have, may need to be performed (e.g., a transwoman may have a "floating prostate" on digital rectal exam indicating that the urethra has been disrupted). Regardless of the timing of disclosure to the health care provider, the provider has a duty to provide medically necessary care according to guidelines and best standards and to communicate the steps of care clearly to the patient.

The priority in all trauma cases in the acute setting is to stabilize hemodynamics, control sources of hemorrhage, and identify injuries that can be immediately treated. People who have experienced trauma often endure a psychological impact that lasts for years. Empathetic, supportive care that minimizes the risk of evoking earlier traumatic experiences is of the utmost importance.

Key Points
- Trauma disproportionately affects LGBTQ patients.
- Complete a primary survey (ABCDE) and then examine the patient from head to toe to ensure that no injuries are missed.
- Trauma assessments must be methodical and thorough to ensure that injuries are not missed, but it is important to communicate clearly to the patient so as not to induce emotional trauma or evoke a past experience of trauma.

Mental Health and Psychiatric Emergencies

Increasing numbers of psychiatric emergencies are treated in EDs across the US. LGBTQ individuals' experiences of violence and discrimination make long-lasting impacts not only on the individuals but also on the broader LGBTQ community. Personal, family, and social attitudes and acceptance of a range of sexual orientations and gender identities are crucial contributing factors to the mental health and personal safety of LGBTQ people. Discrimination, stigmatization, and lack of family acceptance has been associated with increased risk of psychiatric disorders—depression, anxiety, and suicide—as well as increased substance use and dependence.

This section will outline the general physician approach to psychiatric emergencies and psychiatric conditions that disproportionately affect LGBTQ individuals. It is not an exhaustive discussion of psychiatric emergencies.

Patient Assessment

To ensure quality care and prevent alienation, patients with mental health problems should be approached with a nonjudgmental attitude and unconditionally positive regard. Emergency psychiatric assessment is conducted in four steps (Table 10.8):

- Safety and stabilization
- Identification of homicidal, suicidal, or other dangerous behavior
- Psychiatric diagnosis and severity assessment
- Psychiatric consultation

Use of the most minimally confrontational and invasive measures possible is crucial in maintaining the safety of patient, staff, and providers. Patients who are violent toward themselves or staff may require chemical or physical restraint. The clinician should try to deescalate and defuse tense situations if possible—restraints should be a last resort.

Table 10.8 Emergency psychiatric assessment steps

Safety and stabilization	Contain violent and dangerously psychotic persons to help ensure a safe environment for staff, patients, family, and visitors while simultaneously attending to airway, breathing, and circulation.
Identification of homicidal, suicidal, or other dangerous behavior	Determine whether the patient needs to be forcibly detained for emergency evaluation.
Medical evaluation	Determine the presence of any serious organic medical conditions that might cause or contribute to abnormal behavior or thought processes (e.g., hypoglycemia, meningitis, drug withdrawal).
Psychiatric diagnosis and severity assessment	If the behavior change is not the result of an underlying medical condition, it is primarily psychiatric or functional, requiring a psychiatric diagnosis and assessment of the severity of the primary psychiatric problems.
Psychiatric consultation	Determine the need for immediate psychiatric consultation.

Table 10.9 Features associated with organic causes of psychosis

Abnormal vital sign values
Disorientation with clouded consciousness
Abnormal mental status examination findings
Recent memory loss
Age > 40 years without a previous history of psychiatric disorder
Focal neurologic signs
Visual hallucinations
Psychomotor retardation

Table 10.10 Medical conditions that may present as psychiatric emergencies

Medication side effects	Encephalitis
Diabetic ketoacidosis	Meningitis
Hypoglycemia	Hypertensive
Hyperglycemia	encephalopathy
Alcohol intoxication or	Hypocalcemia or
withdrawal	hypercalcemia
Cocaine intoxication	Amphetamine intoxication
Drug withdrawal	Steroid-induced psychosis
Environmental toxins	LSD psychosis
Urinary tract infection	Acute intermittent
Chronic obstructive	porphyria
pulmonary disease	Pheochromocytoma
Myocardial infarction	Multiple sclerosis
Acute liver disease	Cushing's disease
Chronic renal disease	Hypoparathrodism
Hypothyroidism	Syphilis
Hyperthyroidism	AIDS
Metastatic carcinoma or	Systemic lupus
intracranial tumor	erythematosus (SLE)
Subarachnoid or	Wilson's disease
intracranial hemorrhage	Hydrocephalus

Some medical conditions have psychiatric symptoms, including psychosis (Tables 10.9 and 10.10). Medical evaluation should be the same as that for any patient evaluated in the ED, involving a thorough history, including behavioral changes, past medical history and medications, and substance use. When possible, the clinician corroborates historical elements with friends or family members. Physical examination should include a mental status exam and a neurologic exam if any neurologic symptoms are associated with the reported behavioral change.

Depression and Suicide

The prevalence of depression, suicidal ideations, and suicidal behaviors are markedly increased in LGBTQ populations. LGB people have a 1.5 times greater prevalence of depression than do their heterosexual peers. This increased prevalence is associated with experiences of prejudice, lack of family support, and exposure to violence. Some individuals, particularly adolescents who have not come out as LGBTQ, may face debilitating depression as they come to terms with their sexual orientation and gender identity. It is important to provide patients with reassurance, validation, and referral to supportive resources that they can access outside the hospital setting.

The *DSM-5* diagnostic criteria for major depressive disorder are provided in Table 12.1.

When patients are suicidal or homicidal and pose an imminent risk to themselves or others, psychiatric evaluation and hospitalization are needed. Other cases, however, are not so clear.

The "SAD PERSONS" score (Table 10.11) correlates well with the need for hospitalization. Nearly all patients with scores higher than eight require psychiatric hospitalization. Individuals at intermediate risk should be seen by a psychiatrist

Table 10.11 The "SAD PERSONS" system for assessing suicide risk

Risk factor	Score
Male	1
Age (<19 or >45)	1
Depression (or signs or symptoms thereof)	2
Previous suicide attempts or psychiatric care	1
Excessive alcohol or drug use	1
Rational thinking (loss of)	2
Separated/divorced/widowed/single	1
Organized or serious attempt	2
No social support	1
Stated future intent, plan, or mechanism	2

Scoring: >8, high risk; 6–8, intermediate risk; <6, low risk

or other qualified mental health clinician in the ED. If a patient is categorized as low risk under this system but the provider is still concerned about the patient's well-being or future suicide attempts, a mental health provider should be consulted. Nevertheless, safety evaluations cannot be substituted by risk scores. Good safety evaluations also consider contextual features, the modifiability of risk factors, and the presence of protective factors.

A patient with depression must not be discharged to self-care if suicidal with intent, psychotic, demented, or intoxicated. A psychiatry consult should be ordered and appropriate follow-up arranged. Patients should not be started on antidepressants in the ED.

Suicide is the second most common cause of death among individuals younger than 24 years. Overall, it is the ninth leading cause of death in the United States, claiming the lives of 30,000 persons each year. For every death by suicide, there are 20 suicide attempts not resulting in death. As already noted, suicide has a remarkably disproportionate impact on the LGBTQ community. LGB individuals are two or three times more likely to attempt suicide than their heterosexual counterparts, and more than 40% of transgender individuals have attempted suicide at some point in their lives.

Risk factors for suicide include situational crisis, substance use, and psychiatric illness such as major depression, schizophrenia, or panic disorder. Women are three or four times

more likely to attempt suicide than men, but men are three or four times more likely to die by suicide. Access to a firearm increases suicide risk five- to ten-fold. It is important to ask not only whether the patient is having thoughts suicide or non-suicidal self-injury but whether the patient has a plan, the means, and the intent to carry it out.

For virtually any psychiatric complaint, a sensitive and thorough history is warranted. The patient should be asked about current relationship status and whether they have been or are being physically, emotionally, or sexually harmed by anyone. If this is the case, the patient may need hospitalization until safe housing can be arranged, even if a psychiatric admission is not needed.

Anyone who presents after a suicide attempt or with suicidal ideation should undergo a toxicological evaluation as part of the medical evaluation. This includes an electrocardiogram, assessment of aspirin and acetaminophen levels to reveal unreported ingestion, a complete blood count, blood chemistries, an ethanol level, and a urine drug screen. The provider tailors their evaluation if a specific ingestion is confirmed. All ingestion cases should be reported to the Poison Control Center, which can be reached at 800-222-1222.

Key Points
- Discrimination, stigma, and rejection by family of origin are associated with an increased rate of psychiatric disorders among LGBTQ individuals.
- Patient and staff comfort and safety are the primary priorities in ED psychiatric assessments.
- Consider and evaluate the patient for organic causes of depression and psychosis.
- LGBTQ individuals are more likely to die by suicide than are their heterosexual peers. All psychiatric assessments should include screening for suicidality.

Case 10.3

HPI: 25 yo female presents to the ED for depressive symptoms and suicidal ideation. The patient says she feels like she "just cannot go on" and feels "hopeless" and "worthless." She reveals that she is bisexual and just ended a relationship with a woman with whom she continues to live. The patient reports that during the relationship she endured physical and emotional abuse by her partner. She wants to leave their house but is afraid that her partner will come after her. She is estranged from her family and feels that she has nowhere to go. Although she reports feeling depressed and hopeless for the last two months and wishing that she would "go to sleep and not wake up," she denies any specific plan to hurt or kill herself. She is having trouble sleeping and has stopped eating. She is entirely cut off from friends. Goes to work but has trouble concentrating. She feels like everything is in slow motion.

Physical Exam
- Vital signs: HR 80. BP 116/80, RR 17, O_2 sat 100% on RA, T 98.2 °F
- GEN: Awake, alert, and oriented × 3. Appears sad, tearful.
- HEENT: Normocephalic, atraumatic. EOMI, PERRL, moist mucosal membranes, no oropharyngeal erythema, swelling, or exudate.
- CV: RRR, no m/r/g
- PULM: Tachypneic with moderate accessory respiratory muscle use, CTAB, no wheezing
- ABD: Soft, NTND
- MSK: FROM of all extremities. 2+ DP pulses bilaterally.
- Neuro: A&O × 3, no focal neuro deficits, 5/5 strength in all extremities.
- Psych: A&O × 3. Pt appears depressed. Flat affect. Poor concentration. Limited insight. No audio or visual hallucinations, +SI, no HI. No delusions.

- Derm: No rash, no e/o cutting on arms or legs, no linear excoriations or scars on forearms.

A rapid strep test was sent and returned as negative.

Discussion Questions
- Write or present an SBAR for this case. Alternatively, write an assessment and plan for a SOAP note or present a handoff of this patient in your preferred format (e.g., I-PASS, IDEAL).
- How does the history of interpersonal violence (IPV) affect the management of this patient's depression? How does depression affect the management of her IPV?
- Does this person need inpatient psychiatric hospitalization?
- What, if any, safety concerns are there for this patient? What steps can be taken in the ED to ensure her safety?
- What if the patient wants to go home? What are the next steps?

Other Considerations in the Emergency Department

Toxicology and Drug Use, Abuse, and Withdrawal

Higher rates of substance use in the LGBTQ community are strongly tied to an increased prevalence of trauma, discrimination, social stigma, and mental health issues. LGBTQ populations not only have higher rates of tobacco and alcohol use but also use drugs at twice the rate that heterosexuals do. Some estimates indicate that a quarter of LGBT adults abuse alcohol, compared with 5–10% of the general population. Compared with heterosexual women, WSW have a higher prevalence of smoking and excessive drinking. Gay men are 12 times more likely than straight men to use amphetamines and 10 times more likely to use heroin. Poppers (i.e., amyl nitrates) are also commonly used in combination with other substances.

Clinicians should ask about unhealthy substance use and refer patients to appropriate sources of support or addiction resources. Screening, brief intervention, and referral to treatment (SBIRT) has been shown to be an efficacious way to decrease unhealthy substance use and is recommended for use in EDs. SBIRT includes reinforcing healthy behaviors, pointing out potential problems with current substance use to patients who are engaging in low- to medium-risk behaviors, and referring patients with significant dependence or functional impairment to treatment resources.

> **External Resource 10.1**
> **Boston University's Brief Negotiated Interview-Active Referral to Treatment (BNI ART) Institute** created videos on how to use SBIRT in the ED. http://bit.ly/TECe1ch10_01

Intoxication and withdrawal are often treated in the ED. Many recreational substances present as well-described toxidromes. Others, mixed ingestions or new designer drugs, are more difficult to identify. Alcohol withdrawal is a medical emergency and potentially fatal. Signs of alcohol withdrawal include tremulousness, nausea and vomiting, hallucinations, and seizures. Withdrawal from opioids, methamphetamine, and cocaine may be uncomfortable for patients but is not life threatening. Such syndromes are managed symptomatically.

> **Case 10.4**
> HPI: 22yo M brought in by friends after passing out in a club. Pt had been dancing all night, according to his friends he had been drinking a lot of water and they think he took something while they were there, but they aren't sure what. The patient is unable to provide a good history. Lethargic but arousable. History and exam are limited by altered mental status.

Physical Exam
- Vital signs: HR 120 BP 150/90 RR 28 O$_2$ Sat: 96% on RA T 99.9 °F
- GEN: Lethargic, but arousable, laying on stretcher, patient appears diaphoretic.
- HEENT: normocephalic, atraumatic. EOMI, Pupils are dilated in both eyes, equally reactive to light. Moist mucosal membranes, no oropharyngeal erythema, swelling, or exudate.
- CV: tachycardic w/ regular rhythm, no m/r/g
- PULM: tachypneic, CTAB, no wheezing
- ABD: soft, NTND, increased bowel sounds.
- MSK: FROM of all extremities. RLE swelling with mild erythema, calf tender to palpation. 2+ DP pulses bilaterally.
- Neuro: lethargic, oriented only to person, no focal neuro deficits, moves all extremities equally.

Discussion Questions
- Write or present an SBAR for this case. Alternatively, write an assessment and plan for a SOAP note or attempt a handoff of this patient in the most familiar format to you (e.g., I-PASS, IDEAL).
- What type of toxidrome does this patient have? What do you think he took?
- What are you most worried about in this patient?

Emergency Care for Transgender People

Transgender people are one of the most marginalized populations. Despite having unique medical and mental health needs, they experience extreme barriers to care. Transgender people are disproportionately affected by HIV, victimization, mental health issues, and suicide and are less likely to have health insurance than straight or LGB people.

Many transgender patients have had prior difficult experiences in health care settings.

Consequently, fear of stigma and discrimination may prevent them from sharing important information about hormone use, recent surgeries, illicit substances, or suicidality. It is best to avoid assumptions and directly ask each patient their preferred name or title, gender, and pronouns. This information should be documented (if the patient does not object) and shared with the entire clinical team so it is used consistently and coherently during treatment. Using the patient's preferred name and correct pronouns conveys respect and helps build trust between the treatment team and patient. This rapport will enhance the patient's comfort and trust and encourage the patient to more readily share sensitive health information.

When clinically appropriate, transgender persons should be screened for depression, suicidality, substance use, and interpersonal violence. It is more fruitful to ask about specific sexual behaviors than the gender(s) of sexual partners in order to ascertain the risks of pregnancy and sexually transmitted infections.

Most transgender patients will present to the ED for concerns not related to being transgender—c.g., a fall, a motor vehicle accident, or a respiratory infection. However, there are times when the differential diagnosis will depend on what hormones the patient uses, if any. The exact effects of hormone replacement therapy on cardiovascular risk profile are unknown. Oral estrogen may increase the risk for deep vein thrombosis and pulmonary embolism. Some individuals may not be up to date on their cancer screenings because they lack access to or avoidance of preventive care. If a patient does not have a primary care provider, referrals should be made to known LGBTQ-friendly or specialized providers in the area.

Past surgical procedures may also alter the differential diagnosis. For example, a transgender man with lower abdominal pain who has not had his uterus and ovaries removed may have pelvic inflammatory disease or ovarian torsion. A transgender woman with lower abdominal pain who has not had orchiectomy may have testicular torsion. Physical examination is uncomfortable and psychologically difficult for transgender patients, who may experience significant body dysphoria. Clear, respectful communication is paramount when asking what organs are absent or present (the anatomic inventory). It is important to explain why a genital or breast/chest exam is necessary and to obtain explicit consent before proceeding. A sensitive and gentle genital examination is essential to patient-centered care in every patient. In a patient with severe dysphoria or history of abuse, a relaxant or conscious sedation may provide some relief if distress is severe.

Some transgender people take supplements or medications not prescribed by a provider or undergo procedures or surgeries performed by unlicensed practitioners. Postoperative bleeding or infection is a risk with all procedures, especially those performed in unsanitary settings. Some individuals may inject silicone or castor oil for breast or gluteal enhancement. This practice, called *pumping*, can cause disfigurement, sepsis, disseminated intravascular coagulation, and respiratory compromise.

Homelessness and LGBTQ People

Forty percent of homeless adolescents are LGBTQ, indicating that LGBTQ adolescents are far more likely to be homeless than their heterosexual peers. Many LGBTQ adolescents are homeless in order to escape hostile home situations, where they have experienced rejection for their sexual orientation or gender identity or are escaping physical, emotional, or sexual abuse. They may engage in survival sex work after leaving home. They generally have increased risk of STIs, HIV, trauma, abuse, and substance use. All homeless youth should be referred to local support resources. ED-based or hospital social workers are usually the best equipped to assist the patient with additional resources.

Like homeless heterosexual individuals, homeless LGBTQ people are at increased risk for heart disease, cancer, liver disease, kidney disease, skin infections, HIV/AIDS, pneumonia, tuberculosis, tuberculosis, trauma/assault (sexual and physical), and addiction (drug, alcohol, tobacco). They are also at risk for nutritional deficiencies and medical problems related to prolonged environmental exposure, such as chronic wounds, frostbite, hyperthermia, hypothermia, and trench foot.

Key Points

- Rates of substance use, especially tobacco and alcohol, are higher among LGBTQ individuals than among heterosexual ones.
- MSM have a higher rate of use of amphetamines, heroin, and poppers.
- SBIRT is a useful strategy for assessing a patient for substance use in the ED and providing motivational interviewing and referral to treatment.
- Transgender individuals face greater barriers to care than do their cisgender counterparts and are disproportionately affected by HIV, victimization, mental health issues, and suicide and lack of insurance.
- Ask the patient for their correct name and pronouns and use them consistently.
- The differential diagnosis for transgender patients may be impacted by medical and surgical history related to transition. When such information is relevant to a person's care, ask respectful and direct questions about prior surgeries and medications used.
- Homelessness disproportionately affects LGBTQ populations, especially LGBTQ adolescents escaping hostile home environments. The health risks of homelessness are extensive and severe. Social work should be engaged to help the homeless patient gain access to appropriate resources.

Conclusion

Clinicians in the emergency department see a wide variety of patient issues. LGBTQ individuals are at particular risk for trauma, sexually transmitted infection, depression, suicide attempts, suicidal ideation, and substance use disorders. LGBTQ adolescents are also at high risk for homelessness.

Significant research on the LGBTQ experience in the ED remains to be done. Future directions for research and advocacy include disparities in LGBTQ emergency care based on sexual orientation and gender identity and LGBTQ-focused competency training for ED staff.

Sources

Addis S, Davies M, Greene G, Macbride-Stewart S, Shepard M. The health, social care and housing needs of lesbian, gay, bisexual and transgender older people: a review of the literature. Health Soc Care Community. 2009;17(6):647–58.

American College of Surgeons Committee on Trauma. Initial assessment and management. In: Advanced trauma life support for doctors. Chicago: American College of Surgeons; 2008.

Buchmueller T, Carpenter CS. Disparities in health insurance coverage, access, and outcomes for individuals in same-sex versus different-sex relationships, 2000–2007. Am J Public Health. 2010;100(3):489–95.

Centers for Disease Control and Prevention. HIV/AIDS among women who have sex with women. Atlanta: Centers for Disease Control and Prevention; 2006.

Centers for Disease Control and Prevention. National Hospital Ambulatory Medical Care Survey: 2010 emergency department summary tables. Atlanta: Centers for Disease Control and Prevention; 2010. http://www.cdc.gov/nchs/data/ahcd/nhamcs_emergency/2010_ed_web_tables.pdf. Accessed 28 Aug 2014.

Centers for Disease Control and Prevention. CDC Fact Sheet: HIV and AIDS among gay and bisexual men. Atlanta: Centers for Disease Control and Prevention; 2010.

Centers for Disease Control and Prevention. CDC Fact Sheet: syphilis & MSM. Atlanta: Centers for Disease Control and Prevention; 2010.

Centers for Disease Control and Prevention. Monitoring selected national HIV prevention and care objectives by using HIV surveillance data—United States and 6 U.S. dependent areas—2010. HIV Surveill Suppl Rep. 2012;17(No. 3, part A).

Centers for Disease Control and Prevention. CDC Fact Sheet: HPV and men. Atlanta: Centers for Disease Control and Prevention; 2012.

Centers for Disease Control and Prevention. CDC Fact Sheet: viral hepatitis and men who have sex with men. Atlanta: Centers for Disease Control and Prevention; 2012.

Centers for Disease Control and Prevention. Incidence, prevalence, and cost of sexually transmitted infections in the United States. Washington, DC: Centers for Disease Control and Prevention; 2013.

Centers for Disease Control and Prevention. CDC Fact Sheet: HIV among black/African American gay, bisexual, and other men who have sex with men. Atlanta: Centers for Disease Control and Prevention; 2013.

Centers for Disease Control and Prevention. CDC Fact Sheet: HIV and gay, bisexual, and other men who have sex with men. Atlanta: Centers for Disease Control and Prevention; 2018.

Centers for Disease Control and Prevention. CDC Fact Sheet: HIV and transgender people. Atlanta: Centers for Disease Control and Prevention; 2018.

Cochran SD, Sullivan JG, Mays VM. Prevalence of mental disorders, psychological distress, and mental health services use among lesbian, gay, and bisexual adults in the United States. J Consult Clin Psychol. 2003;71(1):53–61.

Cohen MS. Reduction of concentration of HIV-A in semen after treatment of urethritis: implications for prevention of sexual transmission of HIV-1. Lancet. 1997;349:1868–73.

Conron KJ, Mimiaga MJ, Landers SJ. A population-based study of sexual orientation identity and gender differences in adult health. Am J Public Health. 2010;100(10):1953–60.

Crandall ML, Nathens AB, Kernic MA, Holt VL, Rivara FP. Predicting future injury among women in abusive relationships. J Trauma. 2004;56:906–12.

Cunningham RM, Bernstein SL, Walton M, Broderick K, Vaca FE, Woolard R, et al. Alcohol, tobacco, and other drugs: future directions for screening and intervention in the emergency department. Acad Emerg Med. 2009;16(11):1078–88.

Custers EJ, Stuyt PM, DeVries RPF. Clinical problem analysis: a systematic approach to teaching complex medical problem solving. Acad Med. 2000;75(3):291–7.

Denney JT, Gorman BK, Barrera CB. Families, resources, and adult health: where do sexual minorities fit? J Health Soc Behav. 2013;54(1):46–63.

Deutsch MB. Guidelines for the primary and gender-affirming care of transgender and gender nonbinary people. 2nd ed. San Francisco: University of California, San Francisco; 2016. http://transhealth.ucsf.edu/protocols. Accessed 25 Jan 2019.

Diaz RM, Ayala G, Bein E, Henne J, Marin BV. The impact of homophobia, poverty, and racism on the mental health of gay and bisexual Latino men: findings from three US cities. Am J Public Health. 2001;91(6):141–6.

Dilley JA, Simmons KW, Boysun MJ, Pizacani BA, Stark MJ. Demonstrating the importance and feasibility of including sexual orientation in public health surveys: health disparities in the Pacific Northwest. Am J Public Health. 2010;100(3):460–7.

Durso LE, Gates GJ. Serving our youth: findings from a national survey of service providers working with lesbian, gay, bisexual, and transgender youth who are homeless or at risk of becoming homeless. Los Angeles: The Williams Institute with True Colors Fund and The Palette Fund; 2012.

East JA, El Rayess F. Pediatricians' approach to the health care of lesbian, gay, and bisexual youth. J Adolesc Health. 1998;23(4):191–3.

Garofalo R, Wolf RC, Wissow LS, Woods ER, Goodman E. Sexual orientation and risk of suicide attempts among a representative sample of youth. Arch Pediatr Adolesc Med. 1999;153(5):487–93.

Gates GJ. In U.S. LGBT more likely than non-LGBT to be uninsured. Gallup-healthways well-being index. http://www.gallup.com/poll/175445/lgbt-likely-non-lgbt-uninsured.aspx. Accessed 29 Aug 2014.

Grant JM, Mottet LA, Tanis T, Harrison J, Herman JL, Keisling M. Injustice at every turn: a report of the National Transgender Discrimination Survey, executive summary. Washington, DC: National Center for Transgender Equality and National Gay and Lesbian Task Force; 2011.

Gryczynski J, Mitchell SG, Peterson TR, Gonzales A, Moseley A, Schwartz RP. The relationship between services delivered and substance use outcomes in New Mexico's Screening, Brief Intervention, Referral and Treatment (SBIRT) Initiative. Drug Alcohol Depend. 2011;118(2–3):152–7.

Hack JB, Hoffman RS. General management of poisoned patients. In: Tintinalli JE, Stapczynski JS, Ma OJ, Yealy DM, Meckler GD, Cline D, editors. Tintinalli's emergency medicine: a comprehensive study guide. 7th ed. New York: McGraw-Hill; 2011. p. 1187–93.

Herbst JH, Jacobs ED, Finlayson TJ, McKleroy VS, Neumann MS, Crepaz N, HIV/AIDS Prevention Research Synthesis Team. Estimating HIV prevalence and risk behaviors of transgender persons in the United States: a systematic review. AIDS Behav. 2008;12(12):1–17.

Herek GM, Garnets LD. Sexual orientation and mental health. Annu Rev Clin Psychol. 2007;3:353–75.

Ho GYF, Bierman R, Beardsley L, Chang CJ, Burk RD. Natural history of cervicovaginal papillomavirus infection in young women. N Engl J Med. 1998;338(7):423–8.

Hughes TL. Chapter 9: Alcohol use and alcohol-related problems among lesbians and gay men. Annu Rev Nurs Res. 2005;23:283–325.

Ibanez GE, Purcell DW, Stall R, Parsons JT, Gómez CA. Sexual risk, substance use, and psychological distress in HIV-positive gay and bisexual men who also inject drugs. AIDS. 2005;19(suppl 1):49–55.

Kenagy GP. Transgender health: findings from two needs assessment studies in Philadelphia. Health Soc Work. 2005;30(1):19–26.

King M, Semlyen J, Tai SS, Killaspy H, Osborn D, Popelyuk D, Nazareth I. A systemic review of mental disorder, suicide, and deliberate self harm in lesbian, gay, and bisexual people. BMC Psychiatry. 2008;8:70.

Kruks G. Gay and lesbian homeless/street youth: special issues and concerns. J Adolesc Health. 2010;12(7):515–8.

Larkin GL, Beautrais AL. Behavior disorders: emergency assessment. In: Tintinalli JE, Stapczynski JS, Ma OJ,

Yealy DM, Meckler GD, Cline D, editors. Tintinalli's emergency medicine: a comprehensive study guide. 7th ed. New York: McGraw-Hill; 2011.

Larkin GL, Marco CA. Ethical issues in the use of patient restraints. ACEP News. January 2007. p. 20.

Larkin GL, Claassen CA, Emond JA, Pelletier AJ, Camargo CA. Trends in U.S. emergency department visits for mental health conditions, 1992 to 2001. Psychiatr Serv. 2005;56(6):671–7.

Lee GL, Griffin GK, Melvin CL. Tobacco use among sexual minorities in the USA: 1987 to May 2007: a systematic review. Tob Control. 2009;18:275–82.

Lurie S. Identifying training needs of health-care providers related to treatment and care of transgendered patients: a qualitative needs assessment conducted in New England. Int J Transgend. 2005;8(2–3):93–112.

Lyons T, Chandra G, Goldstein J. Stimulant use and HIV risk behavior: the influence of peer support. AIDS Educ Prev. 2006;18(5):461–73.

MacKellar DA, Valleroy LA, Secura GM, et al. Two decades after vaccine license: hepatitis B immunization and infection among young men who have sex with men. Am J Public Health. 2001;91(6):965–71.

Mansergh G, Colfax GN, Marks G, Rader M, Guzman R, Buchbinder S. The circuit party men's health survey: findings and implications for gay and bisexual men. Am J Public Health. 2001;91(6):953–8.

McLaughlin KA, Hatzenbuehler ML, Keyes KM. Responses to discrimination and psychiatric disorders among black, Hispanic, female, and lesbian, gay, and bisexual individuals. Am J Public Health. 2010;100(8):1477–84.

Meckler GD, Elliott MN, Kanouse DE, Beals KP, Schuster MA. Nondisclosure of sexual orientation to a physician among a sample of gay, lesbian, and bisexual youth. Arch Pediatr Adolesc Med. 2006;160(12):1248–54.

National Gay and Lesbian Taskforce. National Transgender Discrimination Survey: preliminary findings. Washington, DC: National Gay and Lesbian Taskforce; 2009. http://www.thetaskforce.org/downloads/reports/fact_sheets/transsurvey_prelim_findings.pdf.

Nobay F, Promes SB. Sexually transmitted diseases. In: Tintinalli JE, Stapczynski JS, Ma OJ, Yealy DM, Meckler GD, Cline D, editors. Tintinalli's emergency medicine: a comprehensive study guide. 7th ed. New York: McGraw-Hill; 2011.

O'Connell JJ. Premature mortality in homeless populations: a review of the literature. Nashville: National Health Care for the Homeless Council; 2005.

Ostrow DG, Stall R. Alcohol, tobacco, and drug use among gay and bisexual men. In: Wolitski RJ, Stall R, Valdiserri RO, editors. Unequal opportunity: health disparities affecting gay and bisexual men in the United States. New York: Oxford University Press; 2008.

Palefsky J, Holly E, Ralston M. High incidence of anal high grade squamous intra-epithelial lesions among HIV-positive and HIV-negative homosexual and bisexual men. AIDS. 1998;12:495–503.

Pitts SR, Pines JM, Handrigan MT, Kellermann AL. National trends in emergency department occupancy, 2001 to 2008: effect of inpatient admissions versus emergency department practice intensity. Ann Emerg Med. 2012;60(6):679–686.e3.

Remafedi G, French S, Story M, Resnick MD, Blum R. The relationship between suicide risk and sexual orientation: results of a population-based study. Am J Public Health. 1998;88(1):57–60.

Roberts AL, Austin SB, Corliss HL, Vandermorris AK, Koenen KC. Pervasive trauma exposure among US sexual orientation minority adults and risk of posttraumatic stress disorder. Am J Public Health. 2010;100(12):2433–41.

Sanchez JP, Hailpern S, Lowe C, Calderon Y. Factors associated with emergency department utilization by urban lesbian, gay, and bisexual individuals. J Community Health. 2007;32(2):149–56.

Sena AC, Miller WC, Hobbs MM, Schwebke JR, Leone PA, Swygard H, Atashili J, Cohen MS. *Trichomonas vaginalis* infection in male sexual partners: implications for diagnosis, treatment and prevention. Clin Infect Dis. 2007;44:13–22.

Smith DM, Mathews WC. Physicians' attitudes toward homosexuality and HIV: survey of a California medical society—revisited (PATHH-II). J Homosex. 2007;52(3–4):1–9.

Su JR, Beltrami JF, Zaidi AA, Weinstock HS. Primary and secondary syphilis among black and Hispanic men who have sex with men: case report data from 27 states. Ann Intern Med. 2011;155(3):145–51.

US Department of Health and Human Services. Healthy people 2010. Washington, DC: US Department of Health and Human Services; 2000. http://www.hhs.gov.

US Preventive Services Task Force. Screening for cervical cancer. Rockville: US Preventive Services Task Force; 2018. https://www.uspreventiveservicestaskforce.org/Page/Document/UpdateSummaryFinal/cervical-cancer-screening2. Accessed 25 Jan 2019.

Van Leeuwen JM, Boyle S, Salomonsen-Sautel S, Baker DN, Garcia JT, Hoffman A, Hopfer CJ. Lesbian, gay, and bisexual homeless youth: an eight-city public health perspective. Child Welfare. 2006;85(2):151–70.

Whitbeck LB, Chen X, Hoyt DR, Tyler KA, Johnson KD. Mental disorder, subsistence strategies, and victimization among gay, lesbian, and bisexual homeless and runaway adolescents. J Sex Res. 2004;41(4):329–42.

World Health Organization Global Health Observatory. HIV/AIDS. http://www.who.int/gho/hiv/en/. Accessed 1 July 2014.

Xavier J, Honnold J, Bradford J. The health, health-related needs, and lifecourse experiences of transgender Virginians: Virginia HIV Community Planning Committee and Virginia Department of Health. Richmond: Virginia Department of Health; 2007.

Zink BJ. Social justice, egalitarianism, and the history of emergency medicine. Virtual Mentor. 2010;12(6):492–4.

HIV/AIDS

11

Brian A. Nuyen, Jennifer L. Glick, Vanessa Ferrel, and W. Christopher Mathews

Overview of Epidemiology, Transmission, Pathophysiology, and Clinical Manifestations of HIV/AIDS

Current Epidemiologic Patterns

When examining HIV epidemiology, it is important to note people and populations are multidimensional, and health disparities tend to follow patterns of marginalization. For example, while HIV incidence and prevalence are high in both gay male and African American populations, they are higher still in communities of gay African American males. Furthermore, it is important to note that data on LGBTQ people are historically limited due to an array of research challenges,

including (1) the shifting understanding of identity and associated challenges in defining and measuring sexual orientation and gender, (2) overcoming reluctance of some LGBTQ people to identify themselves, and (3) obtaining quality samples of a relatively small population. Deep-seated homophobia and transphobia are also at play in the policies and best-practices set by the research community.

Epidemiologic data change rapidly, and the following statistics reflect the most current data at the time of publication. Incidence of HIV infection in the United States has remained relatively stable over the past decade at approximately 50,000 incident cases per year. CDC estimates that approximately 1.1 million people are living with HIV in the US, approximately 16% of whom are unaware of their diagnosis of HIV infection. MSM remain the group with the highest incidence and prevalence of infection. Representing roughly 4% of the US population, in 2017 MSM accounted for 66% and 82% of incident HIV infections among men and overall, respectively. The age range of highest incidence of infection is 25–34 years, but more vulnerable

The first listed author is the chapter's associate editor from The Equal Curriculum Project. The chapter authors are otherwise ordered according to their preference.

B. A. Nuyen (✉)
Stanford University School of Medicine, Stanford, CA, USA

J. L. Glick
Johns Hopkins Bloomberg School of Public Health, Baltimore, MD, USA

V. Ferrel
Montefiore Medical Center, The Bronx, NY, USA

W. C. Mathews
Department of Medicine, University of California San Diego, La Jolla, CA, USA
e-mail: cmathews@ucsd.edu

External Resource 11.1
"Speak Out: Experts Talk Gay Men & HIV/AIDS" – a video by Greater Than AIDS featuring experts from CDC and amfAR who speak about how HIV/AIDS has affected the gay community from epidemiologic, public

health, and cultural viewpoints. The video opened a White House meeting entitled, "Gay and Bisexual Men with HIV/AIDS. Focus. Action. Impact." Total time 7:13. http://bit.ly/TECe1ch11_01

populations tend to have lower ages of infection. Black MSM accounted for 25% of all incident cases in 2017.

Transgender people are at particularly high risk of HIV infection. HIV prevalence in transgender people in the US is around 50 times higher than for other reproductive age adults. From 2009 to 2014, 2351 transgender people were diagnosed with HIV in the United States. Eighty-four percent were transgender women, 15% were transgender men, and less than 1% had another gender identity. Incidence among transgender women is often the highest reported among any population group, in many cases twice that of gay and bisexual men. Further, it is well known that HIV disproportionately impacts people of color in the US, and this trend is also observed in the transgender community. Among transgender women, the highest percentage of incident HIV infection was among blacks (51%) and Latinos (29%). Similar trends in STIs are observed in the transgender population. The high proportion of transgender women who are undiagnosed or unaware that they are infected is more than twice the national average (57% vs. 27%). The prevalence of undiagnosed HIV among transgender men has been estimated at 2–3%, though few studies accounted for or focused on the growing number of transgender men who have sex with gay and bisexual men.

External Resource 11.2
"Against the odds: transgender, black and HIV-positive" – a video by Josh Lederman of Medill News Service/Northwestern News Network featuring Helena Bushong who identifies as MtF transgender and African American. She was diagnosed with HIV in 2002. Total time 4:57. http://bit.ly/TECe1ch11_02

HIV Transmission

HIV is transmitted via intimate sexual contact, injection drug use, vertical transmission from mother to child (in utero, during parturition, or through breast feeding), and contaminated blood products. Epidemiologic studies have identified quantitative HIV viral load in a source patient as a major determinant of transmission risk. For every $\log_{10}$ increase in HIV-1 plasma viral load, there is a 2.4 fold increased risk of HIV transmission. Acute HIV infection is associated with extremely high HIV viremia and is therefore a period of high transmission risk that is compounded by the difficulties of diagnosing acute HIV infection. Reduction of HIV viral load by 0.7 $\log_{10}$ has been associated with a 50% reduction in HIV transmission probability. Transmission risks associated with specific risk behaviors have been recently and comprehensively reviewed, highlighting receptive anal sex without a condom as the sexual behavior associated with highest risk. Co-factors enhancing risk of HIV transmission include sexually transmitted infections (both ulcerative and non-ulcerative) and pregnancy.

Pathophysiology of HIV-1 Infection

External Resource 11.3
"HIV Pathophysiology" by J Levy, University of California San Francisco – a video by World Med School featuring Dr. Jay Levy who reviews the pathophysiology of HIV. Total time 18:27. http://bit.ly/TECe1ch11_03

The primary cellular target of HIV is the CD4 + lymphocyte through interaction with the CD4 receptor and chemokine co-receptors CCR5 and CXCR4. Other cells possessing these receptors can also be infected including monocytes, macrophages, and dendritic cells. It has been established that infection can also occur through CD4-independent mechanisms in the brain (astrocytes) and kidney (renal epithelial cells) and result in organ-specific pathology. Mucosal infection usually occurs through transmission of a single **founder virus** followed by rapidly increasing replication, dissemination, and release of inflammatory cytokines. There is striking depletion of lymphoid tissue in the gastrointestinal tract within days of acute infection, and this depletion is not reversed by subsequent antiretroviral therapy. Several months after the burst of viremia associated with acute infection and in the absence of antiretroviral therapy, a viral setpoint is established that is predictive of the rate of development of opportunistic complications. Both adaptive and innate immune responses are elicited but only in a small minority (<1%) of so-called **elite controllers** (persons infected with HIV who maintain undetectable viral loads in the absence of treatment) is progressive immunodeficiency prevented. During acute HIV infection, CD4 count may drop dramatically with resulting opportunistic infections (OI). After establishment of the viral setpoint and in the absence of treatment, CD4 cells drop, on average, between 50% and 100 cells/µL per year. Immune activation is a

hallmark of active HIV replication and markers of residual immune activation are evident even in patients with suppressed plasma viral load. There is currently great interest in understanding this residual inflammatory immune activation and its demonstrated deleterious associations with mortality, cardiovascular, neurological, oncologic, and hepatic complications.

Clinical Manifestations of HIV Infection

Because of remarkable improvements in antiretroviral therapy and prophylaxis of opportunistic infections, the incidence of major and minor opportunistic infections in developed and some developing country settings has markedly decreased. Comprehensive guidance regarding the natural history of HIV infection and the prevention, diagnosis, and management of HIV-related opportunistic complications is readily available. Figure 11.1 illustrates the typical untreated course of HIV infection.

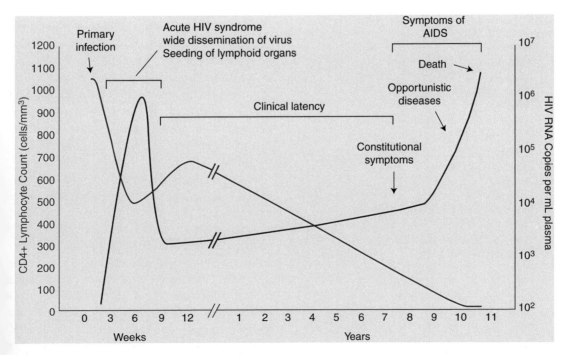

Fig. 11.1 CD4+ Lymphocytes and Viral Load Over Time in Untreated HIV. (Figure made available under the Creative Commons CC0 1.0 Universal Public Domain Dedication. [https://creativecommons.org/publicdomain/zero/1.0/deed.en])

Between 40% and 90% of acutely HIV-infected persons will develop an illness called acute HIV infection that may present similarly to mononucleosis, aseptic meningitis, or an exanthematous viral illness. Rarely, during acute HIV infection the CD4 count may drop sufficiently that an OI develops. However, in the majority, with or without antiretroviral treatment, the acute syndrome resolves and a virological setpoint is achieved by approximately six months after initial infection. Thereafter, depending on the viral setpoint, during the period of so-called **clinical latency**, the CD4 count drops, on average, 78 cells/µL per year. The months to years prior to onset of major opportunistic infections may frequently be accompanied by a variety of clinical manifestations grouped under CDC category B conditions (also known as **AIDS related complex**). These non-AIDS defining conditions include persistent generalized lymphadenopathy (PGL), immune thrombocytopenic purpura (ITP), oral hairy leukoplakia, peripheral neuropathy, herpes zoster, and oral and vaginal candidiasis. Bacterial infections with encapsulated organisms (such as pneumococcus and *Hemophilus influenzae*) and pulmonary tuberculosis also occur with increased frequency at CD4 counts higher than those associated with major opportunistic infections.

Most AIDS defining opportunistic conditions occur, in adults, when the CD4 count has dropped below 200 cells/µL. It is useful to subclassify OIs as early or late based on CD4 count. Late OIs, occurring when the CD4 is less than 50 cells/µL, include primary central nervous system lymphoma, disseminated mycobacterium avium, and CMV end organ disease (e.g., CMV retinitis, encephalitis, colitis). See Table 11.1.

In the setting of concomitant antiretroviral therapy, the clinical presentation of opportunistic infections and malignancies may be altered through what has been referred to as **HIV immune reconstitution inflammatory syndromes (IRIS)**. Two types of immune reconstitution syndromes have been described: paradoxical, in which an already treated OI worsens after starting antiretroviral therapy, and unmasking, in which a subclinical untreated OI manifests earlier and with greater severity than would be expected in the absence of antiretroviral treatment.

As HIV infection has become a chronic manageable infection, other complications have emerged with increasing prevalence including manifestations associated with accelerated aging, certain non-AIDS defining malignancies, metabolic and cardiovascular complications, and neurocognitive disorders. Chap. 7 discusses some cardiac consequences of HIV and HIV treatments. Chap. 12 discusses significant psychiatric and neurologic sequelae of HIV and HIV treatments.

Table 11.1 AIDS-defining opportunistic conditions, early and late

Early
Occur when CD4 count <200 cells/µL
Infections:
Candidiasis of esophagus, bronchi, trachea or lungs
Coccidiomycosis, disseminated or extrapulmonary
Cryptococcal infection, extrapulmonary
Cryptosporidiosis infection, chronic intestinal
Herpes simplex virus infection, chronic ulcers (>1 month duration) or bronchitis, pneumonitis or esophagitis
Histoplasmosis, disseminated or extrapulmonary
Isosporiasis, chronic intestinal (>1 month)
Kaposi sarcoma
Mycobacterium avium complex infection
Mycobacterium tuberculosis of any site
Pneumocystis jiroveci (*P. carinii*) pneumonia
Progressive multifocal leukoencephalopathy
Brain toxoplasmosis
Conditions:
Invasive cervical cancer
HIV-related encephalopathy
Progressive multifocal leukoencephalopathy
Burkitt's lymphoma
Wasting syndrome
Late
Occur when CD4 count <50 cells/µL
Central nervous system lymphoma
Disseminated *Mycobacterium avium* infection
Cytomegalovirus (CMV) end organ disease (CMV retinitis, encephalitis, colitis)

Key Points

- Incidence of HIV infection in the United States has remained relatively stable over the past decade. Men who have sex with men remain the group most heavily affected with incident and prevalent infections. Transgender people are at particularly high risk of HIV infection. HIV also disproportionately impacts people of color in the US.
- HIV is transmitted via intimate sexual contact, injection drug use, vertical transmission from mother to child, and contaminated blood products. Receptive anal sex without a condom is the sexual behavior associated with highest risk. Acute HIV infection is associated with extremely high HIV viremia and is therefore a period of high transmission risk.
- The primary cellular target of HIV is the CD4 + lymphocyte through interaction with the CD4 receptor and chemokine coreceptors CCR5 and CXCR4.
- As HIV infection has become a chronic manageable infection, other complications have emerged with increasing prevalence including manifestations associated with accelerated aging, certain non-AIDS defining malignancies, metabolic and cardiovascular complications, and neurocognitive disorders.

Case 11.1

Riley, a 46-year-old gay male from Cambodia presents in your urgent night clinic with what appears to be a large skin abscess on his inner arm. The charge nurse informs you that he is a "frequent flyer" and has been seen for various infections and moderate trauma. He is a thin appearing man who is oriented to person, place, and time. A 4-cm abscess is present on his left inner forearm. Upon close inspection, you notice track marks in his antecubital

fossa and in both thighs. Physical exam is otherwise unremarkable.

After attending to his wound, what conversation would you have regarding his IV drug use?

What are the most significant risk factors for contracting HIV?

How could a patient be impacted by this diagnosis?

The patient is presenting with one of the common infectious complications of injection drug use, soft tissue infection. His physical examination shows stigmata of chronic injection drug use, specifically needle track marks. In addition, we are told that the patient identifies as gay and has sex with men, thereby calling attention to two major behavioral risk factors for transmission of HIV, hepatitis C, and hepatitis B.

The physician should deal both with the acute problem (a skin abscess) as well as with longer term concerns. Specifically regarding the patient's injection drug use, the following questions should be asked: (1) what drug(s) does he inject? (2) does he share needles and syringes ("works") with others? (3) how often and how much does he inject? (4) when was his last injection? (5) does he have fever, chills, or night sweats? (6) what prior complications of injection drug use has he experienced (e.g., endocarditis, HIV, hepatitis, overdose, seizures, wound botulism, septic thrombophlebitis)? (7) when did he start injecting drugs and what type of treatment, if any, has he received (e.g., methadone, buprenorphine if he is an opiate injector)?(8) has he ever overdosed? and (9) when was he last screened for HIV, hepatitis B and hepatitis C? There are many other issues that should be addressed but the most important thing is to be non-judgmental, establish trust, and try to arrange follow up after acute management of the abscess.

Focusing on potentially transmitting risk behaviors is generally more effective than focusing only on so-called traditional risk groups (gay/bisexual men, injection drug users, recipients of potentially infected blood products, perinatally exposed infants and children). Because of cultural stigma, some patients may not identify as members of a risk group but might acknowledge specific risk behaviors. Furthermore, risk behaviors follow disease transmission pathophysiology, i.e. sharing needles leads to blood borne pathogen transmission, whereas an intravenous drug user identifying as gay does not necessarily share needles.

As mentioned above, the current patient is at particularly high risk because of both injection drug use and sexual contacts. A sexual history was not elicited in the vignette but it is highly important to ask about sexual behaviors [both voluntary and coercive (sex for drugs, money, shelter or food)] to identify and screen for potentially comorbid sexually transmitted infections. As discussed in the chapter, harm reduction approaches to prevention can attenuate risk associated with sexual and drug-related risk behaviors (e.g., pre- and post-exposure prophylaxis, use of condoms and clean works, opiate substitution therapy).

A diagnosis of HIV, even in the current era of very effective treatment, can be psychologically and socially devastating. On the other hand, for some patients suffering from drug addiction (which is frequently associated with involvement with crime, the criminal justice system, violence, homelessness, and stigma), adding HIV is yet another large burden—and maybe not the most important from the patient's perspective. It is important to identify the patient's concerns and priorities and to work within that framework. Motivational interviewing and close follow-up can facilitate engagement in care.

Stigma and Discrimination Inherent in the HIV/AIDS Patient Experience with Emphasis on the LGBTQ Community

History of AIDS and the LGBTQ Community

In June 1981, the inaugural meeting of the Gay and Lesbian Medical Association (now GLMA: Health Professionals Advancing LGBTQ Equality) took place in San Francisco during the same week that the first cases of what was later called Acquired Immune Deficiency Syndrome (AIDS) were reported by the Centers for Disease Control. It was a coincidence that would have profound impact on the LGBTQ community, health care providers, and the entire world. The LGBTQ community was beginning to celebrate its newfound dignity after **Stonewall Riots** and the historic judgment of the American Psychiatric Association in 1973 that removed homosexuality as a diagnosable disorder in its *Diagnostic and Statistical Manual of Mental Disorders*. See Chaps. 1 and 12 for more information. But the next wave of **pathologization of homosexuality** was already well underway. The association of male-with-male sex with the spread of hepatitis B and enteric infections was discussed as "gay bowel syndrome" in the medical literature. Moreover, the early association of the AIDS illness with male-with-male sex was given the syndromic term **gay related immunodeficiency (GRID)**. The first case definition of AIDS was in September 1982. The publication by CDC of the major routes of HIV transmission (excluding casual contact) came a year later, and a new human retrovirus (initially named HTLV-III) was identified as the causative agent of AIDS in 1984.

In 1985, the US Food and Drug Administration licensed the first antibody test to screen the blood supply for HIV. In addition to serologic screening of blood products, potential donors at increased risk of HIV infection were excluded, including men who had sex with men even once since 1977. In March 1987, the first antiretroviral agent, zidovudine (or AZT), was licensed by the FDA for treatment of AIDS after it was shown to prolong life in a randomized controlled trial. In the same month that Larry Kramer started ACT-UP, or AIDS Coalition to Unleash Power, an international direct-action advocacy group working to impact the lives of people with AIDS (PWAs). The group's first action in spring 1987 was a march on Wall Street to protest the high cost and lack of availability of HIV treatment drugs.

The next paradigm-shifting milestone was reported at the 11th International Conference on AIDS in Vancouver in 1996. Combination antiretroviral therapy with HIV protease inhibitors led to prolonged suppression of HIV viral load and could prevent disease progression even in patients previously treated with nucleoside analogue drugs. This inaugurated an era in which HIV came to be seen by some as a chronic manageable disease instead of a death sentence for people who could access and adhere to newer simplified treatment regimens.

Cumulatively, the FDA has approved over three dozen antiretroviral drugs either as single agents or co-formulations. Available drugs target HIV through six different mechanisms of action. Treatment is now successful for most patients who are diagnosed, engaged in care, and treated, and who remain adherent. However, there are many health system challenges for identifying and retaining patients throughout their lifetimes across the **HIV continuum of care**. Failure at any step along the continuum from identification to adherence risks negative consequences for individual patients and for others due to the development of drug resistance.

During the early years of the epidemic, especially prior to highly active antiretroviral therapy (HAART), there was enormous concern in the LGBTQ community regarding the potential personal and professional consequences of an HIV diagnosis. While the CDC mandated that the clinical syndrome of AIDS was reportable to public health authorities in all states, reporting of HIV infection was controversial. Anonymous HIV testing sites provided a mechanism for patients to identify themselves as HIV infected without risking disclosure to public or private third parties.

However, it was recognized that effective use of public health prevention tools required better epidemiological surveillance of HIV infection. Public health advocates, while defending the necessity of confidentiality and legal protections against discrimination, began to argue against **HIV exceptionalism**—policies that prioritized the rights of people living with HIV/AIDS to privacy, confidentiality, and autonomy over public health objectives. Traditional tools of disease control such as routine testing with an opt-out provision, simplified and abbreviated consenting procedures, names-based reporting of HIV infection to public health authorities, contact tracing, and partner notification were gradually implemented during the HAART era. By the end of 2007, names-based reporting of HIV infection had been implemented in all states and territories.

Key Points

- During the early years of the US epidemic, especially prior to the availability of HAART, there was enormous concern in the LGBTQ community regarding the potential personal and professional consequences of an HIV diagnosis.
- In the early 1970s, the LGBTQ community was beginning to celebrate newfound dignity after the Stonewall Riots and the removal of homosexuality from the DSM, but the re-medicalization of homosexuality was underway due to the emergence of HIV and AIDS.
- In March 1987, the first antiretroviral agent, zidovudine (or AZT), was licensed by the FDA for treatment of AIDS after it was shown to prolong life in a randomized controlled trial, the same year ACT-UP was created.
- 1996 inaugurated an era in which HIV came to be seen as a chronic manageable disease instead of a death sentence for the majority of patients able to access and adhere to newer simplified treatment regimens.

- While treatment success is now achievable for the majority of patients diagnosed in the US, engaged in care, treated, and adherent, there remain many health system challenges to assure that patients are identified and retained throughout their lifetimes.

Under different circumstances in which the patient was concerned about exposure to HIV, the patient might be eligible for post-exposure prophylaxis (PEP). PEP is short-term antiretroviral treatment to reduce the likelihood of HIV infection after potential exposure.

Case 11.2

Annalise, a 28-year-old black transgender woman presents to an Emergency Department for non-operative fractured facial bones after a vicious sexual assault. Upon protocol testing for HIV, you discover she has been infected with the virus, and disclose this news to her.

What factors affect Annalise's prognosis following this diagnosis?

What are some resources Annalise can be directed to?

What are the social implications of HIV?

The prognosis for Annalise's HIV infection depends primarily on two factors: (1) the stage of her HIV infection as determined by CD4 and HIV viral load as well as by clinical examination; and (2) initiation and adherence to an antiretroviral regimen to which her virus is fully susceptible. Currently treatment is recommended for all patients with confirmed HIV infection. Annalise should be linked to a clinic that can provide access to the HIV continuum of care, starting with confirmation of the diagnosis, HIV disease staging, and counseling regarding prognosis, treatment, and prevention of secondary HIV transmission.

A diagnosis of HIV, even in the current era of very effective treatment, can be psychologically and socially devastating. It is important to identify the patient's concerns and priorities.

Special HIV/AIDS Risk Factors of LGBTQ People

Any behaviors that put one's blood stream or mucous membranes in contact with the four bodily fluids that carry HIV risk transmission. The most common behaviors are anal and vaginal sex, injection drug use, and, far less commonly in the US, transmission during pregnancy, childbirth, or breast feeding. On an individual level, primary prevention behaviors such as using condoms during sex and knowing one's partner's HIV status, and harm reduction behaviors, such as using clean injecting equipment, reduce the risk of HIV transmission. In a situation where an individual has full agency and access to information and resources, an individual can more often make better choices. However, external factors impact individual choices. Recall that **social determinants of health**—"the conditions in which people are born, grow, live, work and age, including the health system, and which are shaped by the distribution of money, power and resources at global, national and local levels"—weigh more heavily on morbidity and mortality than do attitudes, behaviors, or genetics. This is the case for heart disease, diabetes, and cancer, and it is also true for HIV/AIDS.

Stigma and Discrimination

External Resource 11.4

"Speak Out: Real Voices" – a video by Greater Than AIDS featuring seven Greater Than AIDS ambassadors who speak about their personal experiences with HIV/AIDS in order to raise awareness and reduce stigma. The video opened a White House meeting called "Gay and Bisexual Men with HIV/AIDS. Focus. Action. Impact." Total time 7:19. http://bit.ly/TECe1ch11_04

Stigma and discrimination have interpersonal and institutional forms that can have lifelong impacts on attitudes and behavior. Research shows that stigma and discrimination put people at risk for multiple physical and mental health problems and affect whether they can obtain quality health services. Mistrust or fear of the medical establishment, especially when reinforced by perceived mistreatment across various institutions, has the potential to shape interactions with the medical system, including noncompliance with physician recommendations.

The **minority stress model** was originally developed for lesbians in 1981 and was later expanded to include gay men and bisexuals in 1995 (see Brooks; Meyer). Additional evidence suggests this model also applies to transgender individuals. The minority stress model suggests that members of sexual and gender minorities experience chronic stress due to stigmatization. In the context of LGBTQ health, stigma takes the form of increased societal barriers including reduced employment, limited health care, and reductions in other social benefits. Stress can lead to overall negative health outcomes, including increased use of drugs and alcohol to cope with the stress, and could increase one's HIV vulnerability. Refer to Chap. 12 for a deeper discussion of minority stress and its mechanisms.

Health policies, when informed by transphobic and homophobic belief systems, can exacerbate HIV risk. One example is the lack of LGBTQ-inclusive sexuality education for adolescents, which in LGBTQ youth leads to a lack of knowledge regarding safer sex practices and increased sexual risk-taking. Another example was the New York state policy of using condoms as evidence of prostitution, which was overturned in May 2014. The policy was disproportionately enforced on transgender women, and many civil rights and sex work advocacy organizations claimed the policy led to decreased condom usage in both transactional and non-transactional sex.

MSM & Gay/Bisexual Men

There was a striking and unprecedented behavior change in the gay community in response to the horror of the AIDS epidemic during the 1980s and 1990s. Most MSM acquire HIV through anal sex, which is the riskiest sexual behavior to contract or transmit HIV. Recent studies have quantified the transmission risk of individual sexual risk behaviors, both as risks per episode and cumulatively with repeated exposures over time. Data from these studies may be useful in counseling patients regarding the meaning of *safer sex* (see Chap. 8). For example, the estimated risk of HIV transmission to an anal receptive partner not using condoms is estimated as 138 per 10,000 exposures but can be reduced to 1.1 per 10,000 if the infected partner uses condoms and is on antiretroviral therapy. The effects of safer sex practices compound. One study demonstrated that the one-year risk of HIV transmission among **serodiscordant** male partners practicing both anal receptive and anal insertive sex without condoms was 52%, but that risk could be lowered to 0.3% with correct and consistent condom use combined with antiretroviral therapy for the infected partner and **pre-exposure prophylaxis (PrEP)** for the uninfected partner. PrEP consists of antiretroviral medication taken regularly by a person who does not have HIV but may be at risk. Both ulcerative and non-ulcerative sexually transmitted infections (STIs) have been associated with HIV transmission, and frequent screening and treatment for STIs has been recommended for sexually active MSM as part of an overall prevention strategy.

Concomitant substance use (particularly methamphetamine and crack cocaine) also impacts risk for MSM and other groups. While injection drug use is a direct mode of transmission for HIV, use of other substances has been linked to increased sexual risk taking behavior. Even severe psychiatric disorders, especially bipolar mania have been identified as independent risk factors for HIV risk behaviors. More recently, social networks have been recognized as increasingly important in facilitating HIV transmission. Internet sites and smartphone applications, while remarkable tools for health education and prevention messaging, have also emerged as venues facilitating high risk behaviors.

Decisions that people make regarding sexual behaviors are contextual. One of the contextual determinants of sexual risk behaviors has been termed *serosorting* and *seroadaptation*. These terms refer to sexual behavior decision making conditional on assumed or expressed knowledge of the partner's serostatus and perceived risk of infectivity. For example, a seronegative man might be unwilling to engage in unprotected anal receptive sex with a new partner who says he tested positive for HIV (serosorting) but might modify his decision based on whether his potential partner was on antiretrovirals with an undetectable viral load (seroadaptation).

Transgender

Transgender women experience a host of psychosocial issues such as discrimination, stigmatization, and marginalization. These challenges often limit economic opportunities, affect mental health, and may place members of this population at an increased risk for HIV infection. Factors including needle sharing and substance use, high-risk sexual behaviors, commercial sex work, health care access, lack of knowledge regarding HIV transmission, violence, stigma and discrimination, and mental health issues have been identified in the literature as risk factors for members of this population.

Women

Health care providers need to remember that sexual identity does not necessarily predict behavior and that some women who identify themselves as WSW or lesbian may be at risk for HIV infection through unprotected sex with men. CDC has documented transmission of HIV from an infected woman to her serodiscordant female partner through sexual risk behaviors. High-risk behaviors, such as injection drug use, may play a role in HIV risk in this population.

Key Points
- New trends in understanding the HIV epidemic posit that social determinants of health weigh more heavily in the cause and course of every leading category of illness, including HIV, than do any attitudinal, behavioral, or genetic determinant.
- Stigma and discrimination, both experienced and anticipated, impacts patient interaction with the medical system, including postponement of care seeking and medical adherence and are associated with various negative health outcomes.
- HIV risk factors among MSM include (1) younger cohorts may believe HIV is a chronic condition and therefore less serious, (2) STIs, and (3) substance use.
- Serosorting is a strategy used to reduce HIV risk and is employed largely by MSM.
- HIV risk factors among transgender individuals include: needle sharing and substance use, high-risk sexual behaviors, commercial sex work, health care access, lack of knowledge regarding HIV transmission, violence, stigma and discrimination, and mental health issues.
- HIV risk factors among women include unprotected sex with women *and* men and high risk behaviors such as injection drug use.

Case 11.3

Drew, a 26-year-old white gay man, mentions in a routine visit that he has recently been "hooking up" (loosely defined as participating in casual sexual relationships) anonymously through the internet and a popular smartphone app. He states that he has not been using condoms, stating "it's not really that dangerous to be a top."

What are Drew's risk factors for HIV?

What other information should be elicited?

What advice could you give to Drew regarding future sexual encounters?

What health and social consequences can be foreseen if he ever tests HIV positive?

What are your medical priorities for Drew? How might those compare to Drew's priorities?

Anonymous sex, hook ups through the internet, and condomless sex all place Drew at increased risk of acquiring HIV infection. We do not know if Drew has been tested for HIV previously. He may already be infected and capable of transmitting HIV to his partners, especially if he is not using condoms. Although he states that he only performs anal insertive sex as a "top," it is not true that anal insertive sex without consistent condom use is objectively safe. A recent study by CDC investigators estimated incidence per 10,000 exposures of HIV transmission for anal receptive sex to be 138 and the risk for anal insertive sex to be 11.

Drew should be counseled regarding quantitative risks associated with specific sexual behaviors as well as the uncertainty surrounding those estimates. He should be advised regarding the importance of frequent HIV testing and disclosure of his status to potential sexual partners. If he is found to be negative for HIV infection by sequential testing (to rule out a "window period" infection), the importance of consistent condom use in addition to pre-exposure

prophylaxis (PrEP) should be discussed. It would also be important to discuss drug and alcohol use with Drew since both have been associated with increased risk of potentially transmitting HIV risk.

Some medical consequences of HIV have previously been discussed in section "Overview of Epidemiology, Transmission, Pathophysiology, and Clinical manifestations of HIV/AIDS" of this chapter. A multitude of social consequences may occur including stigma and discrimination by partners, friends, family, coworkers, and health care providers. This can potentially lead to social isolation, mental health concerns, and substance use. Medical priorities should include safer sex counseling, frequent testing, and patient education about PrEP. If HIV testing (including a confirmatory test) were positive, Drew would need to be started on HAART therapy and provided with community support resources. Throughout health care encounters, providers should maintain an empathetic and honest demeanor, participate in patient education opportunities, and develop a trusting relationship with the patient. Follow-up and medication compliance are utmost priority for any HIV positive patient. Providers should be mindful that the typical medical and public health priorities may not be priorities of the patient and strive to understand and work with the patient's competing priorities.

Effective Prevention, Treatment, and Care of HIV/AIDS

Prevention of HIV

In July 2010, the White House released the first National HIV/AIDS Strategy, a comprehensive roadmap for reducing the impact of HIV. The Center for Disease Control and Prevention (CDC) is working to advance the goals of the National

HIV/AIDS Strategy to ensure that HIV prevention efforts have the greatest possible impact through an approach called High-Impact Prevention. CDC is working at both the national level and with state and local partners throughout the United States to identify and implement the most cost-effective and scalable interventions for the most severely affected populations in the geographic areas hardest hit by HIV. This new approach focuses on four main areas: (1) supporting prevention programs, including biological and behavioral interventions, while supporting state and local health departments and community organizations with technical support and capacity building, (2) tracking the epidemic (surveillance), (3) supporting prevention research, and (4) raising awareness, usually through social marketing campaigns.

Biomedical approaches to facilitate earlier diagnosis of HIV as a prevention strategy have included opt-out HIV testing and a modification of the HIV testing algorithm to include a fourth generation HIV antigen-antibody detection assay that shortens the **window period** for detection of acute HIV infection. When discussing an opt-out test, a clinician may say, "We offer HIV testing to everyone at this clinic. We will test you unless you say no."

Additional biomedical tools of proven prevention effectiveness are treatment of HIV infected patients, especially in serodiscordant relationships, as well as the use of PrEP for serodiscordant couples, any sexually-active adult at substantial risk of HIV acquisition, and injection drug users. PrEP has been recommended by CDC and accompanied by a national practice guideline. **Male medical circumcision** has been shown to be a substantive biomedical intervention to reduce HIV acquisition by men (prevention efficacy estimated between 50% and 60%). While there is some evidence that male medical circumcision may reduce HIV acquisition among MSM who practice primarily anal insertive sex, its role for MSM in overall prevention strategies remains unclear. Adequate treatment of HIV in a seropositive person is also prevention. Two recent studies, Opposites Attract and PARTNER2, demonstrated that male-male couples who were

serodiscordant and who did not use condoms or pre-exposure prophylaxis had effectively no risk of transmission if the seronegative partner had viral load below 200 copies per mL. These findings support a philosophy of "treatment as prevention" for HIV.

Targeting prevention efforts using traditional risk factor profiles and venues (e.g., bars, sex parties, and bath houses) have been found to be inadequate both in identification of undiagnosed infection and in reducing HIV transmission in hard to reach and stigmatized populations. Though the use of social media to engage at-risk populations and provide targeted prevention strategies has potential, a review of first-generation smartphone HIV prevention applications found that they were infrequently downloaded and poorly rated.

Clinical Management of HIV Infection

Care of patients with HIV infection demands much more than technical competence in use of antiretroviral medications and management of HIV-related complications. Several models of care have been developed since the beginning of the HIV epidemic in the United States in response to multiple interrelated factors: HIV community prevalence and distribution, geographic setting (urban vs. rural), available insurance coverage and governmental funding (especially the Ryan White care program), HIV provider supply and willingness to treat, special population needs and preferences (e.g., MSM, IVDU, women, children, refugees, and incarcerated persons), and the effects of HIV-related stigma. Among these models of care from the clinician perspective are specialist, generalist, and specialist-generalist co-management models. Both dedicated multidisciplinary HIV clinics and primary care integrated models have been advocated. Whatever the model of care available, it is clear that the solo practitioner will have a great deal of difficulty providing all the required components of care across the **HIV care continuum** without access to numerous **wraparound services**. These services include mental health care, case management, dental care medical specialty referrals, substance use evaluation and treatment, nutritional counseling, and palliative care.

Fortunately many resources are available to assist clinicians in gaining and maintaining expertise in HIV care. Specialty societies including the American Academy of HIV Medicine (AAHIVM), the Gay and Lesbian Medical Association: Health Professionals Advancing LGBT Equality, the HIV Medical Association (HIVMA), and the International Antiviral Society USA (IAS-USA) are particularly useful resources for physicians. Governmentally supported resources for HIV clinicians include AIDSinfo, the AIDS Education and Training Centers (AETC) National Resource Center, and the Clinical Consultation Center ("warm line") operated by HIV experts at the University of California San Francisco.

Being an HIV clinician is both challenging and rewarding. Because of the aging of the first generations of HIV medical providers, there is a projected shortage of HIV clinicians in the US at a time when demand for HIV care is expected to increase due to health care reform and expanded HIV testing and linkage to care.

HIV Treatment and Care in LGBTQ Populations

It is important to note once again that stigma and discrimination impact LGBTQ people in many aspects of their lives and in many settings, including health care environments. Some of the treatment and care barriers stem from the prejudice or lack of competence of HIV and general health care providers. While in the early periods of the epidemic, when HIV providers themselves faced considerable stigma, there is evidence that younger generations of physicians have much less homophobia and HIV phobia. However, research shows that there is still much work to be done to address these issues. In a 2009 study conducted by Lambda Legal using purposive sampling with 4916 LGBT individuals and people living with HIV, more than half of all respondents reported that they experienced at least one of the following types of discrimination in care: being refused needed care; health care professionals refusing to touch them or using excessive precautions; health care professionals using harsh or abusive language; being blamed for their health status; or health care professionals being physically rough or abusive. Almost 56% of lesbian, gay or bisexual (LGB) respondents, 70% of transgender and gender-nonconforming respondents, and 63% of respondents living with HIV had at least one of these experiences. Transgender and gender-nonconforming respondents reported facing barriers and discrimination as much as two to three times more frequently than lesbian, gay or bisexual respondents. A study investigating physician-side barriers to providing transgender health care show that the barriers are multi-faceted. Access barriers impede physicians when referring patients to specialists or searching for reliable treatment information. Clinical management of transgender patients is complicated by a lack of knowledge, and by ethical considerations regarding treatments—which can be unfamiliar or complex to health care providers. The disciplinary division of responsibilities within medicine further complicates care; few practitioners identify transgender health care as an interest area, and there is a tendency to overemphasize transgender status in mental health evaluations. Failure to recognize and accommodate transgender patients within sex-segregated health care systems leads to deficient health policy. Studies show a lack of knowledge, comfort, and skills among health and social service providers who work with transgender clients and patients. This lack of provider competency has resulted in many transgender people avoiding health care services for preventive and urgent/life-threatening conditions, and transgender people having a lower adherence to their HIV medication.

Many resources exist to support doctors and other health care providers in becoming educated about LGBTQ health issues. It is clear that the historical failure to do so has resulted in a wide array of negative health outcomes among this population. It is the responsibility of all health care providers to educate themselves to be culturally and clinically competent in regard to LGBTQ health.

Key Points

- In July 2010, the White House released the first National HIV/AIDS Strategy, a comprehensive roadmap for reducing the impact of HIV.
- Biomedical tools of proven prevention effectiveness include treatment of HIV infected patients, especially in serodiscordant relationships and the use of PrEP for serodiscordant couples, sexually active adults at substantial risk of HIV acquisition, and injection drug users.
- The solo practitioner will have a great deal of difficulty providing all the required components of care across the HIV care continuum without access to numerous wrap around services.
- An overwhelming number of LGBTQ people report stigma and discrimination in health care settings, ranging from refusal of care to verbal and physical harassment. It is the responsibility of all health care providers to educate themselves to be culturally and clinically competent regarding LGBTQ health.

Case 11.4

Oakley, a 23-year-old asexual, agender patient from Ecuador presents in your clinic with flu-like symptoms. During the patient interview, Oakley reports being raped at a social event a few weeks ago. Oakley informs you that they did not report the assault to the authorities due to a fear of retaliation. Physical exam is notable for wheezing and rhinorrhea. Workup indicates a Chlamydia trachomatis infection and an extremely high HIV viral load.

How should this case be managed?

What screenings and/or vaccinations would you offer this patient?

What are some barriers you might foresee in this patient's' care?

There are many things to consider in providing high quality care to this patient.

It is important to recall that systems in general, and medical systems specifically, are not set-up in a way to effectively meet the needs of gender variant patients or patients with non-heterosexual orientations. This could explain why Oakley did not report the sexual assault or immediately seek services, and is only now presenting for treatment weeks later and possibly for a condition that they do not necessarily associate with the assault.

An agender identity is an identity that can be considered under the nonbinary, genderqueer, and transgender umbrellas. Agender individuals have no gender identity and/or no gender expression, while others feel that agender is itself a gender identity. This is similar to and overlaps with the experience of being gender neutral or having a neutral gender identity. Because an agender person's identity label by itself may not provide useful information about anatomy or cultural experiences, providers must carefully think through what information is needed. It will be important to consider what information is actually needed for the patient's treatment, and what is the most sensitive and accurate way of collecting this information. It is up to the professional to practice competent care by asking only appropriate questions and by prefacing potentially sensitive questions with an explanation of why you need the answer. For example, rather than asking, "Are you on hormones?," consider asking, "So that I can consider potential side effects of any medications, could you tell me which medications you're currently using?" This example stresses the importance of asking questions that will assist in treatment and letting the patient know why/how.

As the patient identifies as agender, it will be important to understand what language the patient prefers. The patient should be asked how they choose to be referred to in terms of pronouns and what terms they prefer to use for their body parts. Some agender people may have gender-neutral language for their genitals and other gendered body parts. The patient can also be asked if they have a gender preference for the provider who may be conducting any physical exams.

An asexual is someone who does not experience sexual attraction. For further information see The Asexual Visibility & Education Network (http://www.asexuality. org/home/). Unlike celibacy, which people choose, asexuality is an intrinsic part of a person. There is considerable diversity among the asexual community; each asexual person experiences things like relationships, attraction, and arousal somewhat differently. After a sexual assault an asexual person may face challenges to their identity as an asexual both internally and from others. It is important to affirm Oakley's sexual identity as asexual in the aftermath of a sexual assault. Sexual assault does not impact a person's sexual orientation.

Regarding medical management, the following issues should be addressed.

Forensic evaluation. Generally, forensic evaluation of sexual assault victims should occur within three to seven days of the assault and should be performed by personnel specifically trained to deal comprehensively and sensitively to all details necessary to preserve a chain of custody for evidentiary purposes. Oakley's assault occurred outside the forensic window. Nonetheless, the patient should be encouraged to allow consultation with local sexual assault evaluation experts and authorities.

STI evaluation and treatment. Recommended laboratory evaluation includes testing for pregnancy and sexually transmitted infections (HIV, Chlamydia trachomatis and Neisseria gonorrhoeae using nucleic acid amplification tests (NAAT) of potentially exposed sites, herpes simplex virus, syphilis, hepatitis B and C, and trichomonas). CDC recommends empiric treatment for gonorrhea (ceftriaxone 250 mg IM), Chlamydia (azithromycin 1 g PO), and trichomonas (metronidazole 2 g PO).

Immunization. The patient should be administered hepatitis B vaccine if not known to be immune; if the assailant is known to have hepatitis B, hepatitis B immune globulin (HBIG) should also be administered.

HIV testing and treatment. We are told that Oakley has a very high HIV viral load but we do not know if the patient has been previously tested for HIV. It is very possible that Oakley may now be presenting with acute HIV infection. The finding of a nonreactive HIV antibody test accompanied by a very high HIV plasma viral load would typical be of very recently transmitted HIV infection (a serologic window period infection). If an HIV antibody assay is reactive and the patient has detectable HIV viremia, it cannot be definitively determined whether the infection is recent or chronic. Oakley should be counseled regarding the finding of HIV infection, medically staged (including CD4 count and repeat HIV viral load), and offered antiretroviral therapy according to current guidelines. We are told that Oakley has known infection with HIV and with Chlamydia trachomatis. They should also be screened for gonorrhea, syphilis, trichomonas, hepatitis B and hepatitis C. Oakley already has HIV infection; if Oakley not already immune or actively infected, immunizations for hepatitis A and B, pneumococcus, influenza, and human papillomavirus should be considered.

One challenge in providing exceptional patient care might be identifying a care team that will be able to provide services sensitive to the patient's gender identity *and sexual orientation. It is also important to remember that people with non-normative genders or sexualities are more likely to face social marginalization in other aspects of their lives, such as in employment access which is related to employer provided health insurance access and the ability to purchase independent health insurance.*

Conclusion

HIV/AIDS continues to be a significant focus for the health professions. Understanding HIV prevention and treatment requires attention to biomedical, behavioral, social, and political aspects of the disease. While HIV incidence is unfortunately on the rise in certain populations in the United States, new strategies such as PrEP are becoming available. Early identification and linkage to care for persons living with HIV remains critical. As with many infectious diseases, treating an infected person benefits not just the individual but the community. Both for individual health and for public health, multiple prevention and treatment strategies are needed, addressing stigma, CD4 cell counts, and everything in between.

Boards-Style Application Questions

Question 1. HIV is prevalent in an estimated 1.1 million people living in the United States. Which of the following correctly identifies the virus' primary cell and receptor targets in the human body?

A. CD4 + cell; CCR5 receptor, CXCR4 receptor
B. CD14 + cell; C3b receptor, CXCR8 receptor
C. CD8 + cell; CXCL8 receptor, Fc receptor
D. CD21 + cell; CD56 receptor, CD28 receptor
E. CD16 + cell; CD3 receptor, CXCR4 receptor

Question 2. What is the definitive ranking of incident cases of HIV in the United States in 2010? Note abbreviations: men who have sex with men (MSM); young MSM (YMSM).

A. MSM > black MSM > transgender men > women
B. transgender women > black YMSM > YMSM > MSM
C. transgender women > gay men > bisexual men > transgender men
D. black MSM > black transgender men > women > YMSM
E. transgender women > MSM > YMSM > black YMSM

Question 3. A 41-year-old man presents for a check-up. He denies any current complaints and discloses that unbeknownst to his prior physicians, he regularly engages in sex with male partners. STI and HIV panels are ordered alongside standard labs, and findings are significant for HIV surface antibodies and CD4 count of 500 cells per microliter (normal count is 500–1500 cells per microliter). Given this presentation, which of the following likely identifies the patients' current status and the corresponding clinical recommendations?

	HIV infected	AIDS status	Likely time since infection	HAART recommended?	PrEP recommended?
A	+	+	20 yrs	Yes	No
B	+	+	15 yrs	Yes	No
C	+	−	10 yrs	Yes	No
D	+	−	2 yrs	Yes	Yes
E	−	−	Weeks	No	Yes

Question 4. Which of the following is NOT a mode of HIV transmission?

A. Anal sex
B. Breast feeding
C. Vaginal sex
D. Sharing needles with an HIV positive person
E. Sharing eating utensils with an HIV positive person

Question 5. Which of the following correctly describes the association between viral load, risk of transmission, and CD4+ count in an acute HIV infection?

	Viral load$_1$	Transmission risk	CD4 + count$_2$
A	↑	↑↑	↑
B	↓↓	↓	↓
C	↑↑	↑↑	↓
D	↓	↑	↑
E	↓↓	↑	↓↓

Notes
1. Viral load relative to patient's viral load "set point."
2. CD4 count relative to normal range for an uninfected person.

Question 6. Which of the following correctly ranks the risk of transmission to an HIV negative partner (from highest to lowest) associated with each behavior in an HIV positive patient who:

 I. Participates in mutual masturbation with a HIV negative partner who is using PrEP.
 II. Participates in unprotected anal insertive sex, is not on antiretroviral therapy with viral load >1000 copies/ml, and partner not on PrEP.
 III. Participates in unprotected anal insertive sex, is on antiretroviral therapy with undetectable viral load, and partner not on PrEP.
 IV. Participates in anal insertive sex using a condom, is on antiretroviral therapy with undetectable viral load, and partner not on PrEP.
 V. Participates in anal insertive sex using a condom, is on antiretroviral therapy with an undetectable viral load, and whose partner is using PrEP.

A. I > IV > II > III > V
B. IV > I > II > III > V
C. II > I > IV > V > III
D. II > III > IV > V > I

All risks are equally weighted.

Question 7. Which of the following correctly demonstrate serosorting and seroadaptation?

A. HIV negative patient unwilling to engage in unprotected sex with HIV positive person (serosorting), HIV negative patient more willing to engage in unprotected sex with HIV positive person on antiretroviral therapy (seroadaptation)
B. HIV negative patient more willing to engage in unprotected sex with HIV + person on antiretroviral therapy (serosorting), HIV negative patient unwilling to engage in unprotected sex with HIV + person (seroadaptation)
C. HIV positive patient who is unaware of their status (serosorting), HIV negative patient who is routinely screened for STIs including HIV (seroadaptation)
D. HIV negative patient on PrEP (serosorting), HIV positive patient on antiretroviral therapy (seroadaptation)
E. HIV negative patient on PrEP having solely unprotected sex (serosorting), HIV negative patient with medically circumcised, HIV positive partners (seroadaptation)

Question 8. Individual precautions are an important means of preventing the transmission of HIV. PrEP would LEAST likely be recommended for which of the following patients?

A. A transgender male-to-female patient with an HIV positive partner
B. A young man with many male partners
C. A person who is in a mutually monogamous relationship with an HIV negative partner.
D. A person with a history of injection drug use
E. A sex worker unable to consistently use protective measures

Question 9. During a routine STI screening, your patient is discovered to be HIV positive. What are the reporting guidelines for HIV and how do the guidelines compare to those for AIDS?

A. HIV infection and cases of AIDS must be reported if a patient begins antiretroviral therapy
B. HIV infection and cases of AIDS must be reported on a name-basis by physicians and laboratories offering confidential testing
C. AIDS cases must be reported to the CDC, but HIV cases need not
D. HIV and AIDS case reporting are up to the discretion of the physician
E. Even anonymous HIV testing sites require a patient to disclose their status to the CDC, all AIDS cases must be reported

Question 10. A 24-year-old transgender woman presents to a community clinic for her first wellness visit in several years. Given the impact of stigma and discrimination on the LGBTQ community, what is the appropriate next step to effectively and sensitively screen this patient for HIV risk?

A. Assume that the patient frequents bathhouses and inform her that this is a risky behavior
B. Establish rapport via open-ended, non-judgmental questions that evaluate the possibility of high-risk behaviors
C. Assume that the patient has a history of substance use and counsel her on the dangers of sharing injection equipment
D. Assume that the patient is a sex worker and ask about her clientele
E. Do nothing because this patient is unlikely to contract HIV

Question 11. The patient from the question above is identified as engaging in high-risk behavior. Given the impact of stigma and discrimination on the LGBTQ community, what is the appropriate way to effectively and sensitively counsel this patient?

A. Inform the patient on her HIV risk and educate her on the benefits of safer sex and the benefits of PrEP.
B. Demand that the patient begin PrEP therapy
C. Inform the patient on her HIV risk and demand she use protection at all times
D. Tell the patient she should know better than to engage in risky sex
E. Request that the patient only have sex with people who say they're HIV negative

Question 12. The patient from the question above notes safety and lack of resources as obstacles to care. Given this case scenario, what are the next steps in patient management?

A. Request that the patient follow-up at the clinic with you on a monthly basis
B. Tell the patient to avoid dangerous situations and start keeping all her appointments
C. Let the patient know that getting a real job would fix all her problems
D. Inform the patient that the internet has many resources to help address her concerns
E. Provide information on local resources including case management, support groups, and low-cost health services; assure the patient that you are her advocate and are available to see and support her

Boards-Style Application Questions Answer Key

Question 1. The correct answer is A. The primary cellular target of HIV is the CD4 + lymphocyte through interaction with the CD4 receptor and chemokine co-receptors CCR5 and CXCR4. Other cells possessing these receptors can also be infected including monocytes, macrophages, and dendritic cells.

Question 2. The correct answer is B. Incidence among transgender women is often the highest reported among any population group and in many cases twice that of gay and bisexual men. In 2010, MSM accounted for 78% and 63% of incident

HIV infections among men and overall, respectively. Among young MSM (ages 13–24), black MSM accounted for 55% of all incident cases. Incidence of new HIV infections was 2.1% among transgender persons, 1.2% for males and 0.4% for females. Among transgender persons, the highest percentage of newly identified HIV infection was among blacks (4.1%) and Latinos (3.0%).

Question 3. The correct answer is C. The presence of HIV surface antibodies indicates a chronic state of HIV infection (E is incorrect). Given that the patient denies any current complaints such as recurrent or opportunistic infections, his HIV has not progressed to AIDS (A and B are incorrect). After establishment of the viral set point and in the absence of treatment, CD4 cells drop, on average, between 50% and 100 cells/μL per year – therefore, this patient was infected 8–10 years ago.

Question 4. The correct answer is E. HIV is transmitted via intimate sexual contact, injection drug use, vertical transmission from mother to child (in utero, during parturition, and through breast feeding), and contaminated blood products. Activities such as sharing eating utensils, hugging, kissing, toilet seat contact, and doorknob contact are myths mistakenly associated with HIV transmission.

Question 5. The correct answer is C. Acute HIV infection is associated with extremely high HIV viremia and is therefore a period of high transmission risk that is compounded by the difficulties of diagnosing acute HIV infection. During acute HIV infection, CD4 may drop dramatically with resulting opportunistic infections.

Question 6. The correct answer is D. An HIV infected person with a detectable viral load who participates in unprotected anal insertive sex has the highest risk of transmitting the virus. As precautions such as antiretroviral therapy, reduction of viral load, and PrEP are taken, the risk of transmission decreases. The lowest risk is associated with activities that do not facilitate mucous membrane or bloodstream contact (i.e. mutual masturbation).

Question 7. The correct answer is A. Two of the contextual determinants of sexual risk behaviors have been termed "serosorting" and "seroadaptation". These terms refer to sexual behavior decision making conditional on assumed or expressed knowledge of the partner's serostatus and perceived risk of infectivity. Serosorting is the process of decision making based on partner's HIV status, seroadaptation is the modification of that decision based on partner's HIV management.

Question 8. The correct answer is C. PrEP is recommended for patients at high risk of coming into contact with HIV. High risk factors include HIV positive partners, injection drug use, sex work, and unprotected sex, especially anal receptive sex. The most frequent pattern of transmission is male-to-male, and female-to-female transmission is rare, although the CDC recently documented transmission of HIV from an infected women to her serodiscordant female partner through sexual risk behaviors.

Question 9. The correct answer is B. Since 2007, names-based reporting of HIV infection has been required in all states and territories. In jurisdictions that still sponsor anonymous HIV testing, names of HIV-positive persons are not reported to public health authorities. The health care provider should confirm that testing is indeed anonymous and should disclose this to the patient.

Question 10. The correct answer is B. Taking a thorough sexual history, including past and current partners, protective measures, and history of sexually transmitted infection (STI) are important means of screening for STI risk in all patients. Although substance use, unemployment, bathhouses, and prostitution are associated with some members of the LGBTQ community, not all members participate in these activities. It is unreasonable to assume behaviors or risk based on identity.

Question 11. The correct answer is A. Educating the patient on the risks associated with her behaviors, how risk can be decreased, and encouraging her to modify her behavior is vital not only for benefit, but also for patient rapport. Although the patient should be counseled regarding the benefits of PrEP, it is unreasonable to *demand* she start taking it.

Question 12. The correct answer is E. Although the patient may be eligible for and elect to take PrEP therapy, it is important to deal with the issues of safety and lack of resources identified as concerns. Connecting the patient with local resources such as case management, LGBTQ centers, low-cost alternatives to health care or free clinics, safety hotlines, and anti-violence networks would be effective in meeting these concerns.

Sources

A Timeline of HIV and AIDS. HIV.gov. https://www.hiv.gov/hiv-basics/overview/history/hiv-and-aids-timeline. Accessed February 2, 2019.

Aberg J, Gallant J, Ghanem K, Emmanuel P, Zingman B, Horberg M. Primary care guidelines for the management of persons infected with HIV: 2013 update by the HIV medicine association of the infectious diseases society of America. Clin Infect Dis. 2013;58(1):e1–e34. https://doi.org/10.1093/cid/cit665.

AIDSinfo. https://aidsinfo.nih.gov. National Institutes of Health. Accessed February 2, 2019.

Altman L. New homosexual disorder worries health officials. New York: New York Times; 1982.

American Academy of HIV Medicine. https://aahivm.org/. Accessed February 2, 2019.

Amirkhanian Y. Social networks, sexual networks and HIV risk in men who have sex with men. Curr HIV/AIDS Rep. 2014;11(1):81–92. https://doi.org/10.1007/s11904-013-0194-4.

Angell M. A dual approach to the AIDS epidemic. N Engl J Med. 1991;324(21):1498–500.

Antiretroviral drugs used in the treatment of HIV infection. Fda.gov. https://www.fda.gov/forpatients/illness/hivaids/ucm118915.htm. Published 2018. Accessed February 2, 2019.

Baral S, Poteat T, Strömdahl S, Wirtz A, Guadamuz T, Beyrer C. Worldwide burden of HIV in transgender women: a systematic review and meta-analysis. Lancet Infect Dis. 2013;13(3):214–22. https://doi.org/10.1016/s1473-3099(12)70315-8.

Bavinton B, Pinto A, Phanuphak N, Grinsztejn B, Prestage GP, Zablotska-Manos IB, et al. Viral suppression and HIV transmission in serodiscordant male couples: an international, prospective, observational, cohort study. Lancet HIV. 2018;5(8):e438–47. https://doi.org/10.1016/s2352-3018(18)30132-2.

Bayer R, Fairchild A. Changing the paradigm for HIV testing — the end of exceptionalism. N Engl J Med. 2006;355(7):647–9. https://doi.org/10.1056/nejmp068153.

Bayer R. Public health policy and the AIDS epidemic. N Engl J Med. 1991;324(21):1500–4. https://doi.org/10.1056/nejm199105233242111.

Becasen JS, Denard CL, Mullins MM, Higa DH, Sipe TA. Estimating the prevalence of HIV and sexual behaviors among the US transgender population: a systematic review and meta-analysis, 2006–2017. Am J Public Health. 2018;109(1):e1–8.

Becker G, Newsom E. Socioeconomic status and dissatisfaction with health care among chronically ill African Americans. Am J Public Health. 2003;93(5):742–8.

Becker MH, Joseph JG. AIDS and behavioral change to reduce risk: a review. Am J Public Health. 1988;78(4):394–410.

Bockting WO, Robinson BE, Rosser BR. Transgender HIV prevention: a qualitative needs assessment. AIDS Care. 1998;10(4):505–25.

Bowers JR, Branson CM, Fletcher JB, Reback CJ. Predictors of HIV sexual risk behavior among men who have sex with men, men who have sex with men and women, and transgender women. Int J Sex Health. 2012;24(4):290–302.

Brew B, Chan P. Update on HIV dementia and HIV-associated neurocognitive disorders. Curr Neurol Neurosci Rep. 2014;14(8):468. https://doi.org/10.1007/s11910-014-0468-2.

Brooks V. Minority stress and lesbian women. Lexington: Lexington Books; 1982.

Casagrande S, Gary T, LaVeist T, Gaskin D, Cooper L. Perceived discrimination and adherence to medical care in a racially integrated community. J Gen Intern Med. 2007;22(3):389–95. https://doi.org/10.1007/s11606-006-0057-4.

Cassels S, Katz D. Seroadaptation among men who have sex with men: emerging research themes. Curr HIV/AIDS Rep. 2013;10(4):305–13. https://doi.org/10.1007/s11904-013-0188-2.

Castro H, Pillay D, Cane P, Asboe D, Cambiano V, Phillips A, Dunn DT. Persistence of HIV-1 transmitted drug resistance mutations. J Infect Dis. 2013;208(9):1459–63.

Centers for Disease Control and Prevention. HIV and African American gay and bisexual men. Atlanta: Centers for Disease Control and Prevention; 2018. https://www.cdc.gov/hiv/pdf/group/msm/cdc-hiv-bmsm.pdf. Accessed February 2, 2019.

Centers for Disease Control and Prevention. *HIV and Gay and Bisexual Men*. Atlanta: Centers for Disease Control and Prevention; 2018. https://www.cdc.gov/hiv/pdf/group/msm/cdc-hiv-msm.pdf. Accessed February 2, 2019.

Centers for Disease Control and Prevention. *HIV and young men who have sex with men*. Atlanta: Centers for Disease Control and Prevention; 2014. https://www.cdc.gov/healthyyouth/sexualbehaviors/pdf/hiv_factsheet_ymsm.pdf. Accessed February 2, 2019

Centers for Disease Control and Prevention. *Preexposure prophylaxis for the prevention of HIV infection in the United States – 2017 update: a clinical practice guideline*. Atlanta: Centers for Disease Control and Prevention: US Public Health Service; 2018. https://www.cdc.gov/hiv/pdf/risk/prep/cdc-hiv-prep-guidelines-2017.pdf. Accessed February 2, 2019.

Centers for Disease Control. Changes in sexual behavior and condom use associated with a risk-reduction program–Denver, 1988–1991. MMWR Morb Mortal Wkly Rep. 1992;41(23):412–5.

Centers for Disease Control. Patterns of sexual behavior change among homosexual/bisexual men–selected U.S. sites, 1987–1990. MMWR Morb Mortal Wkly Rep. 1991;40(46):792–4.

Chan P, Brew B. HIV associated neurocognitive disorders in the modern antiviral treatment era: prevalence, characteristics, biomarkers, and effects of treatment. Curr HIV/AIDS Rep. 2014;11(3):317–24. https://doi.org/10.1007/s11904-014-0221-0.

Chan SK, Thornton LR, Chronister KJ, Meyer J, Wolverton M, Johnson CK, et al. Likely female-to-female sexual transmission of HIV–Texas, 2012. MMWR Morb Mortal Wkly Rep. 2014;63(10):209–12.

Chu C, Selwyn P. An epidemic in evolution: the need for new models of HIV care in the chronic disease era. J Urban Health. 2011;88(3):556–66. https://doi.org/10.1007/s11524-011-9552-y.

Cohen J. HIV treatment as prevention. Science. 2011;334(6063):1628–1628. https://doi.org/10.1126/science.334.6063.1628.

Cohen M, Shaw G, McMichael A, Haynes B. Acute HIV-1 infection. N Engl J Med. 2011;364(20):1943–54. https://doi.org/10.1056/nejmra1011874.

Cohen MS. HIV and sexually transmitted diseases: lethal synergy. Top HIV Med. 2004;12(4):104–7.

Cooper F, Barber T. Gay bowel syndrome. Curr Opin Infect Dis. 2014;27(1):84–9. https://doi.org/10.1097/qco.0000000000000032.

De Santis J. HIV infection risk factors among male-to-female transgender persons: a review of the literature. J Assoc Nurses AIDS Care. 2009;20(5):362–72. https://doi.org/10.1016/j.jana.2009.06.005.

Drescher S, von Wyl V, Yang W, Böni J, Yerly S, Shah C, et al. Treatment-naive individuals are the major source of transmitted HIV-1 drug resistance in men who have sex with men in the Swiss HIV cohort study. Clin Infect Dis. 2013;58(2):285–94. https://doi.org/10.1093/cid/cit694.

First report of AIDS. MMWR Morb Mortal Wkly Rep. 2001;50(21):429.

Fischl MA, Richman DD, Grieco MH, et al. The efficacy of azidothymidine (AZT) in the treatment of patients with AIDS and AIDS-related complex. A double-blind, placebo-controlled trial. N Engl J Med. 1987;317(4):185–91.

Gallant JE, Adimora AA, Carmichael JK, Horberg M, Kitahata M, Quinlivan EB, et al. Essential components of effective HIV care: a policy paper of the HIV medicine association of the Infectious Diseases Society of America and the Ryan White Medical Providers Coalition. Clin Infect Dis. 2011;53(11):1043–50. https://doi.org/10.1093/cid/cir689.

Gandhi R, Sax P, Grinspoon S. Metabolic and cardiovascular complications in HIV-infected patients: new challenges for a new age. J Infect Dis. 2012;205(suppl3):S353–4. https://doi.org/10.1093/infdis/jis202.

Gardner E, McLees M, Steiner J, del Rio C, Burman W. The spectrum of engagement in HIV care and its relevance to test-and-treat strategies for prevention of HIV infection. Clin Infect Dis. 2011;52(6):793–800. https://doi.org/10.1093/cid/ciq243.

GLMA: Health Professionals Advancing LGBTQ Equality. http://glma.org/. Accessed February 2, 2019.

Gulick RM, Mellors JW, Havlir D, Eron JJ, Gonzalez C, McMahon D, et al. Treatment with indinavir, zidovudine, and lamivudine in adults with human immunodeficiency virus infection and prior antiretroviral therapy. N Engl J Med. 1997;337(11):734–9.

Hammer SM, Squires KE, Hughes MD, Grimes JM, Demeter LM, Currier JS, et al. A controlled trial of two nucleoside analogues plus Indinavir in persons with human immunodeficiency virus infection and CD4 cell counts of 200 per cubic millimeter or less. N Engl J Med. 1997;337(11):725–33. https://doi.org/10.1056/nejm199709113371101.

Health Resources and Services Administration. Workforce capacity in HIV. Rockville: Health Resources and Services Administration, HIV/AIDS Bureau; 2010.

Herbst JH, Jacobs ED, Finlayson TJ, et al. Estimating HIV prevalence and risk behaviors of transgender persons in the United States: a systematic review. AIDS Behav. 2008;12(1):1–17.

HIV Among Transgender People. cdc.gov. https://www.cdc.gov/hiv/group/gender/transgender/index.html. Published 2018. Accessed February 1, 2019.

HIV Among Transgender People. cdc.gov. https://www.cdc.gov/hiv/group/gender/transgender/index.html. Published 2018. Accessed February 1, 2019.

HIV in the United States and Dependent Areas. cdc.gov. https://www.cdc.gov/hiv/statistics/overview/ataglance.html. Published 2019. Accessed February 2, 2019.

HIV Medicine Association. Hivma.org. https://www.hivma.org/. Published 2019. Accessed February 2, 2019.

Holloway IW, Rice E, Gibbs J, Winetrobe H, Dunlap S, Rhoades H. Acceptability of smartphone application-based HIV prevention among young men who have sex with men. AIDS Behav. 2014;18(2):285–96. https://doi.org/10.1007/s10461-013-0671-1.

Hughes E, Bassi S, Gilbody S, Bland M, Martin F. Prevalence of HIV, hepatitis B, and hepatitis C in people with severe mental illness: a systematic review and meta-analysis. Lancet Psychiatry. 2016;3(1):40–8. https://doi.org/10.1016/s2215-0366(15)00357-0.

International Antiviral Society–USA. IAS-USA. https://www.iasusa.org/. Accessed February 2, 2019.

Kelly J, DiFrancesico W, St Lawrence J, Amirkhanian Y, Anderson-Lamb M. Situational, partner, and contextual factors associated with level of risk at Most recent intercourse among black men who have sex with men. AIDS Behav. 2013;18(1):26–35. https://doi.org/10.1007/s10461-013-0532-y.

Lambda Legal. When health care Isn't caring. Lambda Legal's survey on discrimination against LGBT people and people living with HIV. New York City: Lambda Legal; 2010. http://www.lambdalegal.org/health-care-report. Accessed February 2, 2019.

Lasry A, Sansom S, Wolitski R, et al. HIV sexual transmission risk among serodiscordant couples. AIDS. 2014;28(10):1521–9. https://doi.org/10.1097/qad.0000000000000307.

Lewnard J, Berrang-Ford L. Internet-based partner selection and risk for unprotected anal intercourse in sexual encounters among men who have sex with men: a meta-analysis of observational studies. Sex Transm Infect. 2014;90(4):290–6. https://doi.org/10.1136/sextrans-2013-051332.

Lingappa JR, Hughes JP, Wang RS, Baeten JM, Celum C, Gray GE, et al. Estimating the impact of plasma HIV-1 RNA reductions on heterosexual HIV-1 transmission risk. PLoS One. 2010;5(9):e12598. https://doi.org/10.1371/journal.pone.0012598.

Maartens G, Celum C, Lewin S. HIV infection: epidemiology, pathogenesis, treatment, and prevention. Lancet. 2014;384(9939):258–71. https://doi.org/10.1016/s0140-6736(14)60164-1.

Maiorana A, Koester K, Myers J, Lloyd KC, Shade SB, Dawson-Rose C, Morin SF. Helping patients talk about HIV: inclusion of messages on disclosure in prevention with positives interventions in clinical settings. AIDS Educ Prev. 2012;24(2):179–92. https://doi.org/10.1521/aeap.2012.24.2.179.

Masur H, Brooks J, Benson C, Holmes K, Pau A, Kaplan J. Prevention and treatment of opportunistic infections in HIV-infected adults and adolescents: updated guidelines from the centers for disease control and prevention, national institutes of health, and HIV medicine Association of the Infectious Diseases Society of America. Clin Infect Dis. 2014;58(9):1308–11. https://doi.org/10.1093/cid/ciu094.

Mccusker J, Stoddard AM, Mcdonald M, Zapka JG, Mayer KH. Maintenance of behavioral change in a cohort of homosexually active men. AIDS. 1992;6(8):861–8.

Meade C, Fitzmaurice G, Sanchez A, Griffin M, McDonald L, Weiss R. The relationship of manic episodes and drug abuse to sexual risk behavior in patients with co-occurring bipolar and substance use disorders: a 15-month prospective analysis. AIDS Behav. 2010;15(8):1829–33. https://doi.org/10.1007/s10461-010-9814-9.

Meade C, Sikkema K. HIV risk behavior among adults with severe mental illness: a systematic review. Clin Psychol Rev. 2005;25(4):433–57. https://doi.org/10.1016/j.cpr.2005.02.001.

Meyer IH. Minority stress and mental health in gay men. J Health Soc Behav. 1995;36(1):38–56.

Muessig KE, Pike EC, Fowler B, LeGrand S, Parsons JT, Bull SS, et al. Putting prevention in their pockets: developing mobile phone-based HIV interventions for black men who have sex with men. AIDS Patient Care STDs. 2013;27(4):211–22. https://doi.org/10.1089/apc.2012.0404.

Muessig KE, Pike EC, Legrand S, Hightow-Weidman LB. Mobile phone applications for the care and prevention of HIV and other sexually transmitted diseases: a review. J Med Internet Res. 2013;15(1):e1. https://doi.org/10.2196/jmir.2301.

Mugo N, Heffron R, Donnell D, Wald A, Were EO, Rees H, et al. Increased risk of HIV-1 transmission in pregnancy. AIDS. 2011;25(15):1887–95. https://doi.org/10.1097/qad.0b013e32834a9338.

Mustanski B, Newcomb M, Du Bois S, Garcia S, Grov C. HIV in young men who have sex with men: a review of epidemiology, risk and protective factors, and interventions. J Sex Res. 2011;48(2–3):218–53. https://doi.org/10.1080/00224499.2011.558645.

Mutua F, M'Imunya J, Wiysonge C. Genital ulcer disease treatment for reducing sexual acquisition of HIV. Cochrane Database Syst Rev. 2012; https://doi.org/10.1002/14651858.cd007933.pub2.

Nasrullah M, Wesolowski L, Meyer W, et al. Performance of a fourth-generation HIV screening assay and an alternative HIV diagnostic testing algorithm. AIDS. 2013;27(5):731–7. https://doi.org/10.1097/qad.0b013e32835bc535.

Nemoto T, Operario D, Soma T, Bao D, Vajrabukka A, Crisostomo V. HIV risk and prevention among Asian/Pacific islander men who have sex with men: listen to our stories. AIDS Educ Prev. 2003;15(1 Suppl A):7–20.

Nemoto T, Sausa L, Operario D, Keatley J. Need for HIV/AIDS education and intervention for MTF transgenders. J Homosex. 2006;51(1):183–201. https://doi.org/10.1300/j082v51n01_09.

Okulicz J, Lambotte O. Epidemiology and clinical characteristics of elite controllers. Curr Opin HIV AIDS. 2011;6(3):163–8. https://doi.org/10.1097/coh.0b013e328344f35e.

Önen NF, Overton ET. A review of premature frailty in HIV-infected persons; another manifestation of HIV-related accelerated aging. Curr Aging Sci. 2011;4(1):33–41.

Patel P, Borkowf C, Brooks J, Lasry A, Lansky A, Mermin J. Estimating per-act HIV transmission risk. AIDS. 2014;28(10):1509–19. https://doi.org/10.1097/qad.0000000000000298.

Pathai S, Bajillan H, Landay A, High K. Is HIV a model of accelerated or accentuated aging? J Gerontol Ser A Biol Med Sci. 2013;69(7):833–42. https://doi.org/10.1093/gerona/glt168.

Pearshouse R. U.S.: All states to move to names-based HIV reporting in 2007. HIV AIDS Policy Law Rev. 2007;12(1):37–8.

Centers for Disease Control and Prevention (CDC). Revised surveillance case definition for HIV infection–United States, 2014. MMWR Recomm Rep 2014;63(RR-03):1–10.

Robinson R, Moodie-Mills A. HIV/AIDS inequality structural barriers to prevention, treatment, and care

In: Communities of color. Why we need a holistic approach to eliminate racial disparities in HIV/AIDS. Berkeley: Center for American Progress; 2012.

Rodger AJ. Risk of HIV transmission through condomless sex in MSM couples with suppressive ART: the PARTNER2 study extended results in gay men. Presented at the 22nd international AIDS conference; July 23–27, 2018; Amsterdam, the Netherlands.

Ruan Y, Qian H, Li D, Shi W, Li Q, Liang H, et al. Willingness to be circumcised for preventing HIV among Chinese men who have sex with men. AIDS Patient Care STDs. 2009;23(5):315–21. https://doi.org/10.1089/apc.2008.0199.

Scarce M. Harbinger of plague: a bad case of gay bowel syndrome. J Homosex. 1997;34(2):1–35.

Simoni JM, Pantalone DW. Secrets and safety in the age of AIDS: does HIV disclosure lead to safer sex? Top HIV Med. 2004;12(4):109–18.

Smith D, Mathews W. Physicians' attitudes toward homosexuality and HIV. J Homosex. 2007;52(3–4):1–9. https://doi.org/10.1300/j082v52n03_01.

Snelgrove J, Jasudavisius A, Rowe B, Head E, Bauer G. "Completely out-at-sea" with "two-gender medicine": a qualitative analysis of physician-side barriers to providing healthcare for transgender patients. BMC Health Serv Res. 2012;12(1) https://doi.org/10.1186/1472-6963-12-110.

Sood N, Juday T, Vanderpuye-Orgle J, Rosenblatt L, Romley JA, Peneva D, Goldman DP. HIV care providers emphasize the importance of the Ryan White Program for access to and quality of care. Health Aff. 2014;33(3):394–400. https://doi.org/10.1377/hlthaff.2013.1297.

Tobian A, Kacker S, Quinn T. Male circumcision: a globally relevant but under-utilized method for the prevention of HIV and other sexually transmitted infections. Annu Rev Med. 2014;65(1):293–306. https://doi.org/10.1146/annurev-med-092412-090539.

Tyerman Z, Aboulafia DM. Review of screening guidelines for non-AIDS-defining malignancies: evolving issues in the era of highly active antiretroviral therapy. AIDS Rev. 2012;14(1):3–16.

Vamvakas E. Relative risk of reducing the lifetime blood donation deferral for men who have had sex with men versus currently tolerated transfusion risks. Transfus Med Rev. 2011;25(1):47–60. https://doi.org/10.1016/j.tmrv.2010.08.006.

van den Boom W, Konings R, Davidovich U, Sandfort T, Prins M, Stolte I. Is serosorting effective in reducing the risk of HIV infection among men who have sex with men with casual sex partners? JAIDS J Acquir Immune Defic Syndr. 2014;65(3):375–9. https://doi.org/10.1097/qai.0000000000000051.

Volberding P, Greene W, Lange J, Gallant J. Sande's HIV/AIDS medicine. 2nd ed. Philadelphia: Elsevier Saunders; 2012.

Wagner Z, Wu Y, Sood N. The affordable care act may increase the number of people getting tested for HIV by nearly 500,000 by 2017. Health Aff. 2014;33(3):378–85. https://doi.org/10.1377/hlthaff.2013.0996.

Wang C, Silverberg M, Abrams D. Non-AIDS-defining malignancies in the HIV-infected population. Curr Infect Dis Rep. 2014;16(6):406. https://doi.org/10.1007/s11908-014-0406-0.

Psychiatry and Neurology

12

James R. Lehman, Ashley Rae Martinez,
A. Ning Zhou, and Stephan Carlson

Introduction

While access to competent health care is essential to address LGBTQ health disparities, clinical care accounts for no more than one-quarter the variance of health in populations. The remaining variance is shaped by genetic factors, health behaviors, and social and economic conditions. Consequently, great improvements in mental health outcomes for LGBTQ populations are garnered by changes in the social determinants of health, such as educational and employment achievement; socioeconomic, marital, and housing status; legal rights and governmental policies; and early life experiences. Health professionals who treat patients with mental illness must consider both the biopsychosocial model of individual illness and the broader public health view of prevention and advocacy to address social determinants of health.

History of the Psychiatry of Sexual Orientation and Gender Identity

This section briefly summarizes the pathologization of sexual and gender minorities from a psychiatric context, focusing primarily on the twentieth century. A complimentary historical description is in Chap. 1. Here, the terms *homosexual* and *homosexuality* are used because of their importance in historical context. These terms are now disfavored due to negative connotations. Chap. 1 covers preferred terminology.

Nineteenth century philosophers and physicians progressively argued for the pathologization of same-sex sexual attraction and behavior. They described it as an "insanity" or psychological illness, hypothesizing that it was caused by abnormal development. Comparing it with the belief that these behaviors, identities, and desires were sinful or criminal, the notion that homosexuality could be treated, cured, or changed seemed the lesser of two evils. This **pathologization of homosexuality** was successful, with vestiges of criminalization continuing in the United States until the 1970s.

The first listed author is the chapter's associate editor from The Equal Curriculum Project. The chapter authors are otherwise ordered according to their preference.

J. R. Lehman (✉)
Department of Psychiatry, University of Wisconsin–
Madison, Madison, WI, USA
e-mail: james.lehman@uwalumni.com

A. R. Martinez
University of California, San Diego,
La Jolla, CA, USA

A. N. Zhou
New York-Presbyterian, Columbia and Cornell,
New York, NY, USA

S. Carlson
Brookdale Hospital Medical Center,
Brooklyn, NY, USA

© Springer Nature Switzerland AG 2020
J. R. Lehman et al. (eds.), *The Equal Curriculum*, https://doi.org/10.1007/978-3-030-24025-7_12

Societal and political views criminalizing and pathologizing sexual orientation and gender identity difference continued until the 1950s with a few important exceptions. Sigmund Freud, the father of psychoanalysis, began writing about homosexuality in 1905 and argued that homosexuality was the result of early life experiences but could not be changed. Freud's view of homosexuality was progressive for his time, but his attribution of homosexuality to psychodynamic factors—a proposition that never achieved credibility—is a legacy with some negative consequences for sexual minorities. Later psychoanalysts were more negative in their views of homosexuality and emphasized that it was a condition in need of treatment and conversion.

Alfred Kinsey published research in the 1940s and 1950s documenting that homosexuality is common and that many heterosexual men had had homosexual experiences. In the 1950s, Evelyn Hooker was funded by the National Institute of Mental Health to investigate the psychoanalytic claim that homosexual men were more mentally disturbed than others. She concluded they were as equally well-adjusted as their heterosexual counterparts.

Changes in the American Psychiatric Association's (APA) Diagnostic and Statistical Manual (DSM) paralleled cultural developments leading normalizing the LGBTQ experience from the 1950s to the 1970s. The DSM-I, first published in 1952 and heavily influenced by psychoanalytic thinking, labeled homosexuality as a "sociopathic personality disturbance." Notably, sodomy laws were still widely enforced in the United States at that time. The medicalization of homosexuality also influenced institutional policies in the military, the federal government, and many medical schools, disallowing homosexuals to join, work, or study in these areas. During this time, many mental health professionals attempted to treat or change homosexuals into heterosexuals sometimes by involuntarily committing them to psychiatric hospitals and utilizing psychoanalysis, hormone therapy, castration, and even lobotomy. Attempts to change sexual orientation, called **conversion therapy** or **reparative therapy**, will be discussed later.

The DSM-II (1968) continued to label homosexuality as a mental illness and sexual deviation. The decline of psychoanalysis's influence on psychiatry in the 1950s, the civil rights movement, and activism of LGBTQ people in the late 1960s challenged the assumption that homosexuality was a psychological disorder. The APA removed homosexuality from the DSM-II in 1973 and replaced in the DSM-III with ego-dys-

External Resource 12.1
This American Life episode 204, **"81 Words,"** reports the story of how the American Psychiatric Association decided in 1973 that homosexuality was no longer a mental illness. Total time 59:18. http://bit.ly/TECe1ch12_01

tonic homosexuality, "characterized by guilt, shame, anxiety, and depression," shifting the focus to the individual's reaction to stigma and its effects. Ego-dystonic homosexuality was removed prior to publication of the DSM-IV. These changes corresponded to increasing momentum of the gay civil rights movement.

The history of the pathologization of the transgender community was not mentioned earlier due to its distinct history. That said, into the early twentieth century, sexual orientation and gender identity were conflated in the concept of "sexual inversion," which will not be discussed here. Nonetheless, awareness of and response to **gender discordance** and transgender people advanced slowly in the twentieth century. Experimental sex-change operations began in the 1920s and 30s in Europe. It is unclear when they began in the United States, but they did occur prior to 1950, primarily for persons with **differences of sex development (DSD)**. During the 1930s, endocrinologist Harry Benjamin was one of the first physicians in the United States to treat transgender people with hormone therapy to change their gender appearance. In the 1950s, the term **transsexual** became widely used to describe individuals who desired to change their sex. In 1952, the news media publicized the story of

Christine Jorgensen, born George Jorgensen, who underwent sex reassignment surgery to live as a woman in Denmark. (A contemporary term is *gender affirming surgery*.) This encouraged many transgender people to consider surgical options despite being denied these surgeries in the United States.

In 1979, an interdisciplinary group of health care providers formed the Harry Benjamin International Gender Dysphoria Association, now known as the World Professional Association for Transgender Health (WPATH). Gender dysphoria was defined as serious distress with one's gender identity and thus led to a broader definition of who might be eligible for sex reassignment surgery. In the United States, diagnoses related to gender dysphoria first appeared in the DSM-III (1980) and included gender identity disorder for children, transsexualism (for adolescents and adults), and gender identity disorder of adolescence and adulthood, nontranssexual type (added in the DSM III-R in 1987). With the release of the DSM-IV (1994), the three gender diagnoses were collapsed into gender identity disorder (GID). In 2013, the DSM-5 removed GID but introduced a new diagnosis—**gender dysphoria**. These psychiatric diagnoses have been helpful for many seeking medical and surgical treatments, but many argue for their removal because they may continue to pathologize gender nonconformity. Gender dysphoria and approaches to social transition, hormonal transition, and surgical transition as gender affirmation methods are discussed in Chap. 10.

In the twentieth century, some mental health clinicians offered therapies known as conversion or reparative therapy to change one's sexual orientation. These therapies were often based on religious ideas. Some studies and many interviews showed that these therapies could be harmful. Further, no randomized clinical trials supported the efficacy of reparative therapy, and two poorly designed retrospective studies were refuted. In 1998, the APA approved a position statement on conversion therapy: "…[T]he American Psychiatric Association opposes any psychiatric treatment, such as reparative or conversion therapy which is based upon the assumption that homosexuality *per se* is a mental disorder or based upon the *a priori* assumption that the patient should change his/her sexual orientation."

Social changes accelerated in the 1990s. At many levels of society, from schools, marriage, the military, to adoption, LGBTQ people became more visible. School harassment and bullying based on sexual orientation and gender non-conformity were increasingly recognized. It was acknowledged that LGBTQ students were not only being mentally and physically traumatized, but they were not attending school, not performing as well, and sometimes dropping out. Many schools incorporated LGBTQ support groups to help deal with this bullying.

Chaps. 1 and 2 discuss the rapid shift toward marriage equality as well as other significant legal changes recognizing the equality of LGBTQ persons. Multiple research studies also showed positive health outcomes associated with marriage, such as decreased levels of depression, less substance use, and decreased subjective stress.

Key Points

- Pathologization of homosexuality peaked in the twentieth century, resulting in inhumane treatments such as involuntary commitment to mental hospitals, hormone therapy, castration, and lobotomy.
- A significant turning point was the removal of homosexuality from the DSM in 1973. The American Psychiatric Association opposes reparative or conversion therapy.
- For transgender persons, there are significant tensions around the diagnosis of gender dysphoria. While the diagnosis is helpful for many seeking medical and surgical treatments, it may also be seen as pathologizing gender nonconformity.
- Because of the relatively small role of health care in determining overall health, the greatest improvements in health outcomes for LGBTQ populations are garnered by changes in the

social determinants of health. Civil rights victories and other social and legal advances have been a boon. Nevertheless, LGBTQ people continue to experience shame, guilt, powerlessness and invisibility leading to mental and physical health disparities.

Case 12.1

Mary, 80, presents to Family Medicine clinic today with her partner Barb, 84. Both are lesbian-identifying cisgender women. Mary was added onto the schedule only a couple hours ago. They have been together for 55 years and have been patients of this clinic for over a decade. The resident physician enters the exam room, and after 25 minutes, exits the exam room appearing distraught.

While typing up admission orders, the resident shares that Mary has an extensive cardiovascular disease history and appears to be in acute decompensated heart failure today. He learned that Mary has for several months been struggling with basic activities of daily living (ADLs), specifically functional mobility and self-grooming. Mary now lives exclusively on the first floor of their two-story home and has not been upstairs in over a year. Barb assists Mary with some ADLs but several times has lost balance and fallen while trying to help move Mary into the shower. Barb appears overwhelmed and depressed.

The resident continues by explaining that Mary and Barb were initially resistant to the idea of a hospital admission until the severity of this acute decompensation was reiterated several times. Barb and Mary were receptive to a brief conversation about end of life planning but quickly became frustrated when the resident asked whether they had considered transitioning into an assisted living arrangement like a community-based residential facility (CBRF).

Looking back through Mary's chart in the electronic medical record, the resident finds notes from admission four years ago when Mary was treated for complicated diverticulitis. One of the notes mentions that Mary "fired" one of her nurses and then left against medical advice.

Based on their ages, what experiences may Mary and Barb have had as lesbian women that would differ from an opposite-sex couple of the same generation?

How might the events of the previous hospitalization be explained?

Mary and Barb have been partners for a long time but are not legally married. How does affect them in terms of long-term care and end of life planning?

It is common and understandable that older adults want to stay in their own homes as long as possible. Clinicians are frequently called upon to participate in difficult discussions related to the ability of aging persons to remain in their own homes and to caregiver burnout. The ability of familial and social supports to buffer an aging or sick patient's increasing dependence is an important consideration. As older women who came of age at a time when living openly as lesbians was unlikely to be an option, it is possible that Barb and Mary have relied on each other very heavily for many years. They may have faced difficult circumstances, including social and familial rejection, together. LGBTQ older adults are more likely to be socially isolated than other older adults. Additionally, lesbian women of their time are also far less likely than lesbians of today to have children who may be able and willing to assist in support and care.

With the limited available information, it is difficult to speculate on the events of the previous hospitalization and her extreme reluctance to be hospitalized now. However, it may be worthwhile to spend the time to discuss those events to anticipate how to improve the impending and future hospitalizations. Some suspicions are worth visiting. Firstly, Mary may have had past negative experiences with health care professionals that justify having highly defensive behaviors with staff (this should also be considered as a possible factor for acute compensation if Mary generally avoids health care environments). Secondly, Mary may recall negative experiences she has heard about from friends and acquaintances or even high-profile stories such as that of Lisa Pond and her partner Janice Langbehn, who along with their three adopted children were not allowed to visit Lisa as she lay dying in Miami's Jackson Memorial Hospital. Thirdly, it is possible that Mary or Barb experienced hostile or derogatory treatment by staff during that encounter. Finally, the choice to leave AMA may have had nothing to do with her lesbian identity. In any case, sensitive and open-ended questioning are the most likely to be helpful in the current situation.

There are over a thousand statutory provisions in which marital status is a factor in determining benefits, rights, and privileges. Before the Supreme Court legalized civil marriage equality nationwide in their finding in Obergefell v. Hodges *in 2015, same-sex couples in states without civil marriage equality either had to live without the equal protections or find work-arounds. Many LGBTQ people who are legally married still find it necessary to have additional strategies for legal protections, such as health care powers of attorney, special guardianship arrangements with non-biological parents, etc. Some especially important issues related to civil marriage are insurance eligibility through spouses and parents, immigration sponsorship, family visitation for spouse and non-biological children in care facilities, next-of-kin status for emergency medical decisions and wrongful medical death*

claims, domestic violence interventions, decisions about post-mortem anatomical gifts, survivor benefits, and Medicaid poverty protections applying to certain assets while a spouse is in a care facility. Not all of these can be achieved through mechanisms other than civil marriage. Though every adult, and especially older adults, should have advance directives in place, for Mary and Barb the designation of a health care proxy and the expression of their end of life preferences are especially urgent and may provide significant feelings of safety. Because Mary is competent to prepare these documents, they can be started immediately at this appointment.

By presidential executive order ("Respecting the Rights of Hospital Patients to Receive Visitors and to Designate Surrogate Decision Makers for Medical Emergencies"), patients in hospitals participating in Medicare or Medicaid have the right to designate visitors who shall receive the same visitation privileges as the patient's immediate family members, regardless of whether the visitors are legally related to the patient. Additionally, the order states that all patients' advance directives, such as durable powers of attorney and health care proxies, are to be respected, and that patients' designated representatives otherwise have the right to make informed decisions regarding patients' care.

The protective effects of marriage are thought to be derived from the increased social support and

External Resource 12.2
Drag Queen Panti Bliss's monologue, **"Panti's Noble Call at the Abbey Theatre,"** illustrates minority stress, the evolution of proximal stressors from distal stressors, and internalized homophobia. Total time 10:48.
http://bit.ly/TECe1ch12_02

Table 12.1 Biopsychosocial factors significant to LGBTQ mental health. Factors significant to LGBTQ mental health are listed across domains. Factors listed are not necessarily exclusive to LGBTQ people. Some cross domains. A factor may be harmful, protective, mixed, or irrelevant in a given patient's formulation

Biological	Psychological	Social
Alcohol use	Coming out/"Outness"	Coming out/"Outness"
Health care avoidance	Body image	Community membership
HIV status	Conversion therapy	Employment discrimination
Homelessness	History of abuse	Familial acceptance
Hormonal transition	History of bullying	HIV status
Illicit drug use	Internalized homophobia	Homelessness
Reproductive opportunities	Internalized transphobia	Homophobic community
Risk-taking behaviors	Perceived threats	Housing discrimination
Surgical transition	Positive identity	Insurance status
Violence	Vigilance	Intersectionality
		Intimate partner violence
		Legal partnership
		Romantic partnership
		School climate
		Social transition
		Support groups
		Supportive neighbors
		Transphobic community
		Unsafe neighborhood

legal benefits of marriage. Nevertheless, LGBTQ people continue to experience shame, guilt, powerlessness, and invisibility leading to mental and physical health disparities.

Minority Stress

Two important models of mental illness are the biopsychosocial model and the diathesis-stress model. The **biopsychosocial model** incorporates biological, psychological, and social factors as highly interdependent determinants of mental health and illness. It is a common model used to formulate a working hypothesis for psychopathology in individual patients. Table 12.1 lists some biopsychosocial factors that are common for LGBTQ people. The **diathesis-stress model** conceptualizes that every person has an innate vulnerabilities (diatheses) to mental illness, and psychopathology emerges when these vulnerabilities encounter sufficient stress. As stated before, high prevalence of mental disorders among minority groups may be attributed to greater exposure to social stressors and more limited access to protective psychosocial resources.

A third model, **minority stress theory**, proposes that sexual minority health disparities can be explained in large part by stressors induced by a hostile, homophobic and transphobic dominant culture. It is a useful framework to examine LGBTQ health disparities. Minority stresses are attributable to being a member of a minority group or to being perceived as a member of a minority group. In this model, **distal stressors** are external stimuli (objective stimuli) that are characteristics of an individual's social environment. Distal stressors include harassment, maltreatment, personal and structural discrimination, restricted access to advancement opportunities, and victimization. **Proximal stressors** can be thought of as internal stimuli (subjective stimuli) that rely on individual perceptions. Proximal stressors include expectations of suffering prejudice and the internalization of negative societal attitudes as self-devaluation. Proximal stressors typically arise as a result of distal stressors and may continue even after distal stressors are removed. While some distal and proximal stressors are unique to LGBTQ populations, it is also that many common stressors are simply more prevalent in LGBTQ populations. Although proximal stressors rely on self-identification as a minority, distal stressors usually depend on others' perception that one is a member of a group. **Internalized homophobia** is the conscious or unconscious application of negative societal attitudes and stereotypes about homosexuality to oneself, resulting in self-devaluation or denial.

The minority stress model also incorporates **protective factors**. Sexual minorities may draw upon personal and community-level coping mechanisms and resources to develop resilience. Those who adopt a strong sexual minority identity may be better equipped to manage minority stressors, challenge stereotypes, and address perceived or actual homophobia while affirming a positive self-evaluation. Identity-affirming therapy can mitigate the harms that result from internalizing negative concepts about one's own minority status. Familial and (to a lesser extent) peer supports have the strongest protective potential when they are present and most damaging

potential when they are absent. Unfortunately, compared to other minority groups such as those defined by race or ethnicity, LGBTQ people are more likely to confront negative attitudes from family and peers because they do not share the common minority identity. Figure 12.1 schematizes minority stress in LGBTQ populations.

Understanding minority stress processes can help health professionals and other professionals identify points of intervention to prevent or mitigate harm in individuals and populations. No one health profession can perform all the roles necessary to counteract minority stress for LGBTQ persons. A mental health care team may include psychiatrists, physician assistants, psychologists, pharmacists and/or nurses. Mental health care requires strong coordination with other care providers, particularly the primary care provider. Where access is limited, primary care physicians often act as the sole psychiatric care provider for persons with mental illness.

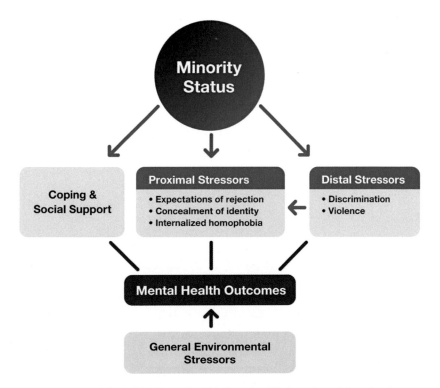

Fig. 12.1 Minority stress model for LGBTQ people. This is a simplified version of the minority stress model. Both protective factors and stressors may be associated with minority status. Proximal stressors can be thought of as internal stimuli (subjective stimuli) that rely on individual perceptions, while distal stressors are external occurrences. Proximal stressors often arise from distal stressors

Effective efforts to combat minority stress must be multi-sectorial and not confined to the clinic. Workers in the health sector need to collaborate with social work and education. Social workers are sometimes available in clinical settings. Social workers may help LGBTQ persons access competent, effective social services. Group support and community-led peer groups may also play a significant role in offering support and coping strategies. In schools and universities, an understanding of minority stress informs the design of homophobia- and transphobia-reducing school-based interventions such as gay-straight alliances. Gay-straight alliances reduce stressors and develop resilience in LGBTQ students. There is

Key Points
- LGBTQ persons are not more innately prone to psychopathology than the general population but are more likely to suffer psychopathology due to a variety of internal and external factors.
- The biopsychosocial model conceptualizes that biological, psychological, and social factors are highly interdependent determinants of mental health and illness.
- The diathesis-stress model conceptualizes that every person has innate vulnerabilities (diatheses) to mental illness. Vulnerability level determines the impact of stressors.
- Minority stress theory proposes that sexual minority health disparities are in large part due in to stressors induced by a homophobic and transphobic dominant culture. Under this model, stressors can be categorized as distal or proximal.
- Distal stressors are objective, external stressors (e.g., discrimination or violence). Proximal stressors are subjective, internal stressors (e.g., concealment of identity or internalized homophobia). Distal stressors largely contribute to proximal stressors.

- Internalized homophobia is the conscious or unconscious application of negative societal attitudes and stereotypes about homosexuality to oneself, resulting in self-devaluation or denial.
- Efforts to counteract minority stress and its psychological effects should draw on interprofessional teams and multi-sectorial interventions.

Case 12.2
An adolescent male who secretly thinks of himself as gay is taunted by classmates and sometimes physically threatened when he walks home from high school. The classmates perceive him as gay and feminine. Over time, the adolescent learns to anticipate and avoid his classmates after school. Avoiding his classmates is a significant source of anxiety.

Later, in college, in the absence of apparent danger, he still feels anxious about walking home from school and pays constant attention to his surroundings while trying to "walk straight." He continues to conceal his gay identity and does not socially integrate with other college students. He regrets being gay. In the absence of social support, he experiences a major depressive episode and generalized anxiety during his second year of college.

What are the distal and proximal stressors in this case? How are they related?

What are the criteria for a major depressive episode?

How common is it for patients to have both major depression and generalized anxiety?

What would have been plausible protective factors or interventions that could have prevented his mental illness?

This case demonstrates internalization of hostile attitudes in his community as inter-

nalized homophobia. The threat of physical harm and negative assumptions about his gender expression are unambiguous distal stressors. The resulting desire to avoid others and to conceal his identity while walking home are proximal stressors. Since high school, this adolescent seems to have lacked protective factors (though we know nothing of his family life).

Table 12.2 lists diagnostic criteria for major depressive disorder (MDD). Take note that the symptoms must be present within the same two-week interval and be different from the individual's prior functionality, causing clinically significant distress or impairments in important areas of functioning.

Studies of outpatients with depression have found that over 40% met criteria for comorbid anxiety. Though medical treatments for depression and anxiety are certainly indicated now that he has developed comorbid depression and generalized anxiety, gay affirmative psychotherapy and identity-affirming social groups should be considered as parts of a comprehensive plan to address the root causes of his mental illness. Family support is one of the most significant factors that may be protective when present and harmful when absent. Peer support is also crucial. A Gay-Straight Alliance (GSA) or similar organization in his high school or community could have prevented or mitigated homophobia in his environment and helped prevent his internalization of negative attitudes about his sexuality.

Table 12.2 DSM-5 diagnostic criteria for major depressive disorder. These symptoms must be present within the same two-week interval and be different from the individual's prior functionality. The symptoms must cause clinically significant distress or impairments in important areas of functioning.

Either or Both	
Depressed mood	Loss of interest or pleasure
And at Least Five of the Following:	
Diminished interest or pleasure in activities, most of the time, verified by subjective account or observation	Diminished concentration or decisiveness, nearly every day, by subjective account or observation
Significant change in weight or appetite (increase or decrease)	Recurrent thoughts of death, recurrent suicidal ideation with or without a specific plan, or suicidal attempt
Insomnia or hypersomnia, nearly every day	Fatigue or loss of energy, nearly every day
Sentiments of guilt or diminished worth	Psychomotor agitation or retardation, beyond subjective restlessness or slowing
Depressed mood most of the day, as observed subjectively by self or others or objectively by provider	

Case 12.3

A 33-year-old Afro-Latina trans woman is referred to a psychiatric clinic after she admits re-experiencing a traumatic event for the last three months. She began hormonal and social transition simultaneously two years ago when she says she "finally came out of the closet as a woman." Her surgical history includes an appendectomy nine years ago and a breast augmentation six months ago. She has a history of alcohol abuse but has not had any alcohol for 5 years. Two weeks after discharge from her recent surgery, she was punched and briefly dragged by her hair after grocery shopping in the late evening. Most injuries were mild, but she suffered a concussion and abrasions her face and arm. She says that she alternates between feeling extremely alert with a sometimes racing heart and feeling exhausted. She now has groceries delivered to her house. She says that she blames herself for going shopping in the late evening. A sexual history and physical exam were omitted because they were irrelevant to the acute presentation.

In addition to the primary diagnosis, what other psychiatric issues should be acknowledged?

What distal stressors are described in this case?

What proximal stressors are described or implied in this case?

How may the current coping strategies be problematic? How can more helpful coping strategies be cultivated?

What areas—including those mentioned above—should be given special attention in her biopsychosocial formulation?

Her history includes traumatic experience, re-experiencing, sympathetic arousal, and avoidance with symptoms lasting at least a month. She has stereotypic post-traumatic stress disorder (PTSD). DSM-5 criteria for PTSD are extensive. Violent victimization itself is a distal stressor. Implied proximal stressors are expectations of victimization and exaggerated negative beliefs about herself—self-blame.

Though the cause and time course of PTSD appear recent, it is important to consider that some anxiety may reflect earlier stresses related to concealing her gender identity until two years ago. It is also important to address her alcohol abuse history because relapse is possible. Recent surgery should be acknowledged as a significant stressor and a potential trauma. While the development of PTSD in this patient can be explained using models that do not incorporate minority status, her heightened risk of victimization and access to viable forms of therapeutic and social support must take into account her gender identity. Transgender women of color are at extremely high risk of violent victimization (review intersectionality).

This patient's primary coping strategy—avoidance—may be effective for preventing distressful situations, but it leaves her unable to participate in society to the extent that she was once able. While medical management of distressing symptoms can lower barriers to resuming normal life activities, coping strategies can be improved through counseling or other positive social relationships.

The biopsychosocial formulation is left to the reader to complete independently. It may be useful to speculate about previous experiences of trauma and current protective factors in the course of the formulation.

unexploited potential for health educators and community health workers to provide tailored, culturally competent services to LGBTQ community members. Chap. 4 explains the high importance of competent social and behavioral health services and programs, with a special emphasis on LGBTQ youth.

LGBTQ Mental Health Disparities

The previous section discussed how minority stress theory explains why LGBTQ individuals are more likely to suffer from psychopathology even though they are not more innately prone to psychopathology than the general population.

Affective, anxiety, and substance use disorders appear to be especially reactive to the effects of social stress. This association may explain why these disorders are so prevalent in the LGBTQ community. Similar to non-LGBT persons, the most frequent presenting problems of LGBT persons include depression, anxiety, and relationship issues.

Epidemiology

As discussed in section "Minority Stress," LGBTQ individuals often face significant trauma and stigma in their lives, generating psychological stress that has been linked to mental health problems. These stressors vary with socioeconomic and demographic factors and are often additive. For example, racial discrimination against African-American, Asian and Pacific Islander, and Latino individuals further increases risk of psychiatric illness in these populations beyond those of white LGBT individuals. Psychiatric illness in LGBTQ populations manifests most commonly as depression, self-harm and suicidality, anxiety, and mixed disorders.

The prevalence of psychiatric morbidity has been shown to range from 42% to 49% among gay, lesbian, and bisexual populations. This prevalence is despairingly high when compared to 12% and 20% of heterosexual men and women, respectively. The situation for LGBT youth is also troubling, with prevalence of suicidal ideation and self-harm reaching 30% and 5% among LGBT high school students compared to 6% and 3% among their non-LGBT peers, respectively. The proportion of LGBT youth considering a suicide attempt within the last year is also double that of their non-LGBT peers (31% vs. 14%, respectively). An analysis of Californian students found a three-fold prevalence of suicidal ideation in the past 12 months for transgender students compared to non-transgender students. LGBTQ youth face these additional risk factors in the context of a high-risk age range for suicidal behavior. Suicide incidence decreases with age in mid-adulthood. Recent data also indicate higher risk of psychiatric illness in bisexual individuals when compared to their gay or lesbian peers, suggesting the presence of risk factors unique to the bisexual experience.

Transgender persons of all ages have been shown to have the highest prevalence of depression, suicidal ideation, death by suicide, anxiety, and other psychiatric illnesses. This especially high prevalence is likely secondary to discrimination, diminished socioeconomic opportunities, increased poverty, lower educational attainment, and higher prevalence of risky sexual behavior and sex work.

Lesser-known psychiatric morbidities among LGBTQ individuals are eating disorders and body dysmorphia. Interestingly, changes in body perception and eating disorders are different among different LGBTQ subgroups, with the most studies comparing lesbian women and gay men to their heterosexual counterparts. Compared to heterosexual men, gay men have greater dissatisfaction with their bodies and higher relative risk of eating disorders, as defined by negative body image and perception leading to body dysmorphia. In contrast, lesbian women exhibit the opposite phenomenon, showing higher prevalence of satisfaction with their bodies and greater likelihood of overweight or obesity. These studies suggest that social and cultural factors significantly contribute to how LGBT individuals view their bodies.

Depression

Depression is common in all populations, but it is especially prevalent in LGBTQ populations. The most common feature of depressive disorders is a sad, empty, or irritable mood, often in the setting of both somatic and cognitive changes. These changes frequently impair the individual's functional capacity but can also present in nonspecific symptoms and complaints. LGB pcople have at least twice the 12-month prevalence and lifetime risk of depression of heterosexual people. Variables associated with depression in gay men include history of suicide attempt, child abuse, and sexual dysfunction. Moreover, some variables associated with depression reflect internal and external homophobia, such as a recent history of anti-gay threats or violence; not identifying as gay, queer, or homosexual; or feeling alienated from the gay community. These issues should be explored in interview in addition to depression symptomatology.

Given its high prevalence in the LGBTQ population, depression is a major public health concern and significant challenge for clinicians treating LGBTQ patients. Therefore, screening for mental illness, especially for anxiety and mood disorders, should be given special priority in LGBTQ patients.

The most frequently studied subtype in LGBTQ epidemiological studies is major depressive disorder, which is defined by the presence of criteria defined in Table 12.2.

Table 12.3 DSM-5 diagnostic criteria for generalized anxiety disorder

Excessive anxiety and worry occurring more often than not for at least 6 months involving many facets of life (e.g. work, school, events, activities)	Association with three or more of the following: restlessness, fatigue, lack of concentration, irritability, muscle tension, sleep disturbance
Inability to control worry	Lack of attributable physiology or other condition
Resultant clinically significant distress or impairment in occupational, social, and other aspects of life	Lack of another mental disorder to better explain the condition

Table 12.4 Warning signs for suicidality. Clinical suspicion should be raised if one or more of the above signs are present via the patient's history or testimony by the patient's friends or family

Hopelessness	Rage, anger, or revenge seeking
Recklessness or engaging in risky behavior	Sensation of being trapped
Increasing substance use	Withdrawal from friends, family, or society at large
Anxiety or agitation	Insomnia or hypersomnia
Dramatic mood changes	Loss of motivation to live or purpose for life

Anxiety/Panic Attacks

Similar to depression, *anxiety* is a blanket term for many anxiety disorders. The common threads among anxiety disorders are features of excessive fear or anticipation of a future threat and related behavioral changes and disturbances. Defining characteristics of anxiety disorders are autonomic surges, thoughts of imminent danger, escape behaviors, muscle tension, and preparation for future danger or caution and avoidance thereof. While risk for anxiety disorders is largely physiological and genetic, environmental triggers are widely prevalent in LGBTQ individuals' communities, involving general life stress, separation from parental figures, and romantic relationships. Sexual minority men and women have at least double risk for having any anxiety disorder. There are subtle gender differences. Gay and bisexual men have a higher prevalence of panic attacks than heterosexual men. Lesbian and bisexual women have a greater prevalence of generalized anxiety disorder than heterosexual women. Criteria for generalized anxiety disorder are provided in Table 12.3.

Suicidal Thoughts and Suicidal Behavior

The coverage of endemic suicides of LGBTQ youth has become popular among news media in the USA. Suicide is often a gradual process, preceded by a state of depression or psychiatric instability and followed by a period of susceptibility to further damage. LGB individuals have twice the prevalence of suicidal ideation as heterosexuals and are six times more likely than heterosexuals to report one or more lifetime suicide attempts by age 21. The lifetime suicide attempt prevalence is higher in gay and bisexual men (about four times the rate of comparable heterosexual men) than in lesbian and bisexual women (about two times the rate of comparable heterosexual women). There is an opposite gender trend for suicidal ideation than for suicide attempts. Lesbian/bisexual women have a higher risk of suicidal ideation whereas gay and bisexual men have a higher risk of suicide attempts. For transgender persons, as high as 47% have considered or attempted suicide in the past three years. Symptoms and behaviors associated with risk of suicide are described in Table 12.4.

Eating Disorders and Body Dysmorphia

Eating disorders include a broad disturbance of eating habits, including any disturbance that impairs physical or psychosocial health. Among the most common eating disorders (and also the most common in LGBT people) are anorexia ner-

Table 12.5 A summary of DSM-5 signs and symptoms of common eating disorders

Disorder	Descriptor	Common symptoms and signs
Anorexia nervosa	Intentional restriction of caloric intake to attain a body low weight, accompanied by an intense fear of gaining weight or disruption of body image	Fear of gaining weight or becoming "fat," weight loss, low BMI, malnutrition, amenorrhea, osteopenia or osteoporosis, nausea, vomiting, metabolic disorders
Bulimia nervosa	Recurrent binge-eating and self-incurred behaviors to prevent weight gain (e.g. vomiting), motivated by an impaired understanding of body image	Nausea, vomiting, medication abuse, normal or overweight BMI, menstrual irregularity or amenorrhea, emotional distress, esophageal tears, gastric rupture, cardiac arrhythmia, skeletal myopathies
Avoidant/ restrictive food intake disorder	An aversion to or lack of interest in the consumption of food	Weight loss, nutritional deficiency, failure to thrive, mood disorders

vosa, bulimia nervosa, and avoidant/restrictive food intake disorder. These disorders are summarized in Table 12.5.

LGBTQ individuals have increased risks of body dysmorphia, especially gay men. Body dysmorphia is defined as impaired functioning, both psychological and social, due to concerns with appearance. The degree of malfunction varies from moderate (avoiding social situations) to severe (avoidance that inhibits work, social interactions, and school). Individuals suffering from severe body dysmorphia are frequently hospitalized in a psychiatric facility. Generally, more severe cases are found in younger individuals, especially adolescents. It is important to recognize that body dysmorphia, an eating disorder, does not equate to gender dysphoria, a term describing a desire to manifest a gender identity that differs from the one assigned at birth. High body dissatisfaction merits diagnostic attention to eating disorders, body dysmorphia, and gender dysphoria.

Special Populations

Child and Adolescent
LGBTQ youth face unique struggles for their mental health. At school, many face increased bullying and victimization, which are significant predictors of depression and suicide attempts. Gender non-conformity in childhood has been associated with the development of an LGBTQ identity and with increased psychological distress, perhaps mediated by bullying and abuse.

LGBT youth have been found to have approximately four times the prevalence of depression, three times the prevalence of anxiety, and four times the prevalence of conduct disorder than other youth. Approximately 20–42% attempt suicide, 30–42% contemplate suicide, and 21% engage in self-harm behaviors.

Geriatric
Most older LGBTQ individuals have experienced discrimination and overt harassment, in addition to a strong fear of discovery and a need to hide one's identity. The mental health consequences of living such a life is not trivial. One-third of elderly LGBT individuals experience some kind of mental health problem in their life. Eleven percent of older LGBT individuals experience suicidal ideation, 4% self-harm, and 83% regular alcohol use. One-fourth of LGBT elders reported needing help for emotional or mental health problems, compared to 14% of aging heterosexual adults.

Ethnic/Racial Minorities
Ethnic/racial minorities who are also sexual and gender minorities experience dual levels of stigma and maltreatment due to both sexuality and race, a result of identity intersectionality. There is a significant association between sexuality-related bullying and depressive symptomatology, history of attempted suicide, and reporting parental abuse. Minority race/ethnicity is associated with a significantly increased risk of suicide attempts in youth. Suicide attempts are especially frequent among African-American LGB adolescents and gay and bisexual adult men of lower socioeconomic status.

Resilience

Despite the mental health challenges and disparities, the majority of LGBTQ individuals do not experience psychopathology despite considerable obstacles, such as extreme homophobia and marginalization. Cultivating the strengths of LGBTQ individuals and communities offers novel opportunities to improve mental health. For example, focusing on the strength of shamelessness can counter homophobia and thereby lead to

External Resource 12.3
In 2012, LGBT students at Brigham Young University (BYU) made a video for the It Gets Better Project, an online video project created to show LGBTQ people that they are not alone and that their lives will get much better if they can just get through their teens. In **"It Gets Better at Brigham Young University,"** Twenty-two students at BYU describe their struggle with their religion and their sexuality. Some of the statistics in the video are sobering: of about 1800 LGBT students at BYU, 74% contemplate suicide, and 24% attempt suicide. http://bit.ly/TECe1ch12_03

Key Points
- LGBTQ individuals are at increased risk for poor mental health.
- Depression and anxiety disorders are more prevalent in LGBTQ populations. This disparity is related to these being stress-sensitive conditions.
- Suicidal behavior is elevated in LGBTQ communities, especially among LGBTQ youth.
- LGBTQ mental health is also impacted by age, gender, and ethnicity.
- Despite the increased risk for poor mental health, LGBTQ individuals and communities are also resilient.

Case 12.4
A 19-year-old lesbian female college student struggles to reconcile her sexual orientation with her religion. She had grown up in a very religious family and many of her closest friends she met at religious events. When it came time to decide on which college to attend, she chose a university that was affiliated with her religion, initially looking forward to meeting many other students who shared her same values. She initially dates several men but soon realizes that she sexually prefers women. The realization terrifies her, as her religion and university are not friendly toward homosexuality. She believes that if she were to tell her friends and family, she would be ostracized and shunned, even expelled from the university.

She initially attempts to repress her sexual feelings, becoming more personally righteous, yet her situation does not improve. She begins entertaining the thought that perhaps it would be easier to end her life, believing that the pain of her death would be less than the pain of her coming out as gay to her family. She develops a plan to kill herself, including a note disclosing her sexual orientation, but decides to call the Trevor Project before acting out her plan. She receives help and is hospitalized at a psychiatric hospital.

When is the most vulnerable time for LGBTQ individuals to attempt suicide?

What is a resource for offer LGBTQ individuals contemplating suicide?

This case highlights the internal struggle that many LGBTQ individuals face when they feel their sexual orientation is not accepted by their religion. The risk for suicide attempts is highest during the adolescent years, and often closely linked to the moment when LGBTQ individuals recognize and disclose their sexual orientation to others. This patient is in an extremely vulnerable moment, nearing the end of her adolescence and just about to come out.

The Trevor Project is an online hotline designed to help LGBTQ individuals who are contemplating suicide or need help immediately. The number is 866-4-U-TREVOR (866-488-7386).

less internalized homophobia and depression. Encouraging sexual creativity may counter HIV risk and provide alternative strategies to create safe sexual expression. Harnessing the strengths and resiliencies of LGBTQ people increases the impact of health promotion efforts.

Substance Use in LGBTQ Populations

LGBTQ individuals are at particular risk for substance use disorders. Many factors are implicated, including the continued popularity of bars and nightclubs for social gatherings for LGBTQ communities, the culture of substance use in the LGBTQ population, and the use of substances to cope with the stresses of reconciling sexual orientation and gender identity with daily life. On average, LGBTQ individuals entering treatment for substance use have more severe substance use problems, greater psychopathology, and greater medical service utilization when compared with heterosexual clients. For LGBTQ adolescents, the number of rejections experienced when first disclosing their sexual orientation is associated with current and subsequent alcohol, cigarette, and marijuana use. This section examines some of the main substances used by the LGBTQ community: alcohol, tobacco, and recreational drugs.

Alcohol

Alcohol use is highly prevalent in the LGBTQ population, but there are notable gender differences. An estimated 85% of urban MSM use

alcohol. For women, it appears that sexual identity is more predictive of alcohol use than sexual behavior. For example, 13% of women identifying as lesbian met criteria for past-year alcohol dependence, compared to 5% of women attracted to women and 4% who have female sex partners. Among gay men, the frequency of alcohol use increased in those who were affluent, resided in urban areas, and had close interpersonal relationships. Mixed results among surveys show adult LGBT populations to have drinking prevalence either equivalent to or higher drinking than the general population. LGBT youth have consistently higher prevalence of alcohol use than the general population, with surveys showing 70% alcohol use prevalence among some populations of LGBT youth compared to 23% in comparable non-LGBT youth. Moreover, drinking behavior increased significantly over time in a linear fashion for LGBT youth, increasing more rapidly for LGBT male youth than female youth. Interestingly, this disparity may not impact long-term alcohol use habits: alcohol use frequency begins to normalize after the age of 18. The risks predisposing LGBTQ individuals to problematic alcohol use are hypothesized to include peer modeling, minority group stigmatization, and experiencing homophobia. Psychological distress and sexual orientation-based victimization are associated with increased alcohol use for female LGBT youth only.

Tobacco

Forty-five percent of LGBT individuals report current use of tobacco, compared to 29% of the general population. In California, gay and bisexual men smoked 50% more than all men, lesbian and bisexual women smoked three times as much as all women, and transgender Californians have double the prevalence of smoking compared to all Californians. LGBT identity predicted any prior cigarette use (about twice the rate of the general population) but not recent use. In addition to smoking more frequently at a younger age, additional risk factors specific to smoking include lower educational attainment, low socio-

Table 12.6 Toxidromes and Withdrawal Syndromes of select substances

Substance	Action	Intoxication symptoms and signs	Withdrawal syndrome
Hallucinogenics (LSD, ecstasy)	Hallucinogen	Hyperthermia, tachycardia, hypertension, tachypnea, euphoria, depersonalization, hallucinations, agitation, nystagmus, seizures	Fatigue, psychiatric and mood disturbances, fatigue, dysphoria
Alkyl nitrites (Poppers)	Stimulant	Hypotension, tachycardia, euphoria, headache, nausea, syncope, skin irritation, tracheobronchitis, allergic reaction, wheezing	Psychiatric and mood disturbances, tremor
Hypnotics (Barbiturates, Benzodiazepines)	Sedative	Hypothermia, bradycardia, hypotension, apnea, bradypnea, hyporeflexia, CNS depression, confusion, stupor, coma	Hypertension, tachycardia, nausea, vomiting, diarrhea, seizures, delirium, death

economic status, depression, stress, victimization by violence, and concurrent alcohol use.

Recreational Drugs

Recreational substance use among LGBTQ people varies among different subgroups. Recreational drug use is common, with weekly drug use in some subgroups of transgender individuals reaching 54%. Among gay men, prevalence can reach 29%. The types of recreational drugs being used are variable, with 28% of LGBT individuals using three or more drugs in the last six months. The most frequently used drug was marijuana, followed (in descending order) by cocaine, amphetamines, ecstasy, hallucinogens, poppers (alkyl nitrate), and barbiturates. Furthermore, the distribution of recreational drug use varies with sexual orientation and gender identity. Transgender individuals tend towards polydrug use, gay and bisexual men towards stimulants, and lesbian and bisexual women towards prescription medications.

Recreational drug use is very common in gay men and MSM. Approximately half of all urban MSM have used recreational drugs in the past six months. Use of club drugs, such as ecstasy, PCP, ketamine, and inhalants are disproportionately higher among gay and bisexual males than among heterosexual men. In Asia, ecstasy (3,4-methylenedioxy-N-methylamphetamine, or MDMA) (8.1%) and Viagra (sildenafil) (7.9%) were the most common recreational drugs used by MSM in the previous six months. HIV-positive MSM report significantly higher levels of individual drug use and polydrug use compared to HIV-negative or serotype unknown MSM. Among LGBT youth, there is nearly double prevalence of marijuana use among youth in neighborhoods with a higher number of LGBT assault hate crimes.

Substance use, particularly alcohol and recreational drugs, can lead to behavioral disinhibition, riskier sexual behavior, and exposure to HIV and other sexually-transmitted infections. For some drugs that have injectable forms, such as methamphetamine, users and their partners are at increased risk for transmission of HIV, hepatitis C, and STIs. The transmission of HIV and hepatitis C can occur sexually, through sharing injection needles, or both.

Table 12.6 summarizes symptoms associated with intoxication and withdrawal from less common illicit drugs.

> **Key Points**
> - LGBTQ individuals are at increased risk for substance use.
> - Different patterns of substance use emerge depending on gender.
> - Lesbian women are far more likely to use tobacco than other women. LGBTQ populations in general have much higher prevalence of tobacco use than the general population.
> - Gay men use more recreational drugs, such as inhalants and marijuana.
> - Increased substance use may put LGBTQ individuals at increased risk for HIV, hepatitis C, and STIs.

Case 12.5

A 32-year-old gay male who was recently introduced to methamphetamine through an acquaintance who promised that the drug would improve his sexual experience. He discovered that it did: sex was much more exhilarating now. He gradually transitioned from intranasal to smoking to injecting. For him, methamphetamine use was always associated with sexual activity. Initially, he would begin by starting on Friday night and ending by Saturday night or Sunday morning. However, eventually the weekend became too short and he began to miss Mondays at work. He would show up to work extremely tired and depressed. Though he recovered by Thursday, he began to have intense cravings again on Friday.

What are the DSM-5 criteria for a substance use disorder?

What are symptoms of methamphetamine intoxication?

What pharmacologic interventions are available to reduce methamphetamine use?

Methamphetamine is a powerful stimulant that markedly increases interest in and pleasure derived from sex. It is an extreme addictive. The prevalence of methamphetamine use in MSM is markedly higher than in the general population—as high as 10.4%.

The DSM-5 criteria for a substance use disorder is as follows: a problematic pattern of use of an intoxicating substance and leading to clinically significant impairment or distress, as manifested by at least two of the following, occurring within a 12-month period: (1) the substance is often taken in larger amounts or over a longer period than was intended; (2) there is a persistent desire or unsuccessful efforts to cut down or control use of the substance; (3) a great deal of time is spent in activities necessary to obtain the substance, use the substance, or recover from its effects; (4) craving, or a strong desire or urge to use the substance; (5) recurrent use of the substance resulting in a failure to fulfill major role obligations at work, school, or home; (6) continued use of the substance despite having persistent or recurrent social or interpersonal problems caused or exacerbated by the effects of its use; (7) important social, occupational, or recreational activities are given up or reduced because of use of the substance; (8) recurrent use of the substance in situations in which it is physically hazardous; (9) use of the substance is continued despite knowledge of having a persistent or recurrent physical or psychological problem that is likely to have been caused or exacerbated by the substance; (10) tolerance, as defined by either of the following: (a) a need for markedly increased amounts of the substance to achieve intoxication or desired effect, (b) a markedly diminished effect with continued use of the same amount of the substance; (11) withdrawal, as manifested by either of the following: (a) the characteristic withdrawal syndrome for other (or unknown) substance, (b) the substance (or a closely related substance) is taken to relieve or avoid withdrawal symptoms.*

*Symptoms of methamphetamine intoxication can mimic symptoms of schizophrenia, with paranoid delusions and hallucinations. In addition, a common symptom of methamphetamine intoxication is **formication**, a tactile hallucination of bugs crawling under one's skin. Methamphetamine users may have multiple skin lesions, which are a result of skin picking in response to formication.*

There are no medications approved by the Food and Drug Administration (FDA) for stimulant dependence. Mirtazapine, an FDA-approved antidepressant, is an attractive option because it has no apparent abuse potential, has an onset of action within two weeks, and is relatively inexpensive. Moreover, less than 1% of patients taking the drug report decreased erectile function, which may lead to greater acceptance in the sexually active MSM community. Mirtazapine is a mixed monoamine agonist/antagonist that facilitates the release of norepinephrine, serotonin, and dopamine. In a randomized controlled trial, the addition of mirtazapine to substance use counseling significantly decreased methamphetamine use among active users and was associated with significant decreases in sexual risk despite low to moderate medication adherence.

Neurology and Psychiatry of HIV

Depression

Depression is the most common psychiatric comorbidity of HIV infection, affecting up to 81% of persons living with HIV. The etiology of clinical depression with HIV infection is multifactorial. Individuals living with HIV and depression often have a history of psychiatric illness which likely predisposes them to depression in later life. This susceptibility can be exacerbated by the social stigmatization often accompanying the diagnosis of HIV infection. Additionally, the HIV infection itself is associated with biologic changes that may account for anxious or depressive symptoms. Studies have demonstrated that persons with a CD4+ T-cell count less than 100 cells/mm^3 have nearly triple the risk for showing signs of clinical depression.

Depression is associated with poorer health outcomes in people affected by both depression and HIV infection, highlighting the importance of screening for and treating depression. The presence of depression is associated with decreased control of viral load, likely due to negative effects of depression on medication adherence. HIV infection with comorbid depression decreases quality of life and increases the risk of substance dependence and unemployment. A patient who has a triple diagnosis of HIV infection, psychiatric illness, and a substance use disorder requires additional clinical consideration and support. Comorbid depression increases mortality in persons living with HIV. Depression is also a public health concern because it is associated with HIV transmission risk behaviors.

Assessing for depression is effective and critical. Populations with HIV/AIDS respond to depression treatment as well as non-HIV populations. Assessing for depression and anxiety symptoms in the health care setting should be regular and thorough for persons with HIV/AIDS. Special attention should be given to individuals who have risk factors for depression. Women and patients identifying a gay or bisexual are at greater risk for depression. Patients lacking social support should be promptly identified and assessed.

Similar to persons without HIV, selective serotonin reuptake inhibitors (SSRIs) are first line treatment of depression within HIV infection. Antiretroviral therapy (ART) itself may benefit depression. Patients who are on ART have significantly lower prevalence of depression. Obtaining and maintaining an undetectable viral load has been linked to depression remission. Unfortunately, evidence shows that depression interferes with psychiatric follow-up and treatment in individuals with HIV. Depression in HIV infection is grossly undertreated. Involving case managers and social workers can maximize continuity of care for patients and help establish financial security through employment or disability income, which are associated with the remission.

HIV-Associated Neurocognitive Disorders (HAND)

HIV-associated neurocognitive disorders (HAND) are a complication of HIV infection and treatment that have become more prevalent as antiretroviral therapies have extended lifespans and transformed HIV/AIDS into a chronic and more manageable illness. Other terms for HAND are HIV encephalopathy, HIV-associated dementia, and AIDS-dementia complex. HAND is characterized by decreased cognitive abilities in individuals with HIV/AIDS. Deficits in memory, attention, and reasoning have been described. Deficits are detectable through special testing even before clinically evident. These cognitive deficits are accompanied by accelerated aging-associated neuron loss in areas of higher cognitive processes in the neocortex. This volume loss is partly mitigated by maintaining higher CD4+ T-cell counts, demonstrating the cognitive benefits of early and sustained pharmacologic treatment of HIV.

However, the clinical picture of HAND is convoluted because neurologic side effects of ART can be difficult to differentiate from those of HIV. Some clinicians advocate for stopping ART for adherent patients with stable CD4+ T-cell counts to reduce potential psychological side effects of the medications. Extensive research is needed to determine the etiology and health consequences of HAND as well as potential treatments and modes of prevention. Cyproheptadine and serotonin reuptake inhibitors have been suggested as affordable and effective mitigators of HAND. In addition to pharmacologic treatment, health care providers should reiterate the importance of physical exercise and social engagement, because both contribute significantly to cognition and general wellbeing.

Distal Sensory Neuropathy

Distal sensory neuropathy (also called HIV-associated peripheral neuropathy) is a disabling, clinically challenging, and common neurologic sequela of HIV infection and treatment. It affects over half of all HIV-positive persons and varies in its clinical presentation. Its most common manifestation is distal neuropathic pain and paresthesia. Peripheral neuropathy is a well-described side effect of nucleoside reverse transcriptase inhibitors (NRTIs) as well as a direct neurologic sequela of HIV infection. It tends to be treatment resistant.

Psychiatric Side Effects of HIV Drugs

NRTIs, particularly zidovudine and abacavir, can cause mania and psychosis. The non-nucleoside reverse transcriptase inhibitor (NNRTI) efavirenz has been repeatedly associated with neurologic and psychiatric side effects amongst patients, with 2–13% of patients discontinuing the medication due to intolerable side effects, most frequently insomnia, irritability, and vivid dreams.

Other Neurologic Conditions

Other noteworthy neurologic sequelae of HIV infection are listed below, with a focus on epidemiology and diagnosis.

- Toxoplasma encephalitis is the most common central nervous system sequela of HIV/AIDS,

usually the result of reactivation of previous infection. Persons with CD4 cells <50 cells/mm^3 are at greatest risk. Typical findings are focal encephalitis, headache, motor weakness, and fever. MRI with contrast usually reveals classic ring-enhancing lesions with some predilection for the basal ganglia. Persons with CD4 cell counts less than 100 cells/mm^3 should be on trimethoprim-sulfamethoxazole (TMP/SMX) prophylaxis for Toxoplasma.

- Viral intracranial opportunistic infections include cytomegalovirus (CMV), varicella zoster virus (VZV), and herpes simplex virus (HSV). In general, clinically apparent encephalitis should prompt empiric treatment with acyclovir. CMV occurs most often at CD4 cells <50 cells/mm^3, causing acute meningo-encephalitis. Diffuse patchy changes are seen on imaging. VZV has diverse presentations; the most important is cerebral vasculitis leading to strokes and transient ischemic attacks. HSV is not common, but classic findings include headache, fever, and seizure. HSV has a predilection for the temporal and inferior frontal lobes. Edema and focal hemorrhage may occur.

- Cryptococcal meningitis may have a long subacute phase before fulminant meningitis. Subacute carriage is common in persons with CD4 cells <50 cells/mm^3. It can occur alongside pulmonary infection. Cryptococcal antigen tests of various fluids (including cerebrospinal fluid) have supplanted the India ink stain. The case-fatality is 10% even with good medical care.

- HIV-associated progressive multifocal leukoencephalopathy (PML) accounts for greater than 80% of PML cases and is associated with the ubiquitous JC virus. It is a demyelinating disease. Extensive white matter lesions can be observed on brain MRI. HIV-associated PML usually occurs below a CD4 count of 200 cells/mm^3. Importantly, initiating ART can cause a rare but extremely dangerous complication called immune reconstitution inflammatory syndrome (IRIS), in which white matter damage is provoked by immune reconstitution.

- AIDS-related non-Hodgkin's lymphoma may spread into the brain.
- Primary central nervous system lymphoma is also a non-Hodgkin's lymphoma that usually presents as a brain tumor. Spinal cord, eyes, and leptomeninges are frequently affected.
- Mononeuropathy multiplex occurs at low CD4 counts and is associated with opportunistic viral infections of nerves. Loss of sensory or motor function corresponds to the anatomy served by a peripheral nerve. Multiple separate peripheral nerves may be affected.
- Progressive polyradiculopathy occurs in advanced immunosuppression (CD4 counts <50 cells/mm^3), almost always affecting lumbosacral nerve roots. It is typically due to CMV, in which case appropriate antiviral treatment may preserve neurologic function. Lumbosacral pain, saddle anaesthesia, and urinary retention are common symptoms.

Key Points
- Depression is a common and debilitating comorbidity within HIV infection requiring active screening and treatment.
- Adequate treatment of depression in the setting of HIV infection produces individual and public health benefits because it reduces morbidity and reduces HIV transmission risk.
- Increasing CD4+ T-cell counts and optimizing ART treatment help control HIV-associated neurocognitive disorders (HAND).
- Sensory neuropathy is a common and often intractable side effect of NRTI medications. It causes significant morbidity in persons living with HIV.
- Several infections and lymphoma may cause diverse and often catastrophic neurologic problems. The differential for nervous system pathology is broad, especially in advanced immunosuppression.

Case 12.6

Dave, a 46-year-old man, presents to HIV clinic. He has been followed by the clinic for a decade since he was diagnosed with HIV and has been adherent to his medications. He is currently taking efavirenz (NNRTI), lamivudine (NRTI), and stavudine (NRTI). His CD4 count from the lab two weeks ago was 280 cells/mm^3. He has a six-year history of neuropathic pain affecting the feet. Other chronic conditions include obesity (BMI 36), type II diabetes mellitus in excellent control (HbA1c<6.4% for many years), and eczema that appears during the winter.

Today, he complains of pain and paresthesia in his right hand that he calls "prickly and sometimes burning." He relates the sensation to what he has felt in both his feet. The pain has worsened gradually over the course of several months. Last week, he also noticed pain and numbness in his lateral right thigh. On neurologic exam, there is diminished sensation to pinprick and vibration of both feet up to the mid-calf. There is mildly diminished sensation to pinprick and vibration throughout the right hand; left hand normal. Strength throughout the upper and lower extremities is 5/5 everywhere tested, including grip strength. All deep tendon reflexes are normal.

What is the most likely explanation for the new symptoms in his right hand?

What is the most likely explanation for the new symptoms in his right thigh?

What are some approaches to distal sensory neuropathy that may be considered in this case?

Distal sensory neuropathy, no matter the source, is typically progressive and noticed first in the lower extremities, beginning from the toes, and has a gradient with the greatest deficits being most distal. The smallest fibers, such as those that carry pinprick, pain, and temperature, are affected first, but eventually motor neurons may be affected with concomitant muscle wasting. As distal neuropathy advances, it begins to affect the hands, resulting in the classic "glove and stockings" distribution. In Dave's case, we cannot easily distinguish between whether HIV or one of his two NRTIs is responsible for the distal neuropathy, which has not progressed to his hands, though the pathophysiology of the two causes appears to differ. Diabetes mellitus may be a contributor, but this seems less likely because Dave has excellent glycemic control.

The finding of numbness in his right thigh is not related to the distal sensory neuropathy. Mononeuropathy multiplex affecting the lateral femoral cutaneous nerve is an anatomically appropriate choice (especially because it is a pure sensory nerve and he has no weakness), but this diagnosis would be more consistent with a lower CD4 cell count. The most likely diagnosis is meralgia paresthetica, pain and sensory loss related to entrapment of the lateral femoral cutaneous nerve as it crosses under the inguinal ligament where it meets the anterior superior iliac spine. This is most often seen in diabetes mellitus or obesity in middle age but can be seen after injuries to the area. The main point is that mononeuropathy multiplex would not be seen with his CD4 cell count.

There is limited research into treatment for HIV-related distal neuropathy. Other potential treatable causes, such as B12, folate, or thiamine deficiency, should be considered and corrected. Likewise, comorbid diabetes mellitus should be adequately controlled if present. Gabapentin has been demonstrated to be better than placebo for treating HIV-associated distal sensory neuropathic pain and sleep interference. Tricyclics have not been shown to be better than placebo for pain but may aid sleep and other comorbid chronic pain. Lidocaine patches have not been shown to

be effective in trials but carry little risk. Capsaicin dermal patches have shown some promise. It may be worthwhile to consider a drug holiday or agents other than what he is currently taking. Stavudine is thought to be a more frequent offender than lamivudine.

Interactions Between Psychiatric Drugs and HIV Drugs

Psychotropic medications are used commonly by HIV-positive persons, with over half of persons living with HIV having used one or more of these medications (compared to 29% of the general population). The increased use of psychotropic medications within this population necessitates a thorough understanding of the safety and effectiveness of these medications in persons with HIV and as well as their interactions with HIV/AIDS therapies. In studies, participants with HIV more frequently reported side effects of SSRIs, the first-line pharmacologic treatment for depression and anxiety. Although the side effects reported were stereotypical to SSRIs (i.e., gastrointestinal upset, sedation, insomnia, anorexia and aggression) HIV-positive individuals were more likely to discontinue SSRIs. This presents additional difficulty adequately treating depression.

Anti-retroviral therapy poses additional potential for medication intolerance. Ritonavir, a cytochrome P450 inhibitor, has been shown to increase the risk of the toxicity of atypical antipsychotics, resulting in confusion and impaired coordination. SNRIs that inhibit cytochrome P450s pose additional risk for medication interactions with ART. Additional research is needed to determine necessary dose adjustments for frequently prescribed psychotropic medications when used with common ART medications. Consistently checking for medication interactions before prescribing new medications is appropriate practice for people with HIV and mental health challenges.

Key Points

- The majority of persons living with HIV report having used a psychotropic medication, necessitating clinician awareness of potential interactions of these medications with ART drugs.
- Persons with HIV are more likely to experience typical SSRI side effects, jeopardizing adherence and adequate treatment of depression in these patients.
- Some ART medications and psychotropic medications are P450 inhibitors, requiring adjustment of medications cleared by the P450 system.

Boards-Style Application Questions

Question 1. A 28-year-old transgender man is referred to psychiatry by his primary care physician. His voice is quiet, he is tearful, and his posture is slumped. He explains that he has been sleeping 11 hours every day and eating little. When you ask what he enjoys in his spare time, he says that he usually likes to bake and play World of Warcraft but has not enjoyed either lately. After admitting a 12-year history of suicidal ideation, he says that he has sometimes thought about using a gun to kill himself, but he does not have access to a gun. His past medical history is significant only for a diagnosis of gender dysphoria and the use of male hormones. His maternal grandmother attempted suicide twice. He admits feeling hopeless. He smokes but does not drink more than two standard drinks of alcohol per week. He works part-time and lives alone. What is the best predictor of suicide attempts?

A. Family history of suicide attempts
B. Hopelessness
C. Hypersomnia
D. Living alone
E. Loss of interest in favorite activities (anhedonia)

Question 2. A 40-year-old lesbian with a history of generalized anxiety disorder presents for health maintenance and influenza vaccination. She remarks that last year her son brought home "the flu" from school, which she thinks she passed on to her partner and friends in her yoga class. She has used escitalopram for three years and shares that her anxiety is "still under control most days." Two first-degree relatives also been diagnosed with generalized anxiety disorder. She shares that her therapist has been working with her on self-monitoring and relaxation techniques. When you ask about stressors in her daily life, she says, "Work is hard, but I like my coworkers. This is a good town. People are really accepting and welcoming. I suppose I'm lucky that I grew up in a pretty tolerant town, too." Which model is the best fit for the pathogenesis of her generalized anxiety disorder?

A. Diathesis-stress model
B. Learned helplessness
C. Minority stress theory
D. Protective factor model
E. Psychodynamic model

Question 3. Alex is a 17-year-old lesbian who has recently come out to her family. Her parents have made it clear that they hope Alex is going through a "phase" and will eventually grow out of her homosexuality. Alex normally does well as a student, earning top grades and earning the respect of her teachers. However, since she has come out to her classmates, she has been increasingly the target of school bullies who make fun of her sexuality. She has become more withdrawn at school, and eventually stops going. Alex has a hard time falling asleep at night, has a poor appetite, finds concentrating on her homework to be difficult, and no longer finds pleasure in her previous hobbies. She sometimes wonders if life is worth living. She often worries, and worries most days of the year. Which of the following is most strongly associated with mood and anxiety disorders in LGBTQ individuals?

A. Age of first romantic relationship
B. Family history
C. Sexual attraction
D. Sexual behavior
E. Sexual orientation

Question 4. LGBTQ populations experience suicidal behavior more frequently than the general population. Please select the one correct statement below:

A. Risk of suicide ideation higher among lesbian/bisexual women; risk of suicide attempts higher among gay/bisexual men
B. Risk of suicide attempts higher among lesbian/bisexual women; risk of suicide ideation higher among gay/bisexual men
C. Risk of suicide ideation is equal between lesbian/bisexual women and gay/bisexual men; risk of suicide attempts higher among gay/bisexual men
D. Risk of suicide ideation higher among lesbian/bisexual women; risk of suicide attempts equal between lesbian/bisexual women and gay/bisexual men
E. Risk of suicide ideation and suicide attempts equal between lesbian/bisexual women and gay/bisexual men

Question 5. Eli is a 24-year-old man is brought in by police to the psychiatric emergency room for assaulting an elderly man and then subsequently getting into a brawl with 12 police officers, injuring 4 of them. When questioned about the event, Eli reports that the voices in his head told him to commit the violent act. He reveals that he hears two distinct alter egos, "sometimes demons, sometimes spirits." When asked if he has experienced other command auditory hallucinations, he replies that the voices told him to drink his own urine, which he did and felt disgusted by the act. He also endorses the ability to insert thoughts into other people's minds as well as telepathic powers. When questioned about his psychiatric history, he reveals that he was diagnosed with bipolar disorder at age 20 and was prescribed valproic acid, risperidone, buspirone, and bupropion, though has not been taking any of his medications for the last month. Eli sometimes drinks a six-pack of beer in one sitting and admits to smoking marijuana and drinking alcohol prior to the violent incident. On exam, his vitals are within normal limits. He appears apologetic and cooperative. He has hematomas around his eyes bilaterally. His speech is at times linear but more often disorganized. He appears to be disturbed by auditory hallucinations and requests help. Of the following choices what is the next best step in management?

A. Check a urine toxicology screen
B. Contact his psychiatrist for details about his psychiatric history
C. Order a face CT scan to evaluate possible facial injuries
D. Order an anti-psychotic medication
E. Restrain to ensure the safety of others

Question 6. Though LGBTQ individuals are at increased risk of using substances, there are different patterns of risk by gender. Which of the following substances are lesbian women more likely to use than gay men?

A. Ecstasy
B. Inhalants
C. Marijuana
D. Methamphetamine
E. Tobacco

Question 7. A 23-year old man with a three-year history of HIV diagnosis reports poor appetite, difficulty concentrating, low mood, and anhedonia for the past month. He states that he has felt run down, avoids going out with friends, and has been taking off from work lately. He denies suicidal and homicidal ideation and denies a history of psychiatric illness. What is the next step in managing this patient?

A. Involuntary hospitalization of the patient
B. Start the patient on 20 mg of fluoxetine and follow-up in two weeks
C. Start the patient on 10 mg nortriptyline and follow-up in two weeks
D. Follow up in two weeks and evaluate for psychotropic medication

Question 8. A 57-year old male with a 17-year history of HIV infection is brought in to his primary care physician's office by his adult daughter who is concerned that he has been having difficulty remembering appointments. She states that he has become increasingly dependent on her for managing his multiple medications and keeping track of social, medical, and work appointments. What is the initial step in evaluating this patient's cognitive complaints?

A. Review his medication list and dosages
B. Refer for formal neuropsychological testing
C. Schedule an MRI scan of the brain
D. Reassure his daughter that this is the normal cognitive decline of aging

Boards-Style Application Questions Answer Key

Question 1. Hopelessness (B) is the strongest predictor of suicide attempts. Personal history of suicide attempts—not family history of suicide attempts—is the strongest predictor of future suicide attempts. Family history of suicide attempts (A) is not a strong predictor of future suicide attempts, but personal history of suicide attempts is. Anhedonia (E) and hypersomnia (C) are diagnostic criteria for major depression but are weakly and indirectly predictive of suicide attempts. Living alone (D) is a contextual factor rather than a prognostic factor for suicide.

Question 2. The diathesis-stress model (A) is the correct answer. Her family history, lack of significant stressors, and wealth of protective factors signals that an underlying genetic vulnerability is more to blame for her GAD than an excess stress load. The psychodynamic model (E) is a non-biological model of psychopathology championed by Freud and his contemporaries. The psychodynamic model attributes mental illness to repressed trauma. This model is old and hard to integrate with medical models of mental illness. There is also no evidence of significant trauma in this patient's past. Learned helplessness (B) is a paradigm most directly applicable to depression. The patient does not report—and we have no reason to suspect—a learned inability to modify controllable factors. In fact, her wellness practices suggest the opposite. Minority stress theory (C) is not obviously applicable. This patient appears fortunate in that she has little subjective

recollection of distal or proximal stressors related to her sexual orientation. This is not to say that objective stressors (e.g., employment discrimination based on her perceived lesbian identity) have not been present. However, underlying genetic vulnerability remains more plausible than heightened stress due to her sexual identity. The protective factor model (D) is a fictitious model. This patient does however have a wealth of protective factors.

Question 3. The correct answer is (E). Mood and anxiety disorders are more strongly linked to LGBTQ identity than to sexual behavior (D) or attraction (C), particularly in women. Though family history (B) is important to consider, sexual orientation is more important in this scenario. Age of first romantic relationship (A) is not associated with mood and anxiety disorders.

Question 4. There is an opposite gender trend for suicide ideation than for suicide attempts. (A) is correct: risk of suicidal ideation is higher among lesbian/bisexual women and risk of suicide attempts is higher among gay/bisexual men. This is in contrast to the overall population, where women are two times more likely than men to make a lifetime suicide attempt.

Question 5. The correct answer is (A). The first action is to order a urine toxicology screen to rule out substance-induced psychosis. Though this patient reports a history of bipolar disorder, which may present with psychotic features, substance-induced psychosis remains suspicious, especially because the patient endorses polysubstance use and admits to using prior to the assault. Although it may be necessary to prescribe an anti-psychotic medication (D) to manage the patient's condition, the first step should be to order a urine toxicology screen. While it would be beneficial to obtain collateral information from the patient's treating psychiatrist (B), this is often not feasible in the acute emergency. Though the patient was brought in due to violent behavior, restraints (E) are not indicated at this time because the patient is cooperative and not agitated. A face CT scan (C) may or may not be indicated depending on the patient's symptoms and physical exam results. A urine toxicology screen can be quickly ordered before the decision about ordering a head CT scan needs to be made.

Question 6. The correct answer is (E). Lesbian women use more tobacco while gay men use more marijuana (C), methamphetamine (D), inhalants (B) and ecstasy (A). In California, lesbian and bisexual women smoke three times as much as all women in the state.

Question 7. The correct answer is (B). This patient meets criteria for clinical depression given his duration of depressed mood, the presence of at least 4 other symptoms of depression, and the impact of his symptoms on his social and work life. The first-line treatment of a patient with depression is an SSRI, regardless of HIV status. This patient does not need to be involuntarily hospitalized (A) at this point given his denial of suicidal and homicidal ideation and general ability to care for himself. Tricyclic antidepressants (C) are not first-line for the treatment of depression in patients with HIV. This patient meets the diagnostic criteria for clinical depression and should be offered pharmaceutical treatment. Delaying treatment (D) is inappropriate.

Question 8. The correct answer is (A). ART medications, in addition to other commonly used chronic medications, can impair memory and should be considered before pursuing further diagnostic testing. This patient's medication list should be reviewed prior to suggesting a referral for formal neurocognitive testing (B). Additionally, brief in-office testing such as the Montreal Cognitive Assessment can be performed by the physician to identify broad areas of memory, attention, or spatial deficits and determine the need for formal neurocognitive testing. Medications should be reviewed and a physical and brief cognitive exam should be performed to determine the need for diagnostic imaging (C). It is inappropriate to dismiss this patient's memory complaints (D) prior to further evaluation.

Sources

Abers MS, Shandera WX, Kass JS. Neurological and psychiatric adverse effects of antiretroviral drugs. CNS Drugs. 2014;28(2):131–45.

Allen DJ, Oleson T. Shame and internalized homophobia in gay men. J Homosex. 1999;37(3):33–43. https://doi.org/10.1300/J082v37n03_03.

Allen VC, Myers HF, Williams JK. Depression among Black bisexual men with early and later life adversities. Cultur Divers Ethnic Minor Psychol. 2014;20(1):128–37. https://doi.org/10.1037/a0034128. Epub 2013 Oct 7. PubMed PMID: 24099486.

Almeida J, Johnson R, Corliss H, Molnar B, Azrael D. Emotional distress among LGBT youth: the influence of perceived discrimination based on sexual orientation. J Youth Adolesc. 2009a;38(7):1001–14. https://doi.org/10.1007/s10964-009-9397-9.

Almeida J, Johnson RM, Corliss HL, Molnar BE, Azrael D. Emotional distress among LGBT youth: the influence of perceived discrimination based on sexual orientation. J Youth Adolesc. 2009b;38(7):1001–14. https://doi.org/10.1007/s10964-009-9397-9.

American Psychiatric Association. Diagnostic and statistical manual of mental disorders. 5th ed. Arlington, VA, US: American Psychiatric Publishing, Inc.; 2013.

Ances BM, Letendre SL, Alexander T, Ellis RJ. Role of psychiatric medications as adjunct therapy in the treatment of HIV associated neurocognitive disorders. Int Rev Psychiatry. 2008;20(1):89–93. https://doi.org/10.1080/09540260701877670. Review. PubMed PMID: 18240065.

Antinori A, Arendt G, Becker JT, Brew BJ, Byrd DA, Cherner M, et al. Updated research nosology for HIV-associated neurocognitive disorders. Neurology. 2007;69(18):1789–99.

Arseniou S, Arvaniti A, Samakouri M. HIV infection and depression. Psychiatry Clin Neurosci. 2014;68(2):96–109. https://doi.org/10.1111/pcn.12097. Epub 2013 Oct 30. PubMed PMID: 24552630.

Ash M, Mackereth C. Assessing the mental health and wellbeing of the lesbian, gay, bisexual and transgender population. Community Pract. 2013;86(3):24–7. Available at: http://www.ncbi.nlm.nih.gov/pubmed/23540015. Accessed 26 Jan 2015.

Aung GL, O'Brien JG, Tien PG, Kawamoto LS. Increased aripiprazole concentrations in an HIV-positive male concurrently taking duloxetine, darunavir, and ritonavir. Ann Pharmacother. 2010;44(11):1850–4. https://doi.org/10.1345/aph.1P139. Epub 2010 Oct 26. PubMed PMID: 20978219.

Benton T, Lynch K, Dubé B, Gettes DR, Tustin NB, Ping Lai J, et al. Selective serotonin reuptake inhibitor suppression of HIV infectivity and replication. Psychosom Med. 2010;72(9):925–32. https://doi.org/10.1097/PSY.0b013e3181f883ce. Epub 2010 Oct 14. PubMed PMID: 20947783; PubMed Central PMCID: PMC2978281.

Berg MB, Mimiaga MJ, Safren SA. Mental health concerns of gay and bisexual men seeking mental health services. J Homosex. 2008;54(3):293–306. https://doi.org/10.1080/00918360801982215.

Bergeron S, Senn C. Body image and sociocultural norms. Psychol Women Q. 1998;22(3):385–401. https://doi.org/10.1111/j.1471-6402.1998.tb00164.x.

Bhatia N, Chow F. Neurologic complications in treated HIV-1 infection. Curr Neurol Neurosci Rep. 2016;16(7):62. https://doi.org/10.1007/s11910-016-0666-1.

Blank MB, Himelhoch S, Walkup J, Eisenberg MM. Treatment considerations for HIV-infected individuals with severe mental illness. Curr HIV/AIDS Rep. 2013;10(4):371–9. https://doi.org/10.1007/s11904-013-0179-3. PubMed PMID: 24158425; PubMed Central PMCID: PMC3857330.

Bockting W, Huang C-Y, Ding H, Robinson B. "Bean", Rosser BRS. Are transgender persons at higher risk for HIV than other sexual minorities? A comparison of HIV prevalence and risks. Int J Transgenderism. 2005;8(2–3):123–31. https://doi.org/10.1300/J485v08n02_11.

Bostwick W. Assessing bisexual stigma and mental health status: a brief report. J Bisex. 2012;12(2):214–22. https://doi.org/10.1080/15299716.2012.674860.

Braet C, Van Vlierberghe L, Vandevivere E, Theuwis L, Bosmans G. Depression in early, middle and late adolescence: differential evidence for the cognitive diathesis-stress model. Clin Psychol Psychother. 2013;20(5):369–83. https://doi.org/10.1002/cpp.1789.

Brew B, Garber J. Neurologic sequelae of primary HIV infection. Handb Clin Neurol. 2018;152:65–74. https://doi.org/10.1016/b978-0-444-63849-6.00006-2.

Centers for Disease Control and Prevention. Compendium of evidence-based interventions and best practices for HIV prevention. 2014. Available at: http://www.cdc.gov/hiv/prevention/research/compendium/.

Cochran BN, Cauce AM. Characteristics of lesbian, gay, bisexual, and transgender individuals entering substance abuse treatment. J Subst Abus Treat. 2006;30(2):135–46. https://doi.org/10.1016/j.jsat.2005.11.009.

Cochran SD, Greer J, Mays VM. Prevalence of mental disorders, psychological distress, and mental health services use among lesbian, gay, and bisexual adults in the United States. J Consult Clin Psychol. 2003;71(1):53–61. https://doi.org/10.1037/0022-006X.71.1.53.

Cochran SD. Emerging issues in research on lesbians' and gay men's mental health: does sexual orientation really matter? Am Psychol. 2001;56(11):931–47. https://doi.org/10.1037/0003-066X.56.11.931.

Colfax GN, Santos G, Das M, et al. Mirtazapine to reduce methamphetamine use: a randomized controlled trial. Arch Gen Psychiatry. 2011;68(11):1168–75. https://doi.org/10.1001/archgenpsychiatry.2011.124.

D'Augelli AR, Hershberger SL, Pilkington NW. Suicidality patterns and sexual orientation-related factors among lesbian, gay, and bisexual youths. Suicide Life Threat Behav. 2001;31(3):250–64.

D'Augelli AR, Hershberger SL. Lesbian, gay, and bisexual youth in community settings: personal challenges and mental health problems. Am J Community Psychol. 1993;21(4):421–48.

Dabaghzadeh F, Khalili H, Ghaeli P, Dashti-Khavidaki S. Potential benefits of cyproheptadine in HIV-positive patients under treatment with antiretroviral drugs including efavirenz. Expert Opin Pharmacother. 2012;13(18):2613–24. https://doi.org/10.1517/14656566.2012.742887. Epub 2012 Nov 10. Review. PubMed PMID: 23140169.

Dal-Bó MJ, Manoel AL, Filho AO, Silva BQ, Cardoso YS, Cortez J, Tramujas L, Silva RM. Depressive symptoms and associated factors among people living with HIV/AIDS. J Int Assoc Provid AIDS Care. 2015;14(2):136–40. [Epub ahead of print] PubMed PMID: 23873218.

Dalmida SG, Koenig HG, Holstad MM, Wirani MM. The psychological well-being of people living with HIV/AIDS and the role of religious coping and social support. Int J Psychiatry Med. 2013;46(1):57–83. PubMed PMID: 24547610.

Drescher J. Queer diagnoses: parallels and contrasts in the history of homosexuality, gender variance, and the diagnostic and statistical manual. Arch Sex Behav. 2010;39(2):427–60. https://doi.org/10.1007/s10508-009-9531-5.

Du Plessis S, Vink M, Joska JA, Koutsilieri E, Stein DJ, Emsley R. HIV infection and the fronto-striatal system: a systematic review and meta-analysis of fMRI studies. AIDS. 2014;28(6):803–11. [Epub ahead of print]. PubMed PMID: 24300546.

Duncan DT, Hatzenbuehler ML, Johnson RM. Neighborhood-level LGBT hate crimes and current illicit drug use among sexual minority youth. Drug Alcohol Depend. 2014;135:65–70. https://doi.org/10.1016/j.drugalcdep.2013.11.001.

Durvasula R, Miller TR. Substance abuse treatment in persons with HIV/AIDS: challenges in managing triple diagnosis. Behav Med. 2014;40(2):43–52. [Epub ahead of print] PubMed PMID: 24274175.

Eggers C, Arendt G, Hahn K, Husstedt IW, Maschke M, Neuen-Jacob E, et al. HIV-1-associated neurocognitive disorder: epidemiology, pathogenesis, diagnosis, and treatment. J Neurol. 2017;264(8):1715–27. https://doi.org/10.1007/s00415-017-8503-2.

Faílde Garrido JM, Lameiras Fernández M, Foltz M, Rodríguez Castro Y, Carrera Fernández MV. Cognitive performance in men and women infected with HIV-1. Psychiatry J. 2013;2013:382126. https://doi.org/10.1155/2013/382126. Epub 2012 Dec 26. PubMed PMID: 24286066; PubMed Central PMCID: PMC3839654.

Fazeli PL, Woods SP, Heaton RK, Umlauf A, Gouaux B, Rosario D, Moore RC, Grant I, Moore DJ, The HNRP Group. An active lifestyle is associated with better neurocognitive functioning in adults living with HIV infection. J Neurovirol. 2014;20(3):233–42. [Epub ahead of print] PubMed PMID: 24554483.

Fergusson DM, Horwood L, Beautrais AL. IS sexual orientation related to mental health problems and suicidality in young people? Arch Gen Psychiatry. 1999;56(10):876–80. https://doi.org/10.1001/archpsyc.56.10.876.

Fredriksen-Goldsen KI, Simoni JM, Kim H-J, et al. The health equity promotion model: reconceptualization of lesbian, gay, bisexual, and transgender (LGBT) health disparities. Am J Orthopsychiatry. 2014;84(6):653–63. https://doi.org/10.1037/ort0000030.

Garcia-Toro M, Aguirre I. Biopsychosocial model in depression revisited. Med Hypotheses. 2007;68(3):683–91. https://doi.org/10.1016/j.mehy.2006.02.049.

Gilman SE, Cochran SD, Mays VM, Hughes M, Ostrow D, Kessler RC. Risk of psychiatric disorders among individuals reporting same-sex sexual partners in the National Comorbidity Survey. Am J Public Health. 2001a;91(6):933–9. Available at: http://www.pubmed-central.nih.gov/articlerender.fcgi?artid=1446471&tool=pmcentrez&rendertype=abstract. Accessed 11 Feb 2014.

Gilman SE, Cochran SD, Mays VM, Hughes M, Ostrow D, Kessler RC. Risk of psychiatric disorders among individuals reporting same-sex sexual partners in the National Comorbidity Survey. Am J Public Health. 2001b;91(6):933–9.

Grassi B, Gambini O, Scarone S. Notes on the use of fluvoxamine as treatment of depression in HIV-1-infected subjects. Pharmacopsychiatry. 1995;28(3):93–4. PubMed PMID: 7568371.

Gruber VA, Rainey PM, Lum PJ, Beatty GW, Aweeka FT, McCance-Katz EF. Interactions between alcohol and the HIV entry inhibitor Maraviroc. J Int Assoc Provid AIDS Care. 2013;12(6):375–7. https://doi.org/10.1177/2325957413495567. Epub 2013 Jul 23. PubMed PMID: 23881910.

Gupta M, Kumar K, Garg PD. Dual diagnosis vs. triple diagnosis in HIV: a comparative study to evaluate the differences in psychopathology and suicidal risk in HIV positive male subjects. Asian J Psychiatr. 2013;6(6):515–20. https://doi.org/10.1016/j.ajp.2013.06.012. Epub 2013 Aug 8. PubMed PMID: 24309864.

Gutiérrez F, García L, Padilla S, Alvarez D, Moreno S, Navarro G, Gómez-Sirvent J, Vidal F, Asensi V, Masiá M. CoRIS. Risk of clinically significant depression in HIV-infected patients: effect of antiretroviral drugs. HIV Med. 2014;15(4):213–23. https://doi.org/10.1111/hiv.12104. Epub 2013 Nov 11. PubMed PMID: 24215356.

Hatzenbuehler ML. How does sexual minority stigma "get under the skin"? A psychological mediation framework. Psychol Bull. 2009;135(5):707–30. https://doi.org/10.1037/a0016441.

Hatzenbuehler ML. The social environment and suicide attempts in lesbian, gay, and bisexual youth. Pediatrics. 2011;127(5):896–903. https://doi.org/10.1542/peds.2010-3020.

Herrick AL, Lim SH, Wei C, Smith H, Guadamuz T, Friedman MS, Stall R. Resilience as an untapped resource in behavioral intervention design for gay men. AIDS Behav. 2011;15(1):25–9. https://doi.org/10.1007/s10461-011-9895-0.

Hightow-Weidman LB, Phillips G, Jones KC, Outlaw AY, Fields SD. Smith for TY of CSISG, Justin C. Racial and sexual identity-related maltreatment among minority YMSM: prevalence, perceptions, and the association with emotional distress. AIDS Patient Care STDs. 2011;25(S1):S39–45. https://doi.org/10.1089/apc.2011.9877.

Hoare J, Carey P, Joska JA, Carrara H, Sorsdahl K, Stein DJ. Escitalopram treatment of depression in human immunodeficiency virus/acquired immunodeficiency syndrome: a randomized, double-blind, placebo-controlled study. J Nerv Ment Dis. 2014;202(2):133–7. https://doi.org/10.1097/NMD.0000000000000082. PubMed PMID: 24469525.

Hooker E. The adjustment of the male overt homosexual. J Proj Tech. 1957;21(1):18–31. https://doi.org/10.1080/08853126.1957.10380742.

Horberg MA, Silverberg MJ, Hurley LB, Towner WJ, Klein DB, Bersoff-Matcha S, Weinberg WG, Antoniskis D, Mogyoros M, Dodge WT, Dobrinich R, Quesenberry CP, Kovach DA. Effects of depression and selective serotonin reuptake inhibitor use on adherence to highly active antiretroviral therapy and on clinical outcomes in HIV-infected patients. J Acquir Immune Defic Syndr. 2008;47(3):384–90. PubMed PMID: 18091609.

Igartua KJ, Gill K, Montoro R. Internalized homophobia: a factor in depression, anxiety, and suicide in the gay and lesbian population. Can J Commun Ment Health. 2003;22(2):15–30. Available at: http://www.ncbi.nlm.nih.gov/pubmed/15868835. Accessed 11 Feb 2014.

Joska JA, Obayemi A Jr, Cararra H, Sorsdahl K. Severe mental illness and retention in anti-retroviral care: a retrospective study. AIDS Behav. 2014;18(8):1492–500. [Epub ahead of print] PubMed PMID: 24515624.

Kabir Z, Keogan S, Clarke V, Clancy L. Second-hand smoke exposure levels and tobacco consumption patterns among a lesbian, gay, bisexual and transgender community in Ireland. Public Health. 2013;127(5):467–72. https://doi.org/10.1016/j.puhe.2013.01.021.

Kaminski P, Chapman B, Haynes S, Own L. Body image, eating behaviors, and attitudes toward exercise among gay and straight men. Eat Behav. 2005;6(3):179–87. https://doi.org/10.1016/j.eatbeh.2004.11.003.

Keltner JR, Fennema-Notestine C, Vaida F, Wang D, Franklin DR, Dworkin RH, CHARTER Group, et al. HIV-associated distal neuropathic pain is associated with smaller total cerebral cortical gray matter. J Neurovirol. 2014;20(3):209–18. [Epub ahead of print] PubMed PMID: 24549970.

Kertzner RM, Barber ME, Schwartz A. Mental health issues in LGBT seniors. J Gay Lesbian Ment Health.

2011;15(4):335–8. https://doi.org/10.1080/19359705.2011.606680.

Kimmel D. Lesbian, gay, bisexual, and transgender aging concerns. Clin Gerontol. 2014;37(1):49–63. https://doi.org/10.1080/07317115.2014.847310.

King M, Semlyen J, Tai SS, et al. A systematic review of mental disorder, suicide, and deliberate self harm in lesbian, gay and bisexual people. BMC Psychiatry. 2008;8:70. https://doi.org/10.1186/1471-244X-8-70.

Kinsey A, Pomeroy W, Martin C, Gebhard P. Sexual behavior in the human female. Philadelphia: W.B. Saunders; 1953.

Kinsey A, Pomeroy W, Martin C. Sexual behavior in the human male. Philadelphia: W. B. Saunders; 1948.

Kristiansen JE, Hansen JB. Inhibition of HIV replication by neuroleptic agents and their potential use in HIV infected patients with AIDS related dementia. Int J Antimicrob Agents. 2000;14(3):209–13. PubMed PMID: 10773489.

L'akoa RM, Noubiap JJ, Fang Y, Ntone FE, Kuaban C. Prevalence and correlates of depressive symptoms in HIV-positive patients: a cross-sectional study among newly diagnosed patients in Yaoundé, Cameroon. BMC Psychiatry. 2013;13:228. https://doi.org/10.1186/1471-244X-13-228. PubMed PMID: 24053612; PubMed Central PMCID: PMC3849101.

Laumann E, Gagnon J, Michael R, Michaels S. The social organization of sexuality: sexual practices in the United States. Chicago: University of Chicago Press; 1994.

Lehavot K, Simoni JM. The impact of minority stress on mental health and substance use among sexual minority women. J Consult Clin Psychol. 2011;79(2):159–70. https://doi.org/10.1037/a0022839.

Letendre S, Ances B, Gibson S, Ellis RJ. Neurologic complications of HIV disease and their treatment. Top HIV Med. 2007a;15(2):32–9. PubMed PMID: 17485785.

Letendre SL, Marquie-Beck J, Ellis RJ, Woods SP, Best B, Clifford DB, Collier AC, Gelman BB, Marra C, McArthur JC, McCutchan JA, Morgello S, Simpson D, Alexander TJ, Durelle J, Heaton R, Grant I, CHARTER Group. The role of cohort studies in drug development: clinical evidence of antiviral activity of serotonin reuptake inhibitors and HMG-CoA reductase inhibitors in the central nervous system. J Neuroimmune Pharmacol. 2007b;2(1):120–7. Epub 2007 Jan 3. PubMed PMID: 18040835.

Levounis P, Drescher J, Barber ME, editors. The LGBT casebook. 1st. ed. Washington, DC: American Psychiatric Pub; 2012.

Lingiardi V, Baiocco R, Nardelli N. Measure of internalized sexual stigma for lesbians and gay men: a new scale. J Homosex. 2012;59(8):1191–210. https://doi.org/10.1080/00918369.2012.712850.

Liu L, Pang R, Sun W, Wu M, Qu P, Lu C, Wang L. Functional social support, psychological capital, and depressive and anxiety symptoms among people living with HIV/AIDS employed full-time. BMC Psychiatry. 2013;13(1):324. https://doi.org/10.1186/1471-244X-13-324. PubMed PMID: 24289721.

Makadon H, Fletcher R, Park, L. Primary care of gay men. UpToDate. 2014. Available at: www.uptodate.com. Accessed 22 Jun 2014.

Manji H, Miller R. The neurology of HIV infection. J Neurol Neurosurg Psychiatry. 2004;75(Suppl 1):i29–35.

Mays VM, Cochran SD. Mental health correlates of perceived discrimination among lesbian, gay, and bisexual adults in the United States. Am J Public Health. 2001;91(11):1869–76. Available at: http://www.pubmedcentral.nih.gov/articlerender.fcgi?artid=1446893&tool=pmcentrez&rendertype=abstract. Accessed 11 Feb 2014.

McCabe SE, Hughes TL, Bostwick WB, West BT, Boyd CJ. Sexual orientation, substance use behaviors and substance dependence in the United States. Addict Abingdon Engl. 2009;104(8):1333–45. https://doi.org/10.1111/j.1360-0443.2009.02596.x.

McCann E, Sharek D, Higgins A, Sheerin F, Glacken M. Lesbian, gay, bisexual and transgender older people in Ireland: mental health issues. Aging Ment Health. 2013;17(3):358–65. https://doi.org/10.1080/13607863.2012.751583.

McKirnan DJ, Peterson PL. Stress, expectancies, and vulnerability to substance abuse: a test of a model among homosexual men. J Abnorm Psychol. 1988;97(4):461–6. Available at: http://www.ncbi.nlm.nih.gov/pubmed/3264559. Accessed 11 Feb 2014.

Mcnair RP, Hegarty K. Guidelines for the primary care of lesbian, gay, and bisexual people: a systematic review. Ann Fam Med. 2010;8(6):533–41.

Meyer IH, Schwartz S, Frost DM. Social patterning of stress and coping: does disadvantaged social statuses confer more stress and fewer coping resources? Soc Sci Med. 2008;67(3):368–79. https://doi.org/10.1016/j.socscimed.2008.03.012.

Meyer IH. Minority stress and mental health in gay men. J Health Soc Behav. 2011;36(1):38–56.

Meyer IH. Prejudice, social stress, and mental health in lesbian, gay, and bisexual populations: conceptual issues and research evidence. Psychol Bull. 2003b;129(5):674–97. https://doi.org/10.1037/0033-2909.129.5.674.

Midanik LT, Drabble L, Trocki K, Sell RL. Sexual orientation and alcohol use: identity versus behavior measures. J LGBT Health Res. 2007;3(1):25–35.

Mills TC, Paul J, Stall R, et al. Distress and depression in men who have sex with men: the urban men's health study. Am J Psychiatry. 2004;161(2):278–85. https://doi.org/10.1176/appi.ajp.161.2.278.

Mustanski BS, Garofalo R, Emerson EM. Mental health disorders, psychological distress, and suicidality in a diverse sample of lesbian, gay, bisexual, and transgender youths. Am J Public Health. 2010;100(12):2426–32. https://doi.org/10.2105/AJPH.2009.178319.

Newcomb ME, Heinz AJ, Mustanski B. Examining risk and protective factors for alcohol use in lesbian, gay, bisexual, and transgender youth: a longitudinal multilevel analysis. J Stud Alcohol Drugs. 2012;73(5):783

Newcomb ME, Mustanski B. Internalized homophobia and internalizing mental health problems: a meta-ana lytic review. Clin Psychol Rev. 2010;30(8):1019–29. https://doi.org/10.1016/j.cpr.2010.07.003.

O'Donnell S, Meyer IH, Schwartz S. Increased risk of suicide attempts among black and latino lesbians, gay men, and bisexuals. Am J Public Health. 2011;101(6):1055–9.   https://doi.org/10.2105/AJPH.2010.300032.

Offen N, Smith EA, Malone RE. Is tobacco a gay issue? Interviews with leaders of the lesbian, gay, bisexual and transgender community. Cult Health Amp Sex. 2008;10(2):143–57. https://doi.org/10.1080/13691050701656284.

Pacek LR, Latkin C, Crum RM, Stuart EA, Knowlton AR. Current cigarette smoking among HIV-positive current and former drug users: associations with individual and social characteristics. AIDS Behav. 2013;18(7):1368–77. [Epub ahead of print] PubMed PMID: 24287787.

Patten SB. Major depression epidemiology from a diathesis-stress conceptualization. BMC Psychiatry. 2013;13:19. https://doi.org/10.1186/1471-244X-13-19.

Paul JP, Catania J, Pollack L, et al. Suicide attempts among gay and bisexual men: lifetime prevalence and antecedents. Am J Public Health. 2002;92(8):1338–45.

Perez-brumer A, Day JK, Russell ST, Hatzenbuehler ML. Prevalence and correlates of suicidal ideation among transgender youth in California: findings from a representative, population-based sample of high school students. J Am Acad Child Adolesc Psychiatry. 2017;56(9):739–46.

Pfefferbaum A, Rogosa DA, Rosenbloom MJ, Chu W, Sassoon SA, Kemper CA, Deresinski S, Rohlfing T, Zahr NM, Sullivan EV. Accelerated aging of selective brain structures in human immunodeficiency virus infection: a controlled, longitudinal magnetic resonance imaging study. Neurobiol Aging. 2014;35(7):1755–68. https://doi.org/10.1016/j.neurobiolaging.2014.01.008. pii: S0197-4580(14)00009-8. [Epub ahead of print] PubMed PMID: 24508219.

Ponce NA, Cochran SD, Pizer JC, Mays VM. The effects of unequal access to health insurance for same-sex couples in California. Health Aff (Millwood). 2010;29(8):1539–48.   https://doi.org/10.1377/hlthaff.2009.0583.

Primeau MM, Avellaneda V, Musselman D, St Jean G, Illa L. Treatment of depression in individuals living with HIV/AIDS. Psychosomatics. 2013;54(4):336–44. https://doi.org/10.1016/j.psym.2012.12.001. Epub 2013 Feb 4. PubMed PMID: 23380671.

Rasmussen L, Obel D, Kronborg G, Larsen C, Pedersen C, Gerstoft J, Obel N. Utilization of psychotropic drugs prescribed to persons with and without HIV infection: a Danish nationwide population-based cohort study. HIV Med. 2014;15(8):458–69. https://doi.org/10.1111/hiv.12135. [Epub ahead of print] PubMed PMID: 24589241.

Reinelt E, Stopsack M, Aldinger M, John U, Grabe HJ, Barnow S. Testing the diathesis-stress model: 5-HTTLPR, childhood emotional maltreatment, and vulnerability to social anxiety disorder. Am J Med

Genet B Neuropsychiatr Genet. 2013;162B(3):253–61. https://doi.org/10.1002/ajmg.b.32142.

Remafedi G, Jurek AM, Oakes JM. Sexual identity and tobacco use in a venue-based sample of adolescents and young adults. Am J Prev Med. 2008;35(6, Supplement):S463–70.   https://doi.org/10.1016/j.amepre.2008.09.002.

Remafedi G. Suicidality in a venue-based sample of young men who have sex with men. J Adolesc Health. 2002;31(4):305–10. https://doi.org/10.1016/S1054-139X(02)00405-6.

Rivers I. Recollections of bullying at school and their long-term implications for lesbians, gay men, and bisexuals. Crisis. 2004;25(4):169–75. Available at: http://www.ncbi.nlm.nih.gov/pubmed/15580852. Accessed 11 Feb 2014.

Roisman GI, Newman DA, Fraley RC, Haltigan JD, Groh AM, Haydon KC. Distinguishing differential susceptibility from diathesis-stress: recommendations for evaluating interaction effects. Dev Psychopathol. 2012;24(2):389–409.   https://doi.org/10.1017/S0954579412000065.

Rosario M, Schrimshaw EW, Hunter J. Disclosure of sexual orientation and subsequent substance use and abuse among lesbian, gay, and bisexual youths: critical role of disclosure reactions. Psychol Addict Behav J Soc Psychol Addict Behav. 2009;23(1):175–84. https://doi.org/10.1037/a0014284.

Ross MW, Rosser BR. Measurement and correlates of internalized homophobia: a factor analytic study. J Clin Psychol. 1996;52(1):15–21.

Rudd M, Berman A, Joiner T, Nock MK, Silverman MM, Mandrusiak M, et al. Warning signs for suicide: theory, research, and clinical applications. Suicide Life Threat Behav. 2006;36(3):255–62. https://doi.org/10.1521/suli.2006.36.3.255.

Russell ST, Joyner K. Adolescent sexual orientation and suicide risk: evidence from a national study. Am J Public Health. 2001;91(8):1276–81. Available at: http://www.pubmedcentral.nih.gov/articlerender.fcgi?artid=1446760&tool=pmcentrez&rendertype=abstract. Accessed 11 Feb 2014.

Russell ST, Ryan C, Toomey RB, Diaz RM, Sanchez J. Lesbian, gay, bisexual, and transgender adolescent school victimization: implications for young adult health and adjustment. J Sch Health. 2011;81(5):223–30. https://doi.org/10.1111/j.1746-1561.2011.00583.x.

Sanchez NF, Rabatin J, Sanchez JP, Hubbard S, Kalet A. Medical students' ability to care for lesbian, gay, bisexual, and transgendered patients. Fam Med. 2006;38(1):21–7. Available at: http://www.ncbi.nlm.nih.gov/pubmed/16378255. Accessed 5 Feb 2015.

Schotte CKW, Van Den Bossche B, De Doncker D, Claes S, Cosyns P. A biopsychosocial model as a guide for psychoeducation and treatment of depression. Depress Anxiety. 2006;23(5):312–24. https://doi.org/10.1002/da.20177.

Silvestre A, Beatty RL, Friedman MR. Substance use disorder in the context of LGBT health: a social work perspective. Soc Work Public Health. 2013;28(3–4):366–76. https://doi.org/10.1080/19371918.2013.7 74667.

Skinner WF. The prevalence and demographic predictors of illicit and licit drug use among lesbians and gay men. Am J Public Health. 1994;84(8):1307–10.

Sloan EP. Retention in psychiatric treatment in a Canadian sample of HIV-positive women. AIDS Care. 2013;26(7):927–30. [Epub ahead of print] PubMed PMID: 24367912.

Stall R, Paul JP, Greenwood G, et al. Alcohol use, drug use and alcohol-related problems among men who have sex with men: the Urban Men's Health Study. Addiction. 2001;96(11):1589–601. https://doi. org/10.1046/j.1360-0443.2001.961115896.x.

Steele LS, Tinmouth JM, Lu A. Regular health care use by lesbians: a path analysis of predictive factors. Fam Pract. 2006;23(6):631–6. https://doi.org/10.1093/ fampra/cml030.

Suicide Prevention Resource Center. Suicide Prevention Resource Center. Suicide risk and prevention for lesbian, gay, bisexual, and transgender youth. Newton: Education Development Center, Inc.; 2009. Available at: http://www.sprc.org/library/.

Suvada J. Neuropathic and neurocongnitive complications of antiretroviral therapy among HIV-infected patients. Neuro Endocrinol Lett. 2013;34(Suppl 1):5–11. PubMed PMID: 24013599.

Tharp AT, DeGue S, Valle LA, Brookmeyer KA, Massetti GM, Matjasko JL. A systematic qualitative review of risk and protective factors for sexual violence perpetration. Trauma Violence Abuse. 2013;14(2):133–67. https://doi.org/10.1177/1524838012470031.

Tsai AC, Karasic DH, Hammer GP, Charlebois ED, Ragland K, Moss AR, Sorensen JL, Dilley JW, Bangsberg DR. Directly observed antidepressant medication treatment and HIV outcomes among homeless and marginally housed HIV-positive adults: a randomized controlled trial. Am J Public Health. 2013a;103(2):308–15. https://doi.org/10.2105/ AJPH.2011.300422. Epub 2012 Jun 21. PubMed PMID: 22720766; PubMed Central PMCID: PMC3558777.

Tsai AC, Mimiaga MJ, Dilley JW, Hammer GP, Karasic DH, Charlebois ED, Sorensen JL, Safren SA, Bangsberg DR. Does effective depression treatment alone reduce secondary HIV transmission risk? Equivocal findings from a randomized controlled trial. AIDS Behav. 2013b;17(8):2765–72. https://doi. org/10.1007/s10461-013-0600-3. PubMed PMID: 23975476; PubMed Central PMCID: PMC3805275.

Vollmayr B, Gass P. Learned helplessness: unique features and translational value of a cognitive depression model. Cell Tissue Res. 2013;354(1):171–8. https:// doi.org/10.1007/s00441-013-1654-2.

Warner J, Mckeown E, Griffin M, Johnson K, Ramsay A, Cort C, King M. Rates and predictors of mental illness in gay men, lesbians and bisexual men and women: results from a survey based in England and Wales. Br J Psychiatry. 2004;185:479–85.

Warriner K, Nagoshi CT, Nagoshi JL. Correlates of homophobia, transphobia, and internalized homophobia in gay or lesbian and heterosexual samples. J Homosex. 2013;60(9):1297–314. https:// doi.org/10.1080/00918369.2013.806177.

Wei C, Guadamuz TE, Lim SH, Huang Y, Koe S. Patterns and levels of illicit drug use among men who have sex with men in Asia. Drug Alcohol Depend. 2012;120(1–3):246–9. https://doi.org/10.1016/j. drugalcdep.2011.07.016.

White P. Biopsychosocial medicine: an integrated approach to understanding illness. USA: Oxford University Press; 2005. p. 256. Available at: http:// www.amazon.com/Biopsychosocial-Medicine-Integrated-Approach-Understanding/dp/019853034X. Accessed 11 Feb 2014.

Woods SP, Hoebel C, Pirogovsky E, Rooney A, Cameron MV, Grant I, Gilbert PE, HIV Neurobehavioral Research Program Group. Visuospatial temporal order memory deficits in older adults with HIV infection. Cogn Behav Neurol. 2013;26(4):171–80. https://doi.org/10.1097/WNN.0000000000000013. PubMed PMID: 24378603; PubMed Central PMCID: PMC3893039.

Data Collection and Research

13

Michael Haymer, Nadejda Bespalova,
Laura Jennings, and Brandyn D. Lau

Introduction: The Importance of Documentation and Meaningful Data

Documenting **sexual orientation**, **sex assigned at birth**, **gender identity, gender expression,** and **sexual behavior** is a necessary component of clinical care and public health in two major ways: (1) documentation is necessary on a patient-specific level to ensure that providers can identify and address patient-specific health needs; and (2) data collection is necessary on a population level to fully identify, track, and address health disparities experienced by LGBTQ people and to improve the value of care and population health

---

The first listed author is the chapter's associate editor from The Equal Curriculum Project. The chapter authors are otherwise ordered according to their preference.

M. Haymer (✉)
David Geffen School of Medicine,
Los Angeles, CA, USA
e-mail: mhaymer@mednet.ucla.edu

N. Bespalova
NYU Langone Medical Center, New York, NY, USA

L. Jennings
University of Pennsylvania Health System,
Philadelphia, PA, USA

B. D. Lau
Johns Hopkins School of Medicine,
Baltimore, MD, USA
e-mail: blau2@jhmi.edu

interventions that are delivered. In this chapter, these major points are discussed:

- The lack of routine collection of sexual orientation and gender identity (SOGI) information has limited the advancement of evidence-based care for LGBTQ individuals' health, negatively affecting medical education and clinical care.
- Many factors within clinical contexts influence if, how, and when disclosure and documentation of SOGI information occur.
- Collecting this information will enable research on LGBTQ health disparities, which has the potential to improve health care and overall health status of LGBTQ persons and populations.
- The act of collecting information from patients raises patient-centered and ethical questions regarding data use, confidentiality, and patient privacy.
- Nationally, there have been successful initiatives to collect this information, and many others are ongoing.

Consequences of Lack of Data Collection at the Interface with Clinician Education and Practice

A lack of population level SOGI information underlies the inadequate understanding of health disparities and the consequent lack of robust evidence-based clinical guidelines for LGBTQ persons and populations. Much of LGBTQ health research has used convenience samples and recruitment methods that limit study designs and generalizability of findings. Without data and research on LGBTQ people, health professionals cannot become fully competent in addressing the health needs of LGBTQ individuals. Research priorities in LGBTQ health have been limited until recently. Between 1989 and 2011, only 0.1% of National Institutes of Health-funded studies addressed LGBTQ health, excluding HIV/AIDS and sexual health.

Health services research demonstrates that clinicians rarely ask patients about their sexual orientation, gender identity, or sexual behaviors. Clinicians often serve as trusted, reliable sources of knowledge and support, but when they do not ask questions about SOGI, patients are less likely to proactively share this information. Research indicates that this is also true of young patients: two-thirds of young LGB adults have never discussed their sexual orientation with a health care provider despite a desire to do so.

Given the personal and medical importance of sexuality, clinicians should be well trained to ask patients in a sensitive and culturally appropriate manner about their sexual orientation, gender identity, sexual behaviors and concerns, and reproductive and family planning needs. Routinely collecting SOGI information strengthens the patient-provider relationship and helps providers assess and respond to risks. Lack of knowledge about or of inquiry into patients' SOGI may make clinicians seem ignorant and dismissive of their LGBTQ patients. Moreover, LGBTQ patients share many of the same life experiences and health risks as cisgender heterosexual individuals, including intimate partner violence, family building, and issues of sexuality. These are important components of all patients' lives, but they are frequently overlooked as a result of stereotyping. Care providers must be aware of limitations in their ability to treat LGBTQ patients and should educate themselves to provide more thorough and targeted education to their patients. Chaps. 3 and 8 should be con-

sulted for more complete discussion of clinical interactions, appropriate history-taking, and satisfactory clinical data collection practices.

A basic understanding of sexual and gender minority (SGM) health on the part of the care provider is critical in removing barriers to collecting information from LGBTQ patients. Clinicians should be able to differentiate data variables of interest. A working knowledge of SGM, and the ability to differentiate them, are important factors in providing care and establishing a rapport. Although terms for gender identity are diverse and constantly evolving, a general understanding of **gender variance** and **gender nonconformity** is crucial. It is important to consider that a willingness to admit to gaps in one's knowledge may improve rapport and decision-making.

False assumptions about sexual orientation (most often the **heterosexual assumption**) may alienate or offend some LGBTQ patients. Health care providers often make erroneous assumptions about patients' SOGI demographics. Gender identity, not natal sex, is considered a key element of an individual's sexual orientation, and patients should be allowed to self-identify both their gender identity and their sexual orientation. For example, a transwoman, having been assigned male sex at birth, may also identify as a lesbian because she is a woman attracted to women. **Health professionals should be prepared to address the circumstance in which legal or technical documents list the patient's natal sex rather than the patient's currently lived gender identity**.

Recall that sexual orientation and sexual behaviors cannot be assumed or inferred from one another. For example, a survey of men in New York City showed that of those who self-identified as heterosexual or straight, 9.4% reported having sex with men within the previous year. A large majority of women who identify as lesbians report past sexual activity with men. **The differences between sexual orientation and sexual behavior affect clinically relevant prevention and treatment considerations**. Sexual orientation is patient-defined. Therefore, a clinician should not label or document a woman as a lesbian because she has recently had sexual partners who are women. Sexual behaviors cannot be inferred from sexual orientation. Therefore, specific forms of sexual contact cannot be assumed from a patient's reported sexual orientation. To provide patient-centered care for all patients, providers should understand that identity is multifaceted and that each patient's expressions of identity are unique, regardless of sexual orientation.

> **Key Points**
> - Because of a lack of SOGI information, clinicians cannot always provide evidence-based care for LGBTQ patients.
> - In addition to providing competent care, health professionals need training to develop competence and comfort with collecting and documenting SOGI information in addition to information about sexual behaviors.
> - SOGI identity terms are defined by the patient.
> - SOGI information and sexual behaviors cannot be assumed or inferred from one another.

Clinical Context of Disclosure and Documentation

Across health care settings, SOGI demographic data are documented by various people, including patients, registrars, medical assistants, nurses, and physicians. Because of the sensitivity of these topics, one must consider patient-centered approaches when collecting and using SOGI information. Multiple methods exist for patients to share their SOGI information, including self-reporting on paper intake forms, online questionnaires through patient portals, or response to verbal inquiry by a registrar, nurse, or clinician. Evidence suggests that patients are most comfortable using non-verbal self-reported approaches for sharing their SOGI information.

The characteristics of health care settings also influence patients' willingness to discuss their SOGI, sexual behavior, and sexual attractions. In outpatient settings, patients with an established patient-provider rapport may be more likely to discuss their SOGI. This contrasts with inpatient or emergency department encounters, during which relationships with providers are often brief and focused on a patient's immediate medical problems. Furthermore, patients can choose their clinicians in outpatient settings and schedule encounters with specific ones, whereas inpatient and emergency settings are more unpredictable and sometimes more threatening to LGBTQ patients. Recent studies have shown that many LGBTQ patients would prefer to select clinicians who are openly LGBTQ or who identify themselves as **allies**. Many clinics have made an active effort to welcome LGBTQ individuals on their websites, which is an important cue to safety and inclusion; however, there has been shown to be great geographic variation in LGBTQ-specific content on websites that may be associated with sociopolitical culture. Patients who are unsure of a provider's beliefs or a hospital's views on LGBTQ patients (often in religiously-affiliated institutions) note reluctance to share their SOGI or relationship status. The demands of the inpatient environment do not remove the need to be cognizant of and sensitive to the existence of LGBTQ people. Likewise, emergency department staff function as the first contact for many patients entering the health care system, making cultural competency critical. Unfortunately, negative experiences in emergency departments are common for LGBTQ patients, and these initial interactions create negative associations with medicine as a whole.

Psychosocial and cultural influences affect a patient's decision to provide their SOGI information. Interviews of gay men have shown that affirmation or rejection on coming out often influences the decision to come out to others. Some men have noted that rejection, or even perceived uneasiness, on the part of a health professional led them to delay or avoid coming out to family members and friends. A professional's position in society, the expectation of a higher level of education, and the history of the **pathologization of homosexuality** make a health professional's reaction especially important. Avoiding heteronormative lines of questioning (e.g., asking a male patient whether he has a girlfriend; asking whether a patient is single, married, widowed, or divorced; or not acknowledging that there are other meaningful forms of partnership) and allowing space for patients to easily offer SOGI information should be part of the clinician's role.

Patients may also withhold information about their SOGI or sexual behaviors because they perceive these personal details as irrelevant to their care. Yet, similar to marital status and religion, this information give providers insight into the values, needs, and lived experiences of the patient. Furthermore, collecting information on sexual orientation is helpful in regard to such medicolegal issues as power of attorney, next of kin rights, and visitation policies. These rationales should be explained to the patient and should guide the documentation and use of these data.

> **Key Points**
> A patient's willingness to share information about their SOGI and sexual behaviors depends on a variety of factors, including the type of health care setting, psychosocial and cultural influences, privacy concerns, and the patient's perception of the information's relevance.

Data's Potential to Improve Health Care and Health Outcomes

Routine SOGI information collection enables researchers to identify and address health disparities experienced by LGBTQ populations and sub-populations. These data can also be used to identify underlying reasons for existing health disparities, including disparities due to health care. These data may in turn lead to effective interventions on the individual or population level. For example, research on health care among lesbian and bisexual women has shown that they face numerous challenges in obtaining

preventive health care services such as routine mammograms. Cost may be a greater concern because of limitations in same-sex–partner health insurance benefits. Mistrust of the health care system and poor relationships with providers often serve as further barriers for lesbian and bisexual women. However, lesbian and bisexual women who report being comfortable with their provider are more likely to seek preventive care.

Patient health illiteracy and misinformation also serve as barriers to quality care. Reports suggest that women who have sex with women (WSW) and transgender men are less likely to seek routine gynecologic care such as Pap smears, in part because of the misperception that these tests are not necessary for them. Although there are conflicting data, providers may be less likely to offer routine gynecologic care to these patients for the same reasons. There are limited data on whether screening mammography is routinely offered to transgender men. Routine and appropriate data collection can reveal barriers and disparities in accessing and utilizing services. Collecting data that are inclusive of SOGI and sexual behaviors enables opportunities for quality improvement, research, and improvement of the evidence base for better practices regarding LGBTQ health.

> **Key Points**
> • Routine SOGI collection in health care settings has the potential to identify barriers to care and drivers of health disparities.
> • The collection of data inclusive of SOGI and sexual behaviors enables opportunities for quality improvement, research, and improvement of the evidence base for better care practices for LGBTQ people.

Storage and Use of Data

There are competing challenges in the documentation of SOGI information, sharing of this information among care providers and care teams whom the patient trusts, and protecting the patient from discrimination by others who may have access to these sensitive data.

Another important consideration is where SOGI data are stored in the patient's medical record and how the information is used. As with all personal information, providers should be prepared to discuss patient privacy concerns, storage of confidential information, and use of personal patient data. One common concern for patients is the disclosure of information to other individuals or entities, including family members, health proxies, other care providers, insurance companies, and employers. For example, a transgender patient may be out to their endocrinologist yet desire to keep this confidential from other providers because of anticipated discrimination or harm within the health care system. Health care professionals should clarify with patients who may see their SOGI information in the record, and when, and take appropriate steps to protect patient privacy. Some practices have adopted electronic health record (EHR) "secret codes" to maintain confidentiality. Health Insurance Portability and Accountability Act (HIPAA) regulations do not formally categorize SOGI as protected health information. Because many states still do not have anti-discrimination laws protecting LGBTQ people, privacy concerns can play a large role in a patient's willingness to share their SOGI information, even when the patient is assured that encounters and the information gathered during them are confidential.

Much of the recent debate about collecting SOGI information centers on clinicians' concerns that collecting such data is burdensome in their clinical workflow and that the questions may offend the patient. Although collecting and documenting SOGI information may take time, the practice empowers the clinician to approach LGBTQ-related issues sensitively, to include partners accompanying the patient in conversations regarding care, and to strengthen the therapeutic alliance between patients and providers. This may require changes in workflow, software, or forms, but it must be emphasized that this information does positively affect care—both interpersonally and biomedically.

Unfortunately, when such information is collected, it is not usually recorded in a standardized format. For example, various EHRs permit documentation of gender identity in social history, as unstructured free text, or in the problem list. Also, the methods of collecting information are diverse: A physician or registrar may ask verbally during intake or the interview; patients may self-report in the clinic, using a questionnaire; or standardized forms may be completed privately at electronic kiosks or at home using a patient health portal. Ideally, SOGI information are joined with the patient encounter and archived in a fashion like that used of other patient demographic characteristics, simplifying the process of aggregating data to detect health and health care disparities. Designated spaces and drop-down menus within EHRs can simplify collection and evaluation of SOGI information.

Key Points

- SOGI collection and documentation raises issues regarding patient confidentiality and privacy. Health professionals should be aware of their patients' desire for specific instances of confidentiality within their medical record, keeping in mind the various health professionals and contexts within which the patient may receive care.
- Debate continues regarding the feasibility and importance of collecting and documenting such identifiers despite opportunities for improvements in care.
- EHRs pose technical difficulties in documentation but can be modified to accommodate SOGI identifiers.

National Strategies and Initiatives for Inclusion

The inclusion of sexual orientation in population health surveys is highly feasible. For example, the Washington State Behavioral Risk Factor Surveillance System (BRFSS) was used to identify health disparities among LGB individuals. The investigators found that lesbian and bisexual women were more likely to have poor physical and mental health and had less access to care and that gay and bisexual men were more likely to have poor mental health and participate in risky health behaviors, including tobacco use. Notably, this study demonstrated that sexual orientation can be captured effectively and routinely as a standard demographic variable in EHRs.

Some large-scale research initiatives that are inclusive of sexual and gender minorities are underway. The *All of Us* Research Program under the National Institutes of Health includes SOGI variables. *All of Us* is a precision medicine initiative seeking to enroll a cohort of over one million diverse Americans. The cohort will serve as a base for specific research protocols for a wide range of diseases with the potential for excellent statistical power. The Population Research in Identity and Disparities for Equality (PRIDE) Study is the first large-scale, prospective longitudinal study of people who identify as LGBTQ, or another sexual or gender minority. Since 2017, the PRIDE Study has enrolled participants from web-enabled devices. Participants complete annual questionnaires on their general health status and focused questionnaires on a variety of health topics.

In 2011, the Institute of Medicine released the report *The Health of LGBT People: Building a Foundation for Better Understanding*, which advocated for the routine collection of SOGI information from patients across a variety of health care settings. The Joint Commission has made recommendations to collect SOGI information for all patients, to identify appropriate processes to collect this information, and to ensure voluntary collection privacy. The Joint Commission has also emphasized the need to collect SOGI information in national and community-based needs assessments aimed at improving LGBTQ health, eliminating health care disparities, and ensuring the delivery of quality health care to LGBTQ patients. In 2013, the National Health Interview Survey (NHIS) began collecting information about sexual orientation. However, gender identity was not included. Requirements

for SOGI data collection were debated as part of Stage II Meaningful Use but were ultimately omitted because of a lack of consensus and provider concerns about clinical relevance, discomfort, and burden. Nevertheless, the Health IT Policy Committee made recommendations to the Office of the National Coordinator for Health Information Technology (ONCHIT) in the fall of 2013 to include available fields and functionality for SOGI information in all certified EHRs.

Several leading health care systems have realized the importance of recording SOGI information. The University of California, Davis was the first academic health system to capture sexual SOGI information in its EHRs. Others are taking similar steps, but numerous challenges and obstacles exist, including the use of multiple EHR systems and information exchange, standardizing provider training, and satisfaction of insurer payment requirements.

The Emergency Department Query for Patient-Centered Approaches to Sexual Orientation and Gender Identity (EQUALITY) Study was funded by the Patient Centered Outcomes Research Institute (PCORI) to engage patients to develop and test patient-centered approaches to collecting sexual orientation and gender identity information in the emergency department. A nationally representative survey conducted by the EQUALITY Study found that the vast majority of clinicians feel that they will offend patients by asking patients about their SOGI information; however, another national survey found that the vast majority of patients were comfortable with providing SOGI information in clinical settings. These findings highly a substantial disconnect between provider and patient beliefs regarding willingness to collect SOGI information. A comparative effectiveness study trialing two different methods of collecting SOGI information found that LGBTQ patients were more comfortable sharing their SOGI information when given a non-verbal self-report option (e.g., questionnaires and forms) compared with clinicians verbally asking during the clinical encounter. This study is one of many across the United States exploring how patients beliefs and preferences regarding the collection of SOGI information affect health care delivery and ultimately affect the health of many LGBTQ populations.

Key Points
- Research shows that the inclusion of SOGI information in population health surveys and clinical settings is feasible and valuable.
- Gender identity is less frequently captured in population health surveys than sexual orientation.

Sources

Allen LB, Glicken AD, Beach RK, Naylor KE. Adolescent health care experience of gay, lesbian, and bisexual young adults. J Adolescent Health. 1998;23:212–20.

Alper J, Feit MN, Sanders JQ, editors. Collecting sexual orientation and gender identity data in electronic health records: workshop summary. Washington, DC: National Academies Press; 2013.

Bauer GR, Scheim AI, Deutsch MB, Massarella C. Reported emergency department avoidance, use, and experiences of transgender persons in Ontario, Canada: results from a respondent-driven sampling survey. Ann Emerg Med. 2014;63(6):713–20.

Bergeron S, Senn CY. Health care utilization in a sample of Canadian lesbian women: predictors of risk and resilience. Women Health. 2003;37(3):19–35.

Brotman S, Ryan B, Meyer E. The health and social service needs of gay and lesbian seniors and their families in Canada. Montreal, Quebec: McGill University School of Social Work; 2006.

Cahill S, Makadon H. Sexual orientation and gender identity data collection in clinical settings and in electronic health records: a key to ending LGBT health disparities. LGBT Health. 2014;1(1):34–41.

Canner JK, Harfouch O, Kodadek LM, Pelaez D, Coon D, Offodile AO 2nd, et al. Temporal trends in gender affirming surgery across the United States. JAMA Surg. 2018;153(7):609–16.

Coulter RW, Kenst KS, Bowen DJ, Scout. Research funded by the National Institutes of Health on the health of lesbian, gay, bisexual, and transgender populations. Am J Public Health. 2014;104:e105–12.

Deutsch MB, Keatley J, Sevelius J, Shade SB. Collection of gender identity data using electronic medical records: survey of current end-user practices. J Assoc Nurses AIDS Care. 2014;25(6):657–63.

Dilley JA, Simmons KW, Boysun MJ, Pizacani BA, Stark MJ. Demonstrating the importance and feasibility of including sexual orientation in public health sur-

veys: health disparities in the Pacific Northwest. Am J Public Health. 2010;100(3):460–7.

Eliason MJ, Streed CG Jr. Choosing "something else" as a sexual identity: evaluating response options on the National Health Interview Survey. LGBT Health. 2017;4(5):376–9.

German D, Kodadek L, Shields R, Peterson S, Snyder C, Schneider EB, et al. Implementing sexual orientation and gender identity data collection in emergency departments: patient and staff perspectives. LGBT Health. 2016;3(6):416–23.

Haider AH, Ranjit A, Vail L, Scott V, Kodadek LM, Shields RY, et al. Emergency department query for patient-centered approaches to sexual orientation and gender identity (EQUALITY): a mixed methods study. JAMA Intern Med. 2017;177(6):819–28.

Haider AH, Adler RR, Schneider E, Leitz TU, Ranjit A, Ta C, et al. Assessment of patient-centered approaches to collect sexual orientation and gender identity information in the emergency department: the equality study. JAMA Netw Open. 2018;1(8):e186506.

Heath M, Mulligan E. Seeking open minded doctors—how women who identify as bisexual, queer or lesbian seek quality health care. Aust Fam Physician. 2007;36(6):469–71.

Human Rights Campaign Foundation. Healthcare equality index, 2014. Washington, DC: Human Rights Campaign; 2014.

Human Rights Campaign Foundation. Healthcare equality index, 2018. Washington, DC: Human Rights Campaign; 2018. ISBN: 1-934765-47-3.

Institute of Medicine Committee on Lesbian, Gay, Bisexual, and Transgender Health Issues: Research Gaps and Opportunities. The health of lesbian, gay, bisexual, and transgender people: building a foundation for better understanding. Bethesda: Institute of Medicine; 2011.

Kodadek LM, Peterson S, Shields RY, German D, Snyder D, Schneider EB, Lau BD, Haider AH. Collecting sexual orientation and gender identity information in the emergency department: the divide between patient and provider perspectives. Emerg Med J. 2019;36(3):136–41.

Kreps GL, Peterkin AD, Willes K, Allen M, Manning J, Ross K, et al. In: Harvey VL, Housel TH, editors. Health care disparities and the LGBT population. Lanham: Lexington Books; 2014.

Krieger N. Embodying inequality: a review concepts, measures, and methods for studying health consequences of discrimination. Int J Health Serv. 1999;29(2):295–352.

Lauver DR, Karon SL, Egan J, Jacobson M, Nugent J, Settersten L, et al. Understanding lesbians' mammography utilization. Womens Health Issues. 1999;9(5):264–74.

Lutwak N. Opportunity also knocks in the emergency room: improved emergency department culture could dramatically impact LGBT perceptions of healthcare. LGBT Health. 2014;1(3):149–50.

Maragh-Bass AC, Torain M, Adler R, Schneider EB, Ranjit A, Kodadek LM, et al. Risks, benefits, and importance of collecting sexual orientation and gender identity in healthcare settings: a multi-method analysis of patient and provider perspectives. LGBT Health. 2017a;4(2):141–52.

Maragh-Bass AC, Torain M, Adler R, Ranjit A, Schneider EB, Shields R, et al. Is it okay to ask: transgender patient perspectives on sexual orientation and gender identity collection in healthcare. Acad Emerg Med. 2017b;24(6):655–67.

Marrazzo JM, Koutsky LA, Kiviat NB, Kuypers JM, Stine K. Papanicolaou test screening and prevalence of genital human papillomavirus among women who have sex with women. Am J Public Health. 2001;91(6):947–52.

National Institutes of Health. All of us research program. U.S. Department of Health & Human Services. Accessed November 19, 2018. Available at allofus.nih.gov.

Nguyen A, Lau BD. Collection of sexual orientation and gender identity information: filling the gaps in sexual and gender minority health. Med Care. 2018;56(3):205–7.

Pathela P, Hajat A, Schillinger J, Blank S, Sell R, Mostashari F. Discordance between sexual behavior and self-reported sexual identity: a population-based survey of New York City men. Ann Intern Med. 2006;145(6):416–25.

Patient Centered Outcomes Research Institute. The pride study. Accessed November 19, 2018. Available at pridestudy.org.

Poteat T, German D, Kerrigan D. Managing uncertainty: a grounded theory of stigma in transgender health care encounters. Soc Sci Med. 2013;84:22–9.

Ruben MA, Blosnich JR, Dichter ME, Luscri L, Shipherd JC. Will veterans answer sexual orientation and gender identity questions? Med Care. 2017;55(suppl 9, suppl 2):S85–9.

Shields RY, Lau BD, Haider AH. Emergency general surgery needs for lesbian, gay, bisexual, and transgender patients: are we prepared? JAMA Surg. 2017;152(7):617–8.

Snelgrove JW, Jasudavisius AM, Rowe BW, Head EM, Bauer GR. "Completely out-at-sea" with "two-gender medicine": a qualitative analysis of physician-side barriers to providing health care for transgender patients. BMC Health Serv Res. 2012;12(1):110.

St Pierre M. Coming out in primary healthcare: an empirical investigation of a model of predictors and health outcomes of lesbian disclosure [doctoral dissertation]. Windsor, Ontario: University of Windsor; 2013.

Streed CG Jr, Makadon HJ. Sex and gender reporting in research. JAMA. 2017;317(9):974–5.

Sue DW. Microaggressions in everyday life: race, gender, and sexual orientation. New York: Wiley; 2010.

Wimberly YH, Hogben M, Moore-Ruffin J, Moore SE, Fry-Johnson Y. Sexual history-taking among primary care physicians. J Natl Med Assoc. 2006;98:1924–9.

Wu HY, Monseur BC, Yin O, Selter JH, Lau BD, Christianson MS. Lesbian, gay, bisexual, transgender (LGBT) content on reproductive endocrinology and infertility clinic websites. Fertil Steril. 2017;108(1):183–91.

Topics in Global LGBTQ Health

14

Shilpen Patel, C. Nicholas Cuneo, John R. Power, and Chris Beyrer

> "We can no longer afford to discriminate against people on the basis of age, sex, ethnicity, migrant status, sexual orientation and gender identity, or any other basis—we need to unleash the full potential of everyone."
> —*Joaquim Chissano, former president of Mozambique, January 2014*

Sex and Gender Across Cultures

Sexual behavior, sexual identity, **sexual orientation**, **gender identity**, and **gender expression** in the United States are discussed in detail in Chap. 1. These constructs—particularly gender

---

The first listed author is the chapter's associate editor from The Equal Curriculum Project. The chapter authors are otherwise ordered according to their preference.

S. Patel (✉)
University of Washington Department of Global Health, Redwood City, CA, USA

C. N. Cuneo
Brigham and Women's Hospital, Boston Children's Hospital, Boston Medical Center, Boston, MA, USA

J. R. Power
Vanderbilt University Medical Center, Nashville, TN, USA

C. Beyrer
Johns Hopkins Bloomberg School of Public Health, Baltimore, MD, USA
e-mail: cbeyrer@jhsph.edu

identity and gender expression—vary from country to country.

Gender identity and expression vary considerably across cultures, affecting sexual behavior and health in diverse and often unpredictable ways. In Myanmar, *ah chawk ma* (broadly feminine) men who have sex with men (MSM) report more sex partners, less consistent condom use, and greater likelihood of a history of sexually transmitted infections than *tha ngwe* (broadly masculine) peers. In India, *kothis* (broadly feminine) MSM have a higher prevalence of human immunodeficiency virus (HIV) infection and other STIs than their *panthi* (broadly masculine) counterparts. Among black South African MSM, gender-nonconforming men experience more discrimination than their gender-conforming peers. Transgender populations living in low-resource settings such as Latin America and Sub-Saharan Africa continue to be understudied.

Third gender is a term sometimes used to describe individuals who are considered neither male nor female and who may occupy a discrete role in a particular society or culture. Third-gender individuals have been known throughout history and around the world. They include the *hijra* of India, the *khawaja sara* of Pakistan, the *kathoeys* of Thailand, the *fa'afafine* of Polynesia, the *two spirits* of Native Americans, the sworn virgins of the Balkans, the *xanith* of Oman, the *mangaiko* of the Democratic Republic of Congo, and the *muxe* of Mexico, among many others. Recent legal rulings in India and Nepal have brought legal recognition to third-gender status in those countries, allowing individuals to designate their genders on government documents such as passports and censuses.

External Resource 14.1
CNN–IBN (Indian Broadcasting Network) examines the **"Story of the 'Third Gender'"** in India, with multiple interviews with members of the *hijra* community in India. Total time 20:42. http://bit.ly/TECe1ch14_01

Human sexual behavior comprises a wide range of physical activities through which human beings experience and express their sexuality, encompassing sexual contact of all forms. Individuals' sexual behavior may or may not be consistent with their expressed sexual orientations, particularly when such behaviors are not culturally embraced (e.g., same-sex, extramarital, or nonprocreative). Sexual mores—the range of what is considered socially acceptable sexual behaviors—are dynamic and vary dramatically both within and across cultures. Even when scope is limited to a specific cultural population, great variation is reported in types and combinations of sexual acts.

Unlike the United States, where sexual orientation is frequently defined as lesbian, gay, or bisexual, it is common in some countries for MSM to distinguish or define themselves on the basis of their sexual roles (e.g., insertive, receptive), particularly when these roles are commonly segregated or adhered to strictly. Within such cultures, MSM who are exclusively insertive partners often consider themselves to have a sexuality that is of negligible distinction from that of their heterosexual peers. As such, these men may be resistant to identifying as gay (or a similar sexual orientation category), because these terms do not maintain this role distinction.

As discussed in Chap. 1, it is important for health professionals to recognize that sexual identity, sexual orientation, and sexual behaviors are all different and to understand how each relates to a patient's overall sexual health. When dealing with patients from diverse cultures, the health professional must be careful to ask questions about sexual identity in an open-ended manner and refrain from pushing patients to define themselves in terms that they do not themselves volunteer.

Key Points
- Gender identity and expression varies considerably across cultures, affecting sexual behavior and health in diverse and often unpredictable ways.
- *Third gender* is a term used to describe individuals who are not considered male or female and who may occupy a discrete role within a particular society.
- Sexual identity, the specific sexuality with which an individual identifies, is culturally influenced and may be based on an individual's attraction to a specific sex, sexual role, or identification with social norms.
- An individual's sexual behavior may vary significantly from the person's reported sexual identity, particularly when that identity is not culturally embraced.

Case 14.1
Sonal, a 28-year old from Mumbai, presents in pain to the outpatient department of the local referral hospital with symptoms of chronic urine retention. At the age of 20, Sonal underwent penectomy and castration ("emasculation") by a local unqualified medical practitioner, or so-called quack doctor. Sonal reports taking approximately 30 minutes under strain in a squatting position to void while urinating. Examination of the external genitalia reveals the findings shown in Fig. 14.1.

Sonal recalls exhibiting gender-nonconforming behavior from an early age and was the object of significant bullying in school by peers. At the age of 11, Sonal was

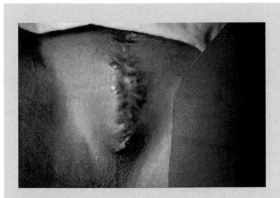

Fig. 14.1 Photo showing urethral stenosis after amputation of the penis by an unskilled practitioner. (From *Indian J Urol*. 2007 23(3):317–318. Reproduced under a Creative Commons Attribution 2.0 Generic (CC BY 2.0) license: https://creativecommons.org/licenses/by/2.0/)

sexually molested by an uncle during a family wedding but never reported the incident. At age 14, Sonal began self-identifying as a *kothi* (a male who selectively adopts female mannerisms and engages in the receptive role during sex) and started regularly sneaking out of the house to have sex with older men. At age 18, Sonal was discovered in bed with a man by a family member and was formally disowned. On leaving the family home, Sonal moved to Mumbai and struggled to find work before becoming introduced to a local *guru*, or *hijra* leader, who took Sonal into her *gharana* (familial house) and began teaching Sonal how to participate in ritual performances for a living as a *hijra*.

What are some of the economic and social factors that may have influenced Sonal's decision to identify as *hijra* and undergo an informal "emasculation" procedure?

What are the risks of undergoing such a procedure? Why are these procedures done by unqualified practitioners?

What are the effects of castration at the age 20 on male secondary sexual characteristics?

What are Sonal's formal surgical options at this point?

Sonal encountered several factors that may have been influential in the decision to identify as hijra *in India. Despite an increasingly marginalized role in Indian society,* hijras *have long held a documented role in the history and cul-*

ture of India, serving a distinct and performative role in many traditional ceremonies, for which they are both tolerated and often compensated by community members (whether out of appreciation or fear, as some believe that hijra *hold mystical powers). In addition to the prospect of economic security offered by* hijra *status, the* hijra *are organized in familial groups that provide love and support to their members, an appealing reality after being disowned by one's family because of one's sexuality. The decision to undergo castration is a complicated one. Sonal may identify as transgender and see "emasculation" as the best option for obtaining gender-affirming surgery. (Gender-affirming surgery is illegal under Section 377 of the Indian Penal Code.) Alternatively, Sonal may have felt pressure to agree to the procedure to continue to participate in the* hijra *community.*

Amputation of the penis and testes by an unskilled provider can lead to any number of complications. Potentially fatal complications include infection resulting in gangrene, sepsis, or both (in the setting of unsterile technique) and uncontrolled bleeding or hemorrhage. Urological complications are numerous. Penile urethral stenosis leading to chronic and painful urine retention is the most common.

Castration after puberty cannot reverse the secondary sexual characteristics acquired during puberty, such as deepening of the voice and male pattern pubic and facial hair. However, it can attenuate some male secondary sexual characteristics, including male muscle mass, body hair, and male pattern baldness. Castration after puberty can reduce a person's libido and has been reported to be associated with changes in mood. Finally, a castrated person who does not take hormone replacement therapy may experience symptoms of menopause such as hot flashes, decreased bone density, and redistribution of adipose tissue.

At this point, Sonal should undergo suprapubic cystostomy to prevent bladder distention, followed by elective perineal urethrostomy to reconstruct the urethral canal. The latter procedure could be coupled with the creation of an artificial vagina and vulva, if Sonal desires.

Table 14.1 The Yogyakarta Principles (2006)

Category	Principle(s)	Interpretation
Rights to Universal Enjoyment of Human Rights, Non-Discrimination and Recognition before the Law	1–3	Defining the principles of the universality of human rights and their application to all persons without discrimination, as well as the right of all people to recognition as a person before the law without sex-reassignment surgery or sterilization
Rights to Human and Personal Security	4–11	Addressing fundamental rights to life, freedom from violence and torture, privacy, access to justice, and freedom from arbitrary detention and human trafficking
Economic, Social and Cultural Rights	12–18	Outlining the importance of nondiscrimination in the enjoyment of economic, social and cultural rights, including employment, accommodation, social security, education, sexual and reproductive health, including the right to informed consent and sex-reassignment therapy
Rights to Expression, Opinion and Association	19–21	Emphasizing the importance of the freedom to express oneself, one's identity, and one's sexuality without State interference based on sexual orientation or gender identity, including the right to participate peaceably in public assemblies and events and otherwise associate in community with others
Freedom of Movement and Asylum	22 and 23	Highlighting the rights of persons to seek asylum from persecution based on sexual orientation or gender identity
Rights of Participation in Cultural and Family Life	24–26	Addressing the rights of persons to participate in family life, public affairs, and the cultural life of their community without discrimination based on sexual orientation or gender identity
Rights of Human Rights Defenders	27	Recognizing the right to defend and promote human rights without discrimination based on sexual orientation and gender identity, as well as the obligation of states to ensure the protection of human rights defenders working in these areas
Rights of Redress and Accountability	28 and 29	Reaffirming the importance of holding rights violators accountable and ensuring appropriate redress for those who face rights violations

Adapted from The Yogyakarta Principles, with permission from ARC International. The Yogyakarta Principles address a broad range of international human rights standards and their application to SOGI issues. On 10 Nov. 2017 a panel of experts published additional principles expanding on the original document reflecting developments in international human rights law and practice since the 2006 Principles, The Yogyakarta Principles plus 10. The new document also contains 111 'additional state obligations' related to areas such as torture, asylum, privacy, health, and the protection of human rights defenders. The full text of the Yogyakarta Principles and the Yogyakarta Principles plus 10 are available at: www.yogyakartaprinciples.org

Human Rights and Legal Status

Yogyakarta Principles

In November 2006, dedicated international human rights authorities gathered in Yogyakarta, Java, to discuss the application of international human rights standards to addressing ongoing abuses to LGBTQ people worldwide. The culmination of this gathering, the Yogyakarta Principles, was agreed upon unanimously. Though these principles have not yet been adopted by the United Nations because of opposition from several countries who violate them, they serve as an important guiding document for interpreting international law as applicable to

LGBTQ individuals. The Yogyakarta Principles are summarized in Table 14.1. In 2017, an additional nine principles were added (Table 14.2).

Criminalization and Legal Rights

The legal rights afforded to individuals of minority sexual orientations and gender identities heavily influence LGBTQ health. Although some countries enforce protections for LGBTQ individuals, at the time of publication of this book over one-third of the world's 196 countries still criminalized same-sex sexual acts between consenting adults. Many such laws are focused on male-male sexual behavior and originated from British colonial anti-sodomy laws. LGBTQ

Table 14.2 The Yogyakarta Principles (2017)

Right	Principle	Explanation
Right to State Protection	30	Everyone, regardless of sexual orientation, gender identity, gender expression or sex characteristics, has the right to State protection from violence, discrimination and other harm, whether by government officials or by any individual or group.
Right to Legal Recognition	31	Everyone has the right to legal recognition without reference to, or requiring assignment or disclosure of, sex, gender, sexual orientation, gender identity, gender expression or sex characteristics. Everyone has the right to obtain identity documents, including birth certificates, regardless of sexual orientation, gender identity, gender expression or sex characteristics. Everyone has the right to change gendered information in such documents while gendered information is included in them.
Right to Bodily and Mental Integrity	32	Everyone has the right to bodily and mental integrity, autonomy and self-determination irrespective of sexual orientation, gender identity, gender expression or sex characteristics. Everyone has the right to be free from torture and cruel, inhuman and degrading treatment or punishment on the basis of sexual orientation, gender identity, gender expression and sex characteristics. No one shall be subjected to invasive or irreversible medical procedures that modify sex characteristics without their free, prior and informed consent, unless necessary to avoid serious, urgent and irreparable harm to the concerned person.
Right to Freedom from Criminalisation and Sanction on the Basis of Sexual Orientation, Gender Identity, Gender Expression or Sex Characteristics	33	Everyone has the right to be free from criminalisation and any form of sanction arising directly or indirectly from that person's actual or perceived sexual orientation, gender identity, gender expression or sex characteristics.
Right to Protection from Poverty	34	Everyone has the right to protection from all forms of poverty and social exclusion associated with sexual orientation, gender identity, gender expression and sex characteristics. Poverty is incompatible with respect for the equal rights and dignity of all persons, and can be compounded by discrimination on the grounds of sexual orientation, gender identity, gender expression and sex characteristics.
Right to Sanitation	35	Everyone has the right to equitable, adequate, safe and secure sanitation and hygiene, in circumstances that are consistent with human dignity, without discrimination, including on the basis of sexual orientation, gender identity, gender expression or sex characteristics.
Right to the Enjoyment of Human Rights in Relation to Information and Communication Technologies	36	Everyone is entitled to the same protection of rights online as they are offline. Everyone has the right to access and use information and communication technologies, including the internet, without violence, discrimination or other harm based on sexual orientation, gender identity, gender expression or sex characteristics. Secure digital communications, including the use of encryption, anonymity and pseudonymity tools are essential for the full realisation of human rights, in particular the rights to life, bodily and mental integrity, health, privacy, due process, freedom of opinion and expression, peaceful assembly and association.
Right to Truth	37	Every victim of a human rights violation on the basis of sexual orientation, gender identity, gender expression or sex characteristics has the right to know the truth about the facts, circumstances and reasons why the violation occurred. The right to truth includes effective, independent and impartial investigation to establish the facts, and includes all forms of reparation recognised by international law. The right to truth is not subject to statute of limitations and its application must bear in mind its dual nature as an individual right and the right of the society at large to know the truth about past events.

(continued)

Table 14.2 (continued)

Right	Principle	Explanation
Right to Practise, Protect, Preserve and Revive Cultural Diversity	38	Everyone, individually or in association with others, where consistent with the provisions of international human rights law, has the right to practise, protect, preserve and revive cultures, traditions, languages, rituals and festivals, and protect cultural sites of significance, associated with sexual orientation, gender identity, gender expression and sex characteristics. Everyone, individually or in association with others, has the right to manifest cultural diversity through artistic creation, production, dissemination, distribution and enjoyment, whatever the means and technologies used, without discrimination based on sexual orientation, gender identity, gender expression or sex characteristics. Everyone, individually or in association with others, has the right to seek, receive, provide and utilise resources for these purposes without discrimination on the basis of sexual orientation, gender identity, gender expression or sex characteristics.

Adapted from The Yogyakarta Principles, with permission from ARC International. The Yogyakarta Principles address a broad range of international human rights standards and their application to SOGI issues. On 10 Nov. 2017 a panel of experts published additional principles expanding on the original document reflecting developments in international human rights law and practice since the 2006 Principles, The Yogyakarta Principles plus 10. The new document also contains 111 'additional state obligations' related to areas such as torture, asylum, privacy, health, and the protection of human rights defenders. The full text of the Yogyakarta Principles and the Yogyakarta Principles plus 10 are available at: www.yogyakartaprinciples.org

criminalization may take the form of increased age of consent for same-sex sexual acts versus those engaged in by people of opposite sexes, illegality of all same-sex sexual acts, or prosecution based on identification (presumed or self-disclosed) as LGBTQ. Legal penalties also vary widely, ranging from corporal punishment to imprisonment to death.

A discriminatory legal environment promotes poor health outcomes among LGBTQ individuals. Apart from the direct consequence of legal penalties, human rights abuses such as blackmail, harassment, and beatings are common experiences in many global LGBTQ communities that are subject to criminalization. Fear of and experience with human rights abuses or criminal prosecution has been associated with avoidance of HIV testing and of seeking health care by MSM.

Criminal statutes also limit service availability. For example, a study of the enforcement of discriminatory Senegalese laws documented that HIV-prevention providers suspend their work with MSM out of fear for their own safety. Decriminalization of minority sexual orientations, gender identities, and sexual behaviors has been identified as a necessary step in combating stigma and promoting health equity.

Criminalization of LGBTQ individuals hampers efforts to conduct research and prevention programs. Criminal statutes limit funding and resources for programs devoted to health issues that affect LGBTQ patients. Fear of identification and prosecution causes reluctance among LGBTQ individuals to participate in research and prevention programs. For this reason, HIV-prevention programs may not be reaching most MSM. **Compared with countries where same-sex sexual acts are not criminalized, African and Caribbean countries that do criminalize such activity have greater HIV prevalence among MSM.** Therefore, outreach efforts must consider the consequences of criminalization and should be conducted in collaboration with community stakeholders.

Stigma

Stigma, which is determined largely by prevailing cultural norms, is often more intense in rural and traditional communities. In many complex ways, stigmatization—in the community, among the general public, in the health care system, and as applied by the makers of policy—negatively affects health outcomes in the global LGBTQ community.

Stigma affects LGBTQ persons directly, contributing to the development of internalized homophobia and affective disorders or maladaptive coping mechanisms such as substance use. Increased sexual risk-taking behavior can be a means of connecting with other LGBTQ individuals or a means of survival, particularly in regions where employment discrimination persists. Stigma is associated with a reluctance to communicate high-risk behaviors to sexual partners and health care workers. It is also associated with avoidance of the health care system. A study of MSM in Swaziland revealed "delayed care-seeking, travel to more distant clinics, and missed opportunities for appropriate services." Globally, this translates to delays in STI testing and initiation of antiretroviral therapy for HIV infection among MSM.

Health professionals around the world often lack understanding and sensitivity toward LGBTQ people. There is a widespread lack of health care facilities and community-based organizations that serve LGBTQ communities, in part because of discrimination in public funding. Efforts to combat stigma include antidiscrimination media campaigns, targeted funding for organizations that facilitate safe and open communication, repeal of criminalizing laws, and training for health professionals on the health care needs of LGBTQ people.

Discrimination and Violence

Discrimination in the form of physical violence can pose a critical threat. Lack of legal protection and pervasive social stigma in many regions encourage targeted mob "justice," including beatings, attacks, and murders. Many LGBTQ communities lack police protection and legal rights. Police in some areas target LGBTQ individuals with blackmail and violence.

Globally, LGBTQ individuals experience a high level of sexual violence. A study in South Africa found that MSM were more than twice as likely to have been sexually assaulted as other men. Further, MSM were found to have experienced a relatively high level of intimate partner violence associated with sex under the influence of drugs or alcohol and unprotected sex. MSM sex workers were more likely to engage in substance use and to have experienced physical and/or sexual violence. Sexual violence puts MSM at greater risk for HIV and other STIs and has been associated with a fear of seeking health care.

LGB women in many regions live with the threat of family violence and "corrective rape," motivated by the belief that rape will cure same-sex sexual attraction or behavior. Such attacks have in many cases led to other forms of torture and even murder. Much LGB-targeted violence occurs in the context of a high level of generalized violence against women (e.g., South Africa, Zimbabwe, Uganda, and Jamaica).

Case 14.2

Obinze is a gay man who lives in central Nigeria. Although he does not live in one of the nine states governed by Sharia law (under which men who engage in same-sex acts are stoned to death), he feels that he must be secretive in finding male partners and has no access to water-based lubricants. In 2014, the Nigerian federal government enacted the Same-Sex Marriage Prohibition Act which, in addition to banning same-sex marriage, banned meetings of the LGBTQ community and imposed a 10-year prison sentence for individuals who "make public show of same-sex amorous relationships."

In what ways might this legislation affect Obinze's health and well-being?

How do these penalties compare to LGBTQ-targeted criminal statutes in other countries?

Criminalization of LGBTQ activity puts individuals such as Obinze at risk for criminal penalties at the hands of law enforcement, as well as human rights abuses outside legal punishment, often exacted by individuals not affiliated with law enforcement. These threats impose myriad barriers to care and prevention services for

LGBTQ people. Criminalization also pro-motes stigma against LGBTQ people that may manifest as discrimination by health care providers or as mental illnesses such as internalized homophobia.

Seventy-five other countries have anti-LGBTQ laws, many of them even more far-reaching or strictly enforced than Nigeria's. Sentencing for LGBTQ identity or behavior in many countries is also more severe, with penalties of longer prison sentences or even death.

Key Points

- The Yogyakarta Principles were estab-lished in 2006 as a guiding document to interpreting international law as appli-cable to LGBTQ individuals. Nine addi-tional principles were added in 2017.
- The legal status of same-sex sexual acts and sexual identities varies significantly from country to country and can have a significant effect on LGBTQ sexual behaviors and health outcomes.
- Stigma, which is largely determined by prevailing cultural norms, affects multi-ple aspects of the LGBTQ experience, contributing to differences in sexual risk behaviors and interactions with the health care system that can lead to adverse health outcomes.
- The experience of discrimination—including harassment, physical vio-lence, and sexual violence—is common in LGBTQ persons and populations around the world.

Health Care Access

Discrimination in Health Care Settings

Discrimination against LGBTQ individuals by health care workers is a major barrier to appropri-ate care worldwide. This discrimination takes a range of forms, from such subtle manifestations as language insensitivity or discomfort in dis-cussing same-sex sexual health topics to direct abuse in the form of derogatory comments, blackmail, denial of care, and violence. In coun-tries where same-sex acts are illegal and provider-patient confidentiality is not protected, patients may go to extensive lengths to conceal their sex-ual orientations and activities in the health care setting for fear that they will be denied care or suffer legal reprisals.

Fear of stigma or discrimination at the hands of health care providers can have devastating effects on individual care and on public health. In Hong Kong, perceived discrimination toward MSM was reported by 39% of respondents and was associated with lower uptake of HIV volun-tary counseling and testing services. This finding was echoed in qualitative interviews of MSM in Chengdu, China, who cited stigma as a major obstacle to obtaining appropriate health care. Transgender persons around the globe are espe-cially vulnerable to discrimination by health care personnel and are often specifically excluded because the stated gender on their official identi-fication documents does not match their gender expression. These and other factors contribute to the disproportionately high burden of HIV/AIDS among transgender women.

In South Africa, where legal protections for LGBTQ individuals exist, MSM in urban areas nonetheless reported disturbing encounters with health care workers that led many to deny their same-sex behaviors or to project a hetero-sexual identity during interviews with provid-ers. In Malawi, Namibia, and Botswana, where same-sex behavior is illegal, only 17% of MSM reported disclosing same-sex practices to a health professional and 19% reporting that they were afraid to seek care. In Lesotho where MSM sex acts became legal in 2012 22% of MSM respondents reported being afraid to seek care in 2011. Studies from south ern Africa reveal a common narrative of dis crimination against and fear among MSM i the health care setting across varying lega backdrops, indicating that legal protections ar a necessary but incomplete step toward greate health equity.

Access to Gender-Affirming Treatment Among Transgender People

Low health system resources in general and stigma affecting trans individuals in specific combine to dramatically limit access to **cross-gender hormone therapy (CGHT)**, also called **gender affirming hormone therapy** or **cross-sex hormone therapy**, and **gender affirming surgery (GAS)** in the developing world. Countries differ dramatically with respect to the availability, legality, cost, and accessibility of CGHT/GAS for transgender people. Access to CGHT/GAS has been correlated with improved mental health among transgender people and is identified as a basic human right in the Yogyakarta principles. Limited access to CGHT/GAS can force individuals identifying as transgender to seek hormones or surgical reassignment on the black market or through medical tourism, with potentially staggering health and economic consequences at the individual level.

Access to CGHT, often involving significant barriers to care and great expense, has been identified as a driver of sex work among transgender women. When CGHT is limited and unsupervised by medical professionals, transgender women are placed at further risk when they take high doses of oral estrogens (rather than sublingual, transdermal, or injectable formulations), a practice that may be harmful. Injectable formulations put users at risk for communicable diseases when the needles are shared.

GAS is offered by a limited number of health care providers who have sought out the specialized training necessary to perform the associated procedures. Access to these providers is often influenced by the standards of care identified by the World Professional Association for Transgender Health (WPATH), such as preceding documentation and clearance by two mental health providers who have worked with the patient over time. As a result of these barriers, there are relatively few trained providers worldwide, and those who do offer GAS often have lengthy waiting lists or have incomplete training. Consequently, transgender persons often journey long distances at considerable cost to get GAS, usually at regional hubs such as Thailand (Asia), Belgium and Serbia (Europe), South Africa (Africa), the United States (Americas) and Iran (Middle East).

Key Points

- Discrimination by health care providers is a major barrier to appropriate care among LGBTQ people worldwide. It ranges from insensitivity to denial of care or even violence.
- Fear of stigma or discrimination at the hands of health care providers influences LGBTQ access and use of health care services, even in countries where legal protections for LGBTQ people exist.
- Trans individuals face particular challenges in accessing gender-confirming treatment, forcing some individuals into the black market for such care or into sex work to pay for such care.
- Gender affirming surgery is a highly specialized service that is unavailable in most countries and out of reach for most trans individuals.

Case 14.3

Daniela, a 32-year-old trans woman who identifies as a *travesti*, is rushed to the hospital in respiratory distress after attending a "pumping party" in Rio de Janeiro. At the party, low-cost injections of silicone were being offered by a *bombadeira* (a person, usually lacking formal medical training, who makes a living offering such injections) for buttock and thigh enhancement. A sex worker, Daniela had been seeing a decline in the rates she was able to negotiate with clients for several months while she had been simultaneously attempting to save money to afford breast implants. The friend who organized the party offered to let her in for a reduced rate (normal admission was about $400). Daniela hoped that with the enhancement(s) she would be able to get back on track in achieving her saving goals for the implants.

What is the most likely explanation for Daniela's respiratory distress?

What are other complications of silicone injections?

What are the major forces driving Daniela's decision to attend the party? What are the major barriers to Daniela's accessing gender affirming treatment in Brazil?

Daniela is most likely suffering from a silicone pulmonary embolism secondary to silicone accidentally being injected into the bloodstream, making its way from the venous system to the right heart to the pulmonary arteries. Another potential explanation would be an acute hypersensitivity reaction to the silicone, which is often not medical-grade but rather industrial-grade (impure).

There are numerous complications of silicone injections in addition to pulmonary embolism and various types of hypersensitivity reactions to the injected material. Because the silicone is injected in liquid form and not confined within an implant, it is potentially mobile and can migrate from the original injection site and into the lower limbs, affecting circulation and leading to edema. Finally, if there is trauma while the silicon is still soft and pliable, it can harden in a permanently disfiguring manner.

As a sex worker, Daniela is reliant on her body for negotiating power with clients and for survival. Silicone implants (either breast or buttock) can cost several thousand dollars. Daniela likely has limited access to credit and will need to save a considerable amount before qualifying for a formal procedure. Furthermore, she could face discrimination while accessing the formal medical system. Pumping parties offer a much cheaper alternative to implants in a more comfortable setting where attendees are more confident that they will not face discrimination due to their gender identity.

Risk Factors

While in many more progressive countries, research on LGBTQ health has evolved to acknowledge health issues beyond sexual behavior, the bulk of global research and research funding has focused on HIV risk in defined MSM populations and to a lesser extent transgender women. Research on transgender men and lesbian and bisexual women is especially lacking globally. This section reflects the existing body of research, which is largely focused on MSM and HIV.

Multiple Partners

Studies of global MSM populations suggest that MSM are more likely to have multiple sex partners (i.e., two or more over a given time period) and concurrent sex partners (i.e., two or more partners at the same time). Although the proportion of MSM who have multiple sex partners varies by context, a sizeable proportion of MSM have multiple sex partners. MSM in urban settings or whose gender expression is more feminine may have higher numbers of sex partners compared to other MSM. Studies in southern Africa show that sex partners of MSM may also be natal women and/or transgender women (the term *MSM* does not exclude men who also have sex with women). MSM commonly have a stable female partner while also having one or more concurrent male sex partners. A study of Chinese MSM showed that having multiple sex partners was just as common among men who had sex with both men and women as it was among men who only had sex with men.

While MSM use condoms more often with irregular partners than with regular partners, simply having multiple sex partners increases the likelihood that MSM will have unprotected anal sex or unprotected vaginal sex. MSM and transgender individuals who have unprotected sex with multiple or concurrent sex partners are at greater risk for HIV compared to those who have unprotected sex with a single partner. This elevated HIV risk is true both when sex partners are men only and when they are both men and women. Similarly, MSM who have multiple sex partners have increased risk for other STIs such as syphilis and HPV.

Sex Work

Studies of global MSM communities indicate that MSM are more likely than non-MSM to be sex workers. In addition, MSM also report higher numbers of commercial male partners and commercial female partners than non-MSM. In addition to exchanging sex for money, sex work includes the exchange of sex for goods or services. Sex workers are generally younger, less educated, and otherwise unemployed. Sex work is often temporary, with continent-wide estimates for duration of sex work ranging from 2.9 years in Asia to 12 years in Latin America. Sex workers often live in environments of pervasive stigmatization and criminalization that further affect their health outcomes.

The rate of condom usage during commercial sex varies by region but is generally below the rate for non-commercial sex, placing sex workers at greater risk for acquiring STIs. Studies show both working as a sex worker and having sex worker partners places LGBTQ individuals at increased risk for HIV infection. In many parts of the world, especially Middle East and North Africa, sex work is one of the principle contributors to new HIV infections. In order to halt the worldwide HIV epidemic, comprehensive strategies to treat and prevent HIV must be inclusive toward sex workers.

Worldwide, transgender women who work as sex workers are at disproportionate risk for HIV infection compared to male or natal female sex workers. In Indonesia, for example, transgender sex workers were observed to have an HIV prevalence of 22% compared to 3.6% among male sex workers or other MSM. Furthermore, a study of newly HIV-diagnosed transgender sex workers in Argentina found that 19% had drug resistant mutations despite reporting not having received antiretroviral treatment. Previous studies showed drug resistance in 4% and 9% of newly diagnosed HIV cases in Argentina's general population and

highlighted the need for careful prevention and treatment among transgender patients. For more information on HIV and sex workers, including MSM and transgender women, see the special 2014 issue of *Lancet* containing Poteat et al.

Substance Use Disorders

Alcohol and substance use disorders are a common mental health concern among global LGBTQ populations. LGBTQ individuals are more likely to report drug and alcohol use and have been observed to have higher rates of alcohol use disorders. Transgender individuals are believed to be at disproportionate risk. A study of Vietnamese MSM showed prevalent alcohol use that was higher among trans-identifying MSM. (Recall from Chap. 1 that the term *MSM* is often problematic for discussing transgender and gender nonconforming people. As here, transgender women are often classified as MSM based on their natal sex.) Substance use among LGBTQ is widely believed to occur as a coping strategy for stigma and discrimination. For example, a study of MSM and transgender women in El Salvador associated decreased binge drinking decreases with increased disclosures of sexual orientation. Substance use among LGBTQ people may also be driven by socioeconomic factors such as poverty, sex work, or urban surroundings. In a study of Chinese MSM sex workers, those who identified as LGBT and those who did not reported similar prevalence of drug and alcohol use when controlling for socioeconomic status.

The use of drugs and alcohol, especially before or during sex, is associated with risk-taking behaviors. Indeed, some LGBTQ communities use psychoactive drugs to enhance sexual comfort or pleasure, e.g., Indonesian transgender sex workers sometimes use the painkiller carisoprodol. Less consistent condom usage is associated with regular drinking and drinking to intoxication and with injection and noninjection drug use (IDU/NIDU). A study of South African MSM showed that drug use led to inconsistent condom use and other high-risk sexual behavior despite a high level of understanding of HIV risks. For this reason, both drug and alcohol use place MSM at risk for HIV, HSV, syphilis, and other STIs.

Drug and alcohol use place LGBTQ individuals at risk for violence, abuse, arrest, and imprisonment. Violence associated with substance use is observed among male sex workers, noncommercial intimate partners, and persons who are not sexual partners. LGBTQ substance users may be more likely to be arrested and imprisoned than non-LGBTQ substance users. One study in Thailand observed that MSM drug users were more likely than other drug users to have been jailed.

In some parts of the world, LGBTQ health is greatly affected by an increased likelihood to engage in IDU. The prevalence and characteristics of IDU depend heavily on local conditions. Continent-level averages for duration of injection drug use range from 5.6 years (Africa) to 21 years (South America). Despite the extreme health risks that individuals with IDU face, accurate population and disease data for IDU are often unavailable, in part because of difficulties posed by widespread criminalization of the injected drugs.

Sharing of nonsterile injection equipment is an efficient mode of transmission that puts individuals with IDU at high risk for bloodborne infections such as HIV and hepatitis C. It may be more common among MSM than in the general IDU population. Among Iranians who engaged in IDU, for example, sharing of non-sterile injection equipment was more common among MSM. In fact, IDU is a major contributor to new HIV cases in many regions and is the single biggest contributor across the Middle East and North Africa. Studies of MSM in Tanzania and Vietnam have confirmed that those with a history of IDU higher prevalence of HIV and hepatitis C. A study of MSM in Zanzibar showed that in addition to greater risk for HIV and HCV, MSM who inject drugs were more likely to engage in risky sexual behavior, to have acquired STIs, and to have been beaten or arrested. Where IDU and MSM health concerns overlap, it is recommended that risk-reduction efforts take integrated approaches that address both risk groups.

Condom Use

Appropriate condom use is one of the most important HIV and STI biomedical prevention interventions for LGBTQ populations. Condom use is often influenced by a complex set of cultural norms and socioeconomic factors, leading studies in different locations to draw mixed conclusions in comparisons of the rates of condom use in MSM and non-MSM. MSM in sub-Saharan Africa with both male and female partners have been shown to use condoms more than MSM who only have male partners. Women who have sex with women (WSW) also face risks in unprotected sex. A study in Cote d'Ivoire showed that 50.7% of LGB women had sex with men and 60% did not practice protected sex. Generally speaking, condom use among LGBTQ people is higher with nonregular or commercial partners and lower with regular partners. In many contexts, transgender MSM (usually female-identifying natal males) are noted to use condoms less often than MSM generally do. A study of transgender women in Jakarta suggested that attitudes toward condom use were the strongest predictor in the behaviors of getting, carrying, and offering condoms, while perceived behavioral control was the strongest predictor of intention for condom use. Tailored transgender-friendly behavioral interventions such as the Sisters program in Pattya, Thailand, have been shown to successfully increase condom use and HIV testing.

Socioeconomic factors dramatically influence condom use. Low access to condoms is often cited as a main reason for inconsistent condom use. Inaccessibility of the condom-compatible water-based lubricants, which are recommended for anal sex, is another barrier. Other factors associated with low condom use include unemployment, younger age, poverty, and migrant status.

Both low education and low HIV-specific knowledge are associated with inconsistent condom use. Similarly, perceptions of high HIV threat and condom efficacy are associated with greater condom use. Experiences with discrimination, not being out to one's family, and negative beliefs in regard to condoms are associated with inconsistent use. Studies show that peer-based communication and communication with one's partner about condoms are effective strategies for increasing condom use. Moreover, positive social norms surrounding condoms are observed to be associated with lower incidence of HIV infection. Nevertheless, there is not a clear association between consistent condom use and HIV testing among MSM, pointing to a need for comprehensive prevention strategies.

Mental Health

As same-sex behavior and gender nonconformity continue to be stigmatized across the globe, **internalized homophobia** (IH; negative prejudice against same-sex attraction or behavior that individuals apply to themselves) is a major issue worldwide and contributes significantly to mental health and risk behaviors. In countries where homophobia is widespread, institutionalized, or criminalized, exceptionally high rates of IH are reported. In Nigeria, a large percentage of MSM reported being affected by IH, which was itself associated with bisexual identity and HIV status. In Uganda, IH was associated with sex while high or drunk and with anal-receptive sex. In China, IH was associated with decreased uptake of HIV testing services. Although evidence on internalized transphobia is currently lacking, poor mental health outcomes in transgender populations suggest a similar phenomenon.

A growing body of evidence supports an increased risk of psychiatric illness, particularly mood and anxiety disorders and suicidal ideation, among LGBTQ individuals worldwide. A major explanation for this association is the **minority stress model**, which attributes health disparities among sexual and gender minority populations in part to the conflict in values these groups face in the dominant social environment. In fact, IH has been found to be associated with mental health disorders, particularly major depressive disorder, on meta-analysis. The minority stress model is explained in Chap. 12.

Major depressive disorder has been reported in high numbers among LGBTQ individuals worldwide, with significant effects on their risk behaviors. Sixty-one percent of MSM in Nepal reported major depressive disorder symptoms (with 47% reporting suicidal ideation), a finding that was also associated with not using condoms during the last incidence of anal sex. Latino and Asian American WSW in the United States reported greater one-year and lifetime histories of depressive disorders. Among several international populations, mental health disorders have been shown to be associated with substance use disorders, sexual risk-taking, and physical violence.

Key Points
- MSM are more likely than non-MSM to have multiple sex partners and concurrent sex partners, increasing their risk for HIV and other STIs.
- Substance use is one of the most common mental health issues among global MSM populations and is linked with sexual risk behavior, violence, and abuse.
- Injection drug use may be more common among LGBTQ individuals than in the general population, but this appears to depend heavily on local context.
- Appropriate condom use is one of the most important HIV and STI biomedical prevention interventions for MSM, but it is influenced dramatically by socioeconomic factors, including education, access, and discrimination.
- Mental health disorders, particularly major depressive disorder, have been shown to be disproportionately higher among LGBTQ populations, in part because of internalized homophobia.

Case 14.4

Lovely is a 24-year-old Zimbabwean who immigrated to South Africa two years ago and has been living in the township of Alexandra. She identifies as a lesbian and became involved with another woman in a nearby neighborhood shortly after arriving in South Africa. She has begun working at a hair salon in Johannesburg. As an undocumented immigrant, she was initially hesitant to be open about her relationship in the community to avoid any unwanted attention but was encouraged by South Africa's progressive legal protections for its LGBTQ citizens and her girlfriend's activism. Three months ago Lovely was approached as she returned home from a bar by three men she had seen from time to time in the community. They challenged her about her relationship with a woman and told her that they were going to "teach her how to enjoy sex the normal way." They forced themselves into her home and took turns raping her. The men did not use condoms. Before leaving, they warned her that if she told anyone they would see that she was deported back to Zimbabwe, where she would be treated even more poorly if she "decided to continue to be a lesbian."

Lovely told no one, including her girlfriend, about what had happened to her, but she visited a local clinic the next day and was able to obtain post-exposure prophylaxis (PEP) for HIV. Today, Lovely has returned to the clinic. She tests negative for HIV but appears tearful and describes a low mood. She reports that over the past seven weeks she has had trouble sleeping, waking early in the morning, many times to panicked memories of the attack. She has lost interest in activities she used to enjoy, such as reading women's magazines and going out with friends and cannot shake feelings of guilt about the attack. Her energy is limited, and she is finding it difficult to take the bus to work each morning. Lovely has lost more than 7 kg since the attack and has little interest in food. She reports that she sometimes has thoughts that life is not worth living, though she has not thought specifically about killing herself. Lovely also notes that she is starting to drink more than usual—as much as a half pint of hard liquor in one night —but now avoids going to bars. She has also started using marijuana on a nightly basis. Her girlfriend is concerned about the changes in behavior and has been asking Lovely to see a mental health professional.

What were the risk factors in this attack? How does Lovely's migrant status contribute to the situation?

What diagnoses should be considered for Lovely's current symptoms?

How does the use of substances factor into Lovely's situation?

Lovely faces multiple risk factors. As an out lesbian, she is a visible target in a community that may not be especially tolerant of alternative sexual identities. As a Zimbabwean, she likely faces additional discrimination, both because of her immigrant status and her ethnic status. Although South Africa has several constitutional and legal protections for LGBTQ-identified citizens, Lovely is undocumented and cannot be assured that she will be able to access these protections.

Lovely meets most of the criteria for a major depressive episode as defined in the DSM-5. Review Chapter 17, Table 1 for criteria. These symptoms are causing clinically significant distress or impairment in function for lovely. Depending on previous history of depression, adjustment disorder with depressed mood may be a more appropriate diagnosis, however.

Lovely also meets criteria for PTSD as defined in the DSM-5, including: (1) the presence of a stressor (the rape); (2) recurrent, involuntary, and intrusive memories; (3) avoidance of trauma-related external reminders (the bar); (4) negative alterations in cognitions and mood (persistent distorted blame, markedly diminished interest in activities); and (5) alterations in arousal and reactivity (self-destructive behavior, sleep disturbance), lasting (6) for more than one month and causing (7) significant symptom-related distress or functional impairment.

Lovely's use of substances is not uncommon in the setting of a recent traumatic event but may be a complicating factor for both diagnosis and treatment of the above. Further, it may constitute a substance use disorder of its own.

Sexual Networks and Epidemiologic Trends

HIV/AIDS

Information on HIV epidemiological trends of MSM populations around the world is imperfect. Most countries in Africa and the Middle East have major gaps in national surveillance data on HIV among MSM, and many other countries have failed to publish recent data. Although net HIV transmission is declining across the general population, HIV transmission among MSM continues to rise in virtually all regions and countries. MSM are disproportionately burdened by HIV, with MSM in Latin American countries 10–100 times more likely to be infected, African MSM two to 20 times more likely, and Asian MSM at least 10 times more likely to be infected. Globally, transgender women are believed to be 49 times more likely to be HIV-positive than members of the general population.

MSM have sexual networks (groups of individuals connected through shared sexual contact) that are generally larger than those of non-MSM, providing more opportunities for MSM to have sex with an HIV-positive partner. Sexual networks can also be shaped by characteristics such as sex between older and younger men; transmission to and from other risk groups, such as sex workers or persons with IDU; and networking through bathhouses, gay clubs, and Internet venues.

HIV's ability to mutate makes drug resistance an important consideration. Drug-resistant mutations can lead to treatment failure, need for second- or third-line treatments, and increased health care costs that constitute a further challenge in resource-poor settings. Mutations are especially problematic when they are transmitted to HIV-naïve individuals, complicating HIV care from an early stage. Drug-resistant HIV is well studied in Asia, where fewer than 5% of new HIV cases have a moderate level of transmitted drug resistance. However, Asian countries have higher rates of transmitted drug resistance among MSM. Studies in other regions suggest that many MSM populations around the globe are also at greater risk for transmitted drug resistance. Furthermore, MSM are at increased risk for infection by two or more HIV variants, further raising the risk for drug resistance.

Sexually Transmitted Infections

More than 1 million STIs transmissions occur every day around the world. Addressing STIs is complicated by the fact that many infections are asymptomatic in their early stages. Cost and geographic barriers make accurate diagnostics inaccessible in resource-poor settings. In addition, high-quality, low-cost rapid diagnostic tests have not yet been developed for many STIs, necessitating burdensome follow-up that complicates the care of hard-to-reach populations. Therefore, STIs are generally treated in low-resource settings only when they become symptomatic.

Although global data on STIs among LGBTQ communities remain limited, studies have documented special risk factors and high prevalence among LGBTQ communities that differ across pathogens and regions. MSM have a higher burden of virtually all STIs and are faced with unique risks of asymptomatic and overlooked oropharyngeal and rectal infections. Both ulcerative and non-ulcerative STIs increase the probability of HIV transmission two- to fivefold. Global studies have further confirmed that STIs are a significant risk factor for HIV in MSM populations. WSW should also undergo regular STI screening despite popular assumptions that this population is at low risk.

Drug resistance is particularly important in gonorrhea, which had developed resistance to all available antibiotics in some regions. MSM are a core group in the emergence and spread of drug-resistant gonorrhea. Rectal gonorrheal infection may facilitate development of resistance through the exchange of genetic material with other rectal coinfections. Drug-resistant gonorrhea is especially difficult to treat in low-resource facilities that cannot culture microbes.

STI care is complicated by a multitude of barriers, including high cost, lack of privacy, inadequate provider training, lack of therapies, and poor syndrome management. Biomedical prevention strategies for STIs are largely limited to condoms and vaccines against HPV. A study of MSM in Hong Kong showed that willingness to use an HPV vaccine varied with the perception of its efficacy, pointing to a need for increased education.

Migrant LGBTQ Populations

Migrants (people who are relocated, voluntarily or involuntarily, across international borders or to other geographic regions within the country of origin) face special health challenges, including insecure citizenship status, inconsistent or limited access to health care, and past exposures such as violence, malnutrition, poverty, infectious disease, and sex work. The **intersectionality** of migrant status and LGBTQ identities produces some complicated health challenges. For example, health-related efforts to reach out to migrant populations through the provision of comprehensive services (e.g., interpretation) in mobile clinics or patient-centered homes could backfire among LGBTQ individuals who avoid interacting with people from their own ethnic backgrounds out of fear of having their sexuality disclosed to friends and relatives.

Even after resettling in well-resourced countries, LGBTQ migrants may be the victims of discrimination that is harmful to health. This phenomenon has been well documented among Asian and Pacific Islander MSM in the United States, among whom racism and anti-immigrant discrimination have been linked to depression and unprotected secondary-partner anal sex. LGBTQ migrants face not only the conflicts of identity associated with assimilating into a new culture but also the challenges of navigating sexual identity within a completely new environment, often without the ability to turn to family members or close friends for support. If the new environment proves hostile, prejudicial experiences can quickly be internalized and transformed into self-destructive or self-injurious behaviors.

> **Key Points**
> - Although total HIV incidence is declining in the world population, HIV transmission among MSM continues to rise in virtually all regions and countries.
> - MSM populations around the globe are at greater risk for drug-resistant HIV.
> - Globally, LGBTQ individuals have a higher burden of virtually all STIs and are faced with special risks of asymptomatic and overlooked rectal infections.
> - The intersectionality of migrant status and LGBTQ identities produces some complicated health challenges, often involving isolation and the internalization of prejudicial experiences.

> **Case 14.5**
> Esther is a straight cisgender woman who lives in Nairobi, Kenya, with her husband, Simon, a bisexual cisgender man. Unbeknownst to Esther, who is now only sexually active with Simon, Simon has several other concurrent male sexual partners. He rarely uses condoms or other prevention modalities, saying that condoms cause him discomfort.
>
> Esther presents to the clinic with vaginal itching accompanied by a thick yellow discharge. Although the clinic doesn't have culturing facilities, Esther's provider diagnoses gonorrhea and prescribes a norfloxacin injection (considered first-line in Kenya), along with a course of oral doxycycline. Esther chooses not to tell Simon about her diagnosis and completes the full course of medication. Two weeks later, Esther is surprised to see her symptoms return.
>
> **Considering what you know of Simon and Esther's sexual history, what are some conditions for which Esther may be at increased risk?**

As the symptoms persist, Esther and Simon immigrate to England. How might their new circumstances affect their health, Esther's current condition in particular?

Because Simon is having unprotected sex with other men, he is at higher risk for virtually all STIs, including gonorrhea. As in most countries, HIV prevalence among Kenyan MSM is higher than among the general population, putting Simon and his contacts at greater risk for transmission. Even though gonorrhea is generally non-ulcerative, it still heightens the risk of HIV transmission. Also, because the prevalence of drug-resistant gonorrhea and HIV is higher among Kenyan MSM, Esther is at increased risk for acquiring these strains as well.

Although Esther and Simon's move to England may improve their access to diagnostic facilities and second- or third-line medications, their presence as immigrants and Simon's bisexual identity may make them uniquely vulnerable to prejudice. This could lead to Simon to engage in further sexual risk-taking or self-destructive behavior that could complicate Esther's condition.

Global Interventions Affecting LGBTQ Individuals

Male Circumcision

Male circumcision is a cost-effective HIV-prevention strategy. A landmark 2006 study showed that circumcision reduces a man's risk of acquiring HIV from a female partner by 60%. However, circumcision is uncommon in many areas of the world, prompting voluntary medical male circumcision (VMMC) campaigns targeting adult males, especially in sub-Saharan Africa. New nonsurgical circumcision devices enable men to undergo VMMC without the need for sutures or access to a surgeon.

Although male circumcision is believed to have a preventive effect on HIV transmission during insertive anal sex, research so far has been inconclusive. Nevertheless, because many global MSM have female sex partners, circumcision may still be a preventive option for some MSM. There is little evidence of increased sexual risk behavior or decreased sexual satisfaction among MSM who have undergone VMMC.

Willingness to undergo adult circumcision is generally low among men and, more specifically, among MSM. MSM and transgender individuals attending voluntary testing and counseling sessions in Thailand expressed low interest in circumcision compared with other interventions; 86% were interested in taking PrEP and 70% in HIV vaccine trials, but only 30% were interested in VMMC. Obstacles to engagement are often culturally influenced: a belief that circumcision is not for adults, fear of side effects, and doubts about the procedure's effectiveness are all cited as reasons for refusal. Studies of Chinese MSM show that knowledge of the HIV-prevention effects of circumcision in vaginal or anal sex increases the willingness of MSM to undergo VMMC.

Microbicides

Microbicides are medicines that are applied topically inside the rectum or vagina to prevent disease transmission. They come in a range of formulations—gels, creams, or suppositories—and work by blocking the entry, replication, and/or spread of microbes. Some microbicides are combined with spermicides.

Although many microbicide clinical trials are ongoing, no microbicides have been approved at the time of this book's publication. If effective, microbicides could provide an alternative to condoms as a contraception and disease-prevention technology. Unlike condoms, microbicides do not rely on an insertive partner's cooperation. This is especially advantageous in sexual relationships in which the power dynamic limits one partner's agency, as is often the case with male-female partnerships or with sex workers.

In 2012, the landmark CAPRISA microbicide trial showed that antiretroviral-based microbicide was 39% effective in reducing women's risk for sexual HIV transmission. Epidemiological analyses have suggested that a microbicide of this level of efficacy could have a dramatic impact on the global HIV epidemic. Mathematical modeling of a hypothetical microbicide scale-up in 73 low-income countries predicted that 6 million infections could be prevented if 30% of women used microbicides. Nevertheless, the uptake of microbicides among global LGBTQ communities necessitates further population-specific research and will likely require special initiatives to combat barriers to access, stigma, and discrimination.

Condoms and Water-Based Lubricants

Using condoms with condom-compatible lubricants (CCLs) during anal sex prevents condom breaks and epidermal trauma that facilitate HIV and STI transmission. Water-based lubricants are compatible with latex condoms, whereas petroleum-based lubricants, though commonly used by MSM in sub-Saharan Africa and other regions, cause condoms to break. Some recent studies have even suggested that certain types of water-based lubricants actually facilitate STI transmission. More research is needed to determine which water-based lubricants are safe, but the use of condoms with a CCL during anal sex is still recommended.

Lack of availability, interrupted supply, and poor quality of lubricants make access a major barrier to CCL use in many areas around the globe. Even when CCLs are available, many MSM do not know that water-based lubricants are recommended for use with condoms. This and other factors lead to alarmingly low levels of CCL use by MSM. Lubricant use is generally more common than condom use and may be influenced by different factors. Although urban and rural Vietnamese MSM both have high rates of condom use, rural MSM were found in one study to be less likely to use CCLs. Nevertheless,

exclusive use of water-based lubricants among MSM has been shown to be associated with a lower rate of unprotected anal sex, defined as sex without a condom or condom failure.

Pre-Exposure Prophylaxis (PrEP)

Pre-exposure prophylaxis, or PrEP, refers to the use of antiretroviral drugs by HIV-negative people before engaging in high-risk activities such as unprotected sex to prevent transmission of HIV. The landmark Preexposure Prophylaxis Initiative (iPrEx) study, published in the *New England Journal of Medicine* in 2010, was conducted with 2499 HIV-seronegative men and transgender women who had sex with men across Peru, Ecuador, South Africa, Brazil, Thailand, and the United States and were randomized to receive the combination drug emtricitabine and tenofovir disoproxil fumarate (FTC-TDF) or placebo daily. The study documented a 44% reduction in the incidence of HIV among those taking FTC-TDF, with a 95% reduction in relative risk of acquiring HIV when adherence was taken into account. Based on the results of iPrEx and other trials (including Partners PREP, which involved 4758 HIV-serodiscordant heterosexual couples), the United States Food and Drug Administration approved FTC-TDF for use as PrEP in July 2012.

PrEP has several key advantages in the global context. As a once-daily medication, it does not rely on behavior change at the time of sex and does not necessitate the permission or awareness of the sexual partner, unlike barrier methods of protection. This quality has particular implications for sex workers and receptive partners, who may not always be able to negotiate condom use. Although PrEP has been heralded as a major advance in prevention for high-risk individuals, it has had only limited uptake thus far and remains a controversial approach, with critics citing ethical allocation of drugs (in the context of countries that have not yet achieved universal antiretroviral coverage for HIV-positive individuals), potential issues of adherence and resistance, drug toxicity, cost-effectiveness, and behavioral repercussions. Although several ongoing clinical trials are exploring these potential issues, PrEP remains one of few effective available strategies for curbing the epidemic in the high-risk MSM population and has, furthermore, been adopted by the World Health Organization in its *Consolidated Guidelines for HIV Prevention, Diagnosis, Treatment, and Care for Key Populations.*

Harmful Interventions

Homosexuality has not been classified by the American Psychiatric Association as a disorder since 1973. It was also removed from the World Health Organization's *International Classification of Diseases* (ICD-10) in 1990. **Conversion therapy**, also known as *reparative therapy*, comprises a diverse set of nonstandard interventions that approach homosexuality as a mental disorder that can be treated. These interventions are often religious in nature and are based on the assumption that a person's sexuality is mutable and can be reoriented through extensive therapy and/or prayer.

Several studies have documented the harmful effects of conversion therapy, including self-hatred, depression, sexual dysfunction, anxiety, low self-esteem, drug use, and suicidal ideation. Furthermore, conversion therapy has not been shown to be successful in changing the sexual orientations of participants. Many well-respected international professional societies—including the American Psychiatric Association, the American Counseling Association, the Psychological Society of South Africa, and the Pan-American Health Organization—oppose the practice. In recent years, a small but growing number of US states have enacted legislation forbidding the practice of conversion therapy on minors.

In the global context, conversion therapy is still being endorsed by evangelical Christian groups across Latin America, Asia, and sub-Saharan Africa. In countries where minors have limited legal rights, minors may be subjected against their will to these harmful interventions at length, with potentially devastating consequences. In June 2013, an apology was issued by the former chairman of Exodus International, and the organization was shuttered. Exodus International was one of the largest sponsors of conversion therapy, operating hundreds of ministries across 19 countries in Africa, Asia, Europe, and Latin America. However, many other organizations remain in existence, unregulated by regional medical boards, continuing to pose a threat to the health and well-being of LGBTQ individuals worldwide.

Case 14.6

Aditya is a 17-year-old MSM sex worker who lives in Jakarta, Indonesia. Although he works various jobs, none allows him to support his family as well as his job as a sex worker does. Most of Aditya's clients prefer to be the insertive partner and do not like using condoms, and a few have threatened violence when he has suggested condom use. He is lucky to get an appointment at one of the few community-based providers that is both MSM-friendly and able to provide the latest prevention modalities. Aditya reveals his situation to his provider, who decides to test him for HIV. Although the test comes back negative, the provider recognizes Aditya's risk for HIV infection and decides to recommend preventive measures.

What are the benefits and drawbacks of different prevention options?

Which option is best suited to reduce Aditya's risk for HIV infection?

Because Aditya cannot leave sex work and is not in a position to negotiate condom use, recommending behavior change or condom use will likely be ineffective. Although VMMC is believed to be preventive for the insertive partner, its benefits for the receptive partner are unknown, making it an imperfect recommendation for Aditya. Microbicides have yet to be approved by the FDA and are unavailable in the global context. Pre-exposure prophylaxis is one prevention option that does not require behavior change or partner consent. Although there are questions regarding PrEP's role in drug toxicity, resistance, adherence, and behavior, worries about these issues have yet to be confirmed, making PrEP a well-suited intervention for preventing HIV transmission in high-risk individuals such as Aditya.

Key Points
- Voluntary medical male circumcision is believed to prevent HIV transmission in anal sex (as it does in penile-vaginal sex), but uptake is limited.
- In the future, microbicides may provide an alternative to condoms that do not rely on an insertive partner's full cooperation.
- Studies have found that global MSM populations have alarmingly low levels of condom-compatible lubricant use, in large part because of a lack of access.
- Pre-exposure prophylaxis (PrEP), a recently developed biomedical prevention strategy, has been endorsed by the World Health Organization as an effective approach to curbing the HIV epidemic in high-risk MSM populations.
- Despite its proven harmful effects, conversion therapy—a diverse set of nonstandard interventions that approach homosexuality as a mental disorder that can be treated—is still being practiced in some settings.

Conclusion

At a time when availability and quality of health care continue to expand around the world, LGBTQ people are a uniquely vulnerable population affected by complex issues at the intersection of health, access to care, and human rights.

Although important steps forward have been made in the fight against HIV worldwide, MSM and transgender women are still a key population with a rising incidence of infection. Discrimination, both individual and institutionalized, present exceptional barriers to care in addition to restricting human rights. Moreover, interpersonal violence and harmful attempts at conversion therapy still plague LGBTQ people, especially in sub-Saharan Africa.

Although these issues are not unique to LGBTQ individuals in low- and middle-income countries, these populations bear an exceptional burden that is further compounded by the unjust realities of living in resource-limited settings. However, innovative approaches to prevention and therapeutic treatment have shown promise. Cultural humility and awareness must always be exercised while working within the global context, particularly across the disparate identities and groups that make up LGBTQ communities.

Boards-Style Application Questions

Question 1. A 23-year-old recent immigrant from Brazil presents for a mental status examination after experiencing depressed mood, anhedonia, and reduced energy in the wake of a breakup with his girlfriend of seven years back in Brazil. During the interview the patient reveals a recent same-sex sexual experience with a man he met at a local bar. When asked about his sexual orientation, he states that he is "straight" but wanted to "try something new," though he is now confident after the experience that he prefers women. As you write your note, which of the following observations regarding the man's sexuality do you conclude is the most accurate?

A. The patient is bisexual
B. The patient is an ego-dystonic homosexual
C. The patient has an ambiguous sexual identity
D. The patient is homosexually active but claims to be heterosexual
E. The patient identifies as heterosexual but reports a recent sexual experience with a man

Question 2. A 26-year-old man presents to an HIV clinic in Kano State, Nigeria, for enrollment in HIV care after receiving a positive result on a rapid test followed by confirmatory ELISA. You are providing care at the clinic as a visiting faculty member of the local university medical school. During your interview, the patient discloses that he has been involved in a yearlong exclusive relationship with a male partner whose HIV status is unknown. They have had unprotected anal sex. You are aware that under Nigerian law, homosexual acts are a criminal offense punishable by life imprisonment. What is the most appropriate course of action?

A. Reporting the patient to local authorities for violating local laws and ending the encounter
B. Documenting the patient's sexuality in his medical record, enrolling him in care, and encouraging him to tell his partner to get tested
C. Refraining from documenting the patient's sexuality in his medical record but enrolling him in care and encouraging him to tell his partner to get tested
D. Documenting the patient's sexuality in his medical record, enrolling him in care, and notifying his partner's family that the man may have been exposed to HIV
E. Refraining from documenting the patient's sexuality in his medical record but enrolling him in care and notifying his partner's family that the man may have been exposed to HIV

Question 3. A 20-year-old Jamaican woman presents to you for a forensic physical evaluation after being vaginally raped outside her home in Kingston by a group of five men a month ago. She identifies as a lesbian and reports that she was attacked after speaking out about her sexuality on a local radio show. She is now applying for asylum in the United States. In addition to collecting photographic documentation of the patient's nongenital injuries to support her asylum case, a comprehensive examination should include:

A. A pregnancy test and counseling
B. Acyclovir for herpes simplex virus prophylaxis
C. A rectal swab for DNA identification of the woman's assailants

D. Minimal discussion of the specifics of the assault to avoid retraumatizing the patient
E. Initiation of tenofovir and emtricitabine therapy plus raltegravir for postexposure prophylaxis against HIV infection

Question 4. A 28-year-old preoperative transgender woman who recently immigrated from Costa Rica presents for a consultation regarding hormone therapy. She says that she is a sex worker and reports using condoms for receptive anal sex with clients but not for oral sex. She asks for a prescription for hormone replacement because her supply from a "friend" in Costa Rica is running out. She does not know the dosage or type of pills she has been taking, which are unmarked and supplied in a plastic bag. The patient also expresses interest in prophylaxis against HIV. She does not smoke and has no history of blood clots.

Blood tests reveal:
HIV: negative
HBsAg: negative
Anti-HBc (total and IgM): negative
Anti-HBs: negative
Creatinine: 0.5
ALT: 16 IU/L
AST: 12 IU/L

Which of the following medications is not appropriate for the patient at this time?

A. Hepatitis B vaccine
B. Spironolactone tabs
C. Sublingual estradiol
D. Medroxyprogesterone
E. Estrogen/progestin tabs
F. Tenofovir and emtricitabine tabs

Question 5. An investigator is attempting to study HIV prevalence and risk behaviors among men who have sex with men (MSM) in Dakar, Senegal, where same-sex sexual activity is punishable by one to five years of imprisonment and very few MSM are "out." Study resources are limited but the results will be used to inform rollout of a targeted treatment and prevention campaign for MSM around the country. Which of these study designs is the most appropriate for accomplishing the investigator's goals?

A. Randomized controlled trial
B. Longitudinal prospective cohort study
C. Cross-sectional survey involving respondent-driven sampling
D. Ecological study
E. Retrospective cohort study of patients at an HIV clinic
F. None, because any study would be unethical

Question 6. A 42-year-old Ghanaian-Dutch man presents to your clinic alone, complaining of tender bumps in his groin and a newly developed lesion on his penis. He and his wife have lived in Amsterdam for the past 15 years and report no recent travel to tropical countries. On physical examination, you note tender inguinal lymphadenopathy and palpate a thin, ropy cord on the dorsal side of his penis. You suspect lymphogranuloma venereum (LGV). You read in a recent journal article that the LGV epidemic is almost completely concentrated in men who have sex with men (MSM) in Holland. What is the appropriate way of eliciting the patient's sexual history?

A. "I'm a very gay-friendly provider so please be comfortable sharing any details as I now ask you some questions about your sexual past."
B. "With your permission, I am now going to ask some questions about your sexual activity which are important given the nature of your symptoms – please be as honest as possible. Everything you tell me will remain completely confidential."
C. "Does your wife know that you are bisexual?"
D. "Are you sexually attracted to men, women, or both?"
E. "When is the last time you had sex with a man?"

Question 7. A 23-year-old man presents to you complaining of a sore throat that he is afraid he caught on the plane back from a recent trip to Cambodia and Thailand. The patient's vacation was significant for multiple episodes of unprotected insertive and receptive oral and anal sex with several different men. At one point the man experienced dysuria but says he got "antibiotic pills" at a local pharmacy shortly thereafter that "cleared it up." Other than this episode, the young man's recent history is unremarkable. He has been taking doxycycline 100 mg daily for malaria prophylaxis and will continue it for 25 more days. On examination he is mildly febrile; his tonsils are inflamed and coated with a green discharge. The best treatment for his condition is:

A. Ceftriaxone
B. Penicillin V
C. Azithromycin
D. Ciprofloxacin
E. Amoxicillin/clavulanate

Question 8. A 16-year-old boy presents for HIV/STI testing and a general physical examination to a clinic in Durban, South Africa. He is asymptomatic. The patient reports having multiple concurrent male and female partners and says that he engages exclusively in insertive anal and vaginal sex. The patient says that he uses condoms inconsistently, claiming, "I live in the moment," and "I hate routine." Genitourinary examination reveals a normal uncircumcised penis with no lesions or discharge. The result of a whole-blood HIV rapid test is negative. Which of the following interventions is most appropriate to reduce the patient's risk of acquiring and transmitting HIV in the future?

A. Female condoms
B. Nonoxynol-9 microbicide
C. Abstinence-centered education
D. Tenofovir and emtricitabine
E. Voluntary medical male circumcision

Boards-Style Application Questions Answer Key

Question 1. This patient has clearly identified himself as heterosexual with a preference for women, a declaration that is not negated by his recent same-sex sexual experience (option E). Sexual experimentation is not uncommon throughout adulthood, particularly young adulthood (<25 years). Bisexual (option A) is an identity that the patient has not claimed and is therefore an inappropriate way of describing the patient. "Ambiguous sexual identity" (option C) D implies that the patient has not clearly stated his sexual identity, which he has. "Ego-dystonic homosexual" (option B) and "Homosexually active but claims to be heterosexual" (option C) are both phrased judgmentally and inaccurate.

Question 2. The most important things to do are enroll the patient in treatment and get his partner tested by empowering the patient to notify his partner (option C). The first duty is to do no harm. Without knowing how the medical record is stored, accessed, and used, it is potentially dangerous to the patient for you to document information about his sexuality that could be used against him in a court of law (options B and D). Telling the partner's family that the man has been exposed to HIV is a blatant violation of patient confidentiality (options D and E) and is not acceptable.

Question 3. The correct answer is option A. A pregnancy test is indicated because the victim was vaginally raped and is of reproductive age; if the result is positive, she should be counseled in regard to her available options, including termination of the pregnancy. Because the episode occurred a month ago, there is little hope that any DNA evidence remains in or on the victim's body (option C). This woman has been the victim of so-called corrective rape and is now applying for asylum, for which she requires physical and written documentation of evidence, including specific details of the traumatic event, by a trained health care provider. Avoiding discussion of the specifics (option D) would be harmful to her

case. Initiation of postexposure prophylaxis (options B and E) is not warranted more than 72 hours after exposure, although an HIV test is indicated.

Question 4. The correct answer is F, estrogen/progestin tabs. This woman has already been undergoing hormone therapy, but it was likely a suboptimal regimen of estrogen by mouth, which can cause liver damage. A standard preoperative hormone regimen includes an antiandrogen (e.g., option B, spironolactone), sublingual estrogen (option C), and a progestogen (option D). Her bloodwork reveals no liver or kidney damage that would contraindicate hormone replacement or HIV pre-exposure prophylaxis (F), for which she qualifies in light of her expressed interest, a negative HIV blood test, and her high level of risk as a sex worker. This patient lacks hepatitis B surface antibody, so immunization for hepatitis B is indicated (option A).

Question 5. The correct answer is option F. The most economical and efficient way to assess prevalence among this population is a cross-sectional survey; because of the difficulties in gaining access to this population, participants are often recruited through respondent-driven sampling, sometimes known as the "snowball" method. Options A, B, D, and E are all prohibitively expensive, and there are no guarantees that the population of interest would be accessed by their methods. African MSM are an understudied and at-risk population that is in need of targeted and data-driven efforts at HIV prevention and treatment. Although the substantial legal restrictions and stigma against MSM populations in countries such as Senegal highlight the need for well-informed study designs that provide the assurance of utmost confidentiality to participants, they should not serve as a deterrent to working with this vulnerable group (option D, no study).

Question 6. The correct answer is E, asking the patient's permission before asking probing questions about the patient's sexual activity and reassuring the patient of the confidentiality of his answers. It is best to preface the sensitive questions posed during a sexual history with some framing statement and a reminder of patient confidentiality. Options A, B, and D (assuming that the patient is bisexual or gay) are all presumptive and will likely undermine any existing rapport you have built with the patient. Although epidemiological context can be helpful in clinical decision-making, you must never make individual assumptions about a patient before you on the basis of population-level data. This man has identified himself as being married to a woman. Option C, immediately asking when the patient last had sex with another man had is too abrupt without any sort of preceding statement.

Question 7. This patient's history is most indicative of pharyngeal gonorrhea, which would likely have been unresponsive to any oral antibiotic. The only recommended treatment for pharyngeal gonorrhea is injectable ceftriaxone (option A). Azithromycin (option C) or doxycycline is often administered with ceftriaxone to treat possible concomitant chlamydial infection but is not the main treatment for gonorrhea. Pharyngeal Chlamydia is more difficult to acquire (particularly while the patient is taking daily doxycycline) and is less common among MSM populations.

Question 8. This patient is living in a country with a significant adult HIV prevalence (both female and MSM) and is routinely engaging in risky sexual behavior. Voluntary medical male circumcision (option E) has been shown to significantly and substantially reduce the risk of acquiring HIV in males who engage in opposite-sex intercourse and has been shown in pooled meta-analyses to have a protective effect on men who engage in insertive anal sex with other men. The history indicates that the patient would probably not use (A) the female condom (which would only be protective to some of his partners anyway) or (B) nonoxynol-9 microbicide during sex and would not be receptive to (C) abstinence education. Nor is he likely to be compliant with a PrEP regimen (option D), and incomplete adherence to the regimen could leave him more susceptible to antiretroviral resistance if he were to contract the virus in the future.

Sources

Adebajo SB, Eluwa GI, Allman D, Myers T, Ahonsi BA. Prevalence of internalized homophobia and HIV associated risks among men who have sex with men in Nigeria. Afr J Reprod Health. 2012;16(4):21–8.

Africa: new report on how HIV/AIDS programming is failing LGBT people. HIV AIDS Policy Law Rev. 2007;12(1):37–8.

Aung T, McFarland W, Paw E, Hetherington J. Reaching men who have sex with men in Myanmar: population characteristics, risk and preventive behavior, exposure to health programs. AIDS Behav. 2013;17(4): 1386–94.

Auvert B, Taljaard D, Lagarde E, Sobngwi-Tambekou J, Sitta R, Puren A. Randomized, controlled intervention trial of male circumcision for reduction of HIV infection risk: the ANRS 1265 trial. PLoS Med. 2005;3(5):e226.

Baral S, Adams D, Lebona J, Kaibe B, Letsie P, Tshehlo R, et al. A cross-sectional assessment of population demographics, HIV risks and human rights contexts among men who have sex with men in Lesotho. J Int AIDS Soc. 2011;14:36.

Baral S, Burrell E, Scheibe A, Brown B, Beyrer C, Bekker LG. HIV risk and associations of HIV infection among men who have sex with men in peri-urban Cape Town, South Africa. BMC Public Health. 2011;11:766.

Baral S, Holland CE, Shannon K, Logie C, Semugoma P, Sithole B, et al. Enhancing benefits or increasing harms: community responses for HIV among men who have sex with men, transgender women, female sex workers, and people who inject drugs. J Acquir Immune Defic Syndr. 2014;15(66):S319–28.

Baral S, Trapence G, Motimedi F, Umar E, Iipinge S, Dausab F, Beyrer C. HIV prevalence, risks for HIV infection, and human rights among men who have sex with men (MSM) in Malawi, Namibia, and Botswana. PLoS One. 2009;4(3):e4997.

Baral SD, Ketende S, Mnisi Z, Mabuza X, Grosso A, Sithole B, et al. A cross-sectional assessment of the burden of HIV and associated individual- and structural-level characteristics among men who have sex with men in Swaziland. J Int AIDS Soc. 2013;16(Suppl 3):18768.

Baral SD, Poteat T, Stromdahl S, Wirtz A, Guadamuz TE, Beyrer C. Worldwide burden of HIV in transgender women: a systematic review and meta-analysis. Lancet Infect Dis. 2013;13(3):214–22.

Berry MC, Go VF, Quan VM, Minh NL, Ha TV, Mai NV, et al. Social environment and HIV risk among MSM in Hanoi and Thai Nguyen. AIDS Care 2013;25(1):38–42.

Beyrer C, Baral S, Kerrigan D, El-Bassel N, Bekker LG, Celentano DD. Expanding the space: inclusion of most-at-risk populations in HIV prevention, treatment, and care services. J Acquir Immune Defic Syndr. 2011;57(Suppl 2):S96–9.

Beyrer C, Baral S, van Griensven F, Goodreau SM, Chariyalertsak S, Wirtz AL, Brookmeyer R. Global epidemiology of HIV infection in men who have sex with men. Lancet. 2012;380(9839):367–77.

Beyrer C, Jittiwutikarn J, Teokul W, Razak MH, Suriyanon V, Srirak N, et al. Drug use, increasing incarceration rates, and prison-associated HIV risks in Thailand. AIDS Behav. 2003;7(2):153–61.

Beyrer C, Sripaipan T, Tovanabutra S, Jittiwutikarn J, Suriyanon V, Vongchak T, et al. High HIV, hepatitis C and sexual risks among drug-using men who have sex with men in northern Thailand. AIDS. 2005;19(14):1535–40.

Beyrer C, Trapence G, Motimedi F, et al. Bisexual concurrency, bisexual partnerships, and HIV among southern African men who have sex with men. Sex Transm Infect. 2010;86(4):323–7.

Beyrer C, Wirtz A, Walker D, Johns B, Sifakis F, Baral SD. The global HIV epidemics among men who have sex with men. Washington, DC: The World Bank; 2011.

Beyrer C. LGBT Africa: a social justice movement emerges in the era of HIV. SAHARA J. 2012;9(3):177–9.

Bhatta DN. HIV-related sexual risk behaviors among male-to-female transgender people in Nepal. Int J Infect Dis. 2014;22:11–5.

Bianchi FT, Reisen CA, Zea MC, Vidal-Ortiz S, Gonzales FA, Betancourt F, et al. Sex work among men who have sex with men and transgender women in Bogota. Arch Sex Behav. 2014;43(8):1637–50.

Brahmam GN, Kodavalla V, Rajkumar H, Rachakulla HK, Kallam S, Myakala SP, et al. Sexual practices, HIV and sexually transmitted infections among self-identified men who have sex with men in four high HIV prevalence states of India. AIDS. 2008;22(Suppl 5):S45–57.

Calkin J. The silicone sisterhood. The Independent. Arts + Entertainment; 1994.

Carobene M, Blocic F, Farias MS, Quarleri J, Avila MM. HIV, HBV, and HCV molecular epidemiology among trans (trasvenstites, transsexuals, and transgender) sex workers in Argentine. J Med Virol. 2014;86(1):64–70.

Chakrapani V, Newman PA, Shunmugam M, McLuckie A, Melwin F. Structural violence against Kothi-identified men who have sex with men in Chennai, India: a qualitative investigation. AIDS Educ Prev. 2007;19(4):346–64.

Chakrapani V, Newman PA, Shunmugam M. Secondary HIV prevention among kothi-identified MSM in Chennai, India. Cult Health Sex. 2008;10(4):313–27.

Chakrapani V. Hijras/transgender women in India: HIV, human rights and social exclusion. Mumbai: United Nations Development Programme (UNDP), India; 2010.

Chariyalertsak S, Kosachunhanan N, Saokhieo P, Songsupa R, Wongthanee A, Chariyalertsak C, et al. HIV incidence, risk factors, and motivation for biomedical intervention among gay, bisexual men, and transgender persons in Northern Thailand. PLoS One. 2011;6(9):e24295.

Chng CL, Wong FY, Park RJ, Edberg MC, Lai DS. A model for understanding sexual health among Asian American/Pacific Islander men who have sex with men (MSM) in the United States. AIDS Educ Prev. 2003;15(1 suppl A):21–38.

Cochran SD, Mays VM, Alegria M, Ortega AN, Takeuchi D. Mental health and substance use disorders among Latino and Asian American lesbian, gay, and bisexual adults. J Consult Clin Psychol. 2007;75(5):785–94.

Colby D, Minh TT, Toan TT. Down on the farm: homosexual behaviour, HIV risk and HIV prevalence in rural communities in Khanh Hoa province, Vietnam. Sex Transm Infect. 2008;84(6):439–43.

Colton Meier SL, Fitzgerald KM, Pardo ST, Babcock J. The effects of hormonal gender affirmation treatment on mental health in female-to-male transsexuals. J Gay Lesbian Ment Health. 2011;15(3):281–99.

Consolidated guidelines on HIV prevention, diagnosis, treatment and care for key populations. Geneva: World Health Organization; 2014.

Cook SH, Sandfort TGM, Nel JA, Rich EP. Exploring the relationship between gender nonconformity and mental health among black South African gay and bisexual men. Arch Sex Behav. 2013;42(3):327–39.

Daryani P. Differentiating the vulnerability of kothis and hijras to HIV/AIDS: a case study of Lucknow, Uttar Pradesh. [study abroad thesis.]. Brattleboro, VT: SIT Graduate Institute, Study Abroad; 2011.

De Boni R, Veloso VG, Grinsztejn B. Epidemiology of HIV in Latin America and the Caribbean. Curr Opin HIV AIDS. 2014;9(2):192–8.

Deuba K, Ekstrom AM, Shrestha R, Ionita G, Bhatta L, Karki DK. Psychosocial health problems associated with increased HIV risk behavior among men who have sex with men in Nepal: a cross-sectional survey. PLoS One. 2013;8(3):e58099.

Dunkle KL, Wong FY, Nehl EJ, Lin L, He N, Huang J, Zheng T. Male-on-male intimate partner violence and sexual risk behaviors among money boys and other men who have sex with men in Shanghai, China. Sex Transm Dis. 2013;40(5):362–5.

Fay H, Baral SD, Trapence G, Motimedi F, Umar E, Iipinge S, et al. Stigma, health care access, and HIV knowledge among men who have sex with men in Malawi, Namibia, and Botswana. AIDS Behav. 2011;15(6):1088–97.

Fazito E, Cuchi P, Mahy M, Brown T. Analysis of duration of risk behaviour for key populations: a literature review. Sex Transm Infect. 2012;88(Suppl 2):i24–32.

Feng Y, Wu Z, Detels R. Evolution of men who have sex with men community and experienced stigma among men who have sex with men in Chengdu, China. J Acquir Immune Defic Syndr. 2010;53(suppl 1):S98–S103.

Fethers K, Marks C, Mindel A, Estcourt CS. Sexually transmitted infections and risk behaviours in women who have sex with women. Sex Transm Infect. 2000;76(5):345–9.

Finneran C, Chard A, Sineath C, Sullivan P, Stephenson R. Intimate partner violence and social pressure among gay men in six countries. West J Emerg Med. 2012;13(3):260–71.

Gao MY, Wang S. Participatory communication and HIV/AIDS prevention in a Chinese marginalized (MSM) population. AIDS Care. 2007;19(6):799–810.

Goodreau SM, Goicochea LP, Sanchez J. Sexual role and transmission of HIV type 1 among men who have sex with men in Peru. J Infect Dis. 2005;191(suppl 1):S147–58.

Gostin LO, Kim SC. Ethical allocation of preexposure HIV prophylaxis. JAMA. 2011;305(2):191–2.

Gouws E, Cuchi P. Focusing the HIV response through estimating the major modes of HIV transmission: a multi-country analysis. Sex Transm Infect. 2012;88(suppl 2):i76–85.

Grant RM, Lama JR, Anderson PL, McMahan V, Liu AY, Vargas L, et al. Preexposure chemoprophylaxis for HIV prevention in men who have sex with men. N Engl J Med. 2010;363(27):2587–99.

Gu J, Lau JT, Tsui H. Psychological factors in association with uptake of voluntary counselling and testing for HIV among men who have sex with men in Hong Kong. Public Health. 2011;125(5):275–82.

Guo Y, Li X, Song Y, Liu Y. Bisexual behavior among Chinese young migrant men who have sex with men: implications for HIV prevention and intervention. AIDS Care. 2012;24(4):451–8.

Habib T. A long journey towards social inclusion: initiatives of social work for hijra population. Gothenburg: Department of Social Work, University of Gothenburg; 2012.

Hardon A, Idrus NI. On Coba and Cocok: youth-led drug-experimentation in Eastern Indonesia. Anthropol Med. 2014;21(2):217–29.

Hidaka Y, Ichikawa S, Koyano J, Urao M, Yasuo T, Kimura H, et al. Substance use and sexual behaviours of Japanese men who have sex with men: a nation-wide internet survey conducted in Japan. BMC Public Health. 2006;6:239.

Hoyos J, Fernandez-Balbuena S, de la Fuente L, Sordo L, Ruiz M, Barrio G, et al. Never tested for HIV in Latin-American migrants and Spaniards: prevalence and perceived barriers. J Int AIDS Soc. 2013;16:18560.

Inoue Y, Yamazaki Y, Kihara M, Wakabayashi C, Seki Y, Ichikawa S. The intent and practice of condom use among HIV-positive men who have sex with men in Japan. AIDS Patient Care STD. 2006;20(11): 792–802.

Itaborahy LP, Zhu J. State-sponsored homophobia. A world survey of laws: criminalization, protection and recognition of same-sex love. Geneva: International Lesbian Gay Bisexual Trans and Intersex Association; 2013.

Jobson GA, Theron LB, Kaggwa JK, Kim HJ. Transgender in Africa: invisible, inaccessible, or ignored? SAHARA J. 2012;9(3):160–3.

Johnston LG, Alami K, El Rhilani MH, Karkouri M, Mellouk O, Abadie A, et al. HIV, syphilis and sexual risk behaviours among men who have sex with men in Agadir and Marrakesh, Morocco. Sex Transm Infect. 2013;89(suppl 3):iii45–8.

Kaplan RL, Wagner GJ, Nehme S, Aunon F, Khouri D, Mokhbat J. Forms of safety and their impact on health: an exploration of HIV/AIDS-related risk and resilience among trans women in Lebanon. Health Care Women Int. 2014;36(8):917–35.

Kennedy CE, Baral SD, Fielding-Miller R, Adams D, Dludlu P, Sithole B, et al. "They are human beings, they are Swazi": intersecting stigmas and the positive health, dignity and prevention needs of HIV-positive men who have sex with men in Swaziland. J Int AIDS Soc. 2013;16(suppl 3):18749.

Khan SI, Hussain MI, Parveen S, Bhuiyan MI, Gourab G, Sarker GF, et al. Living on the extreme margin: social exclusion of the transgender population (hijra) in Bangladesh. J Health Popul Nutr. 2009;27(4):441–51.

Konan YE, Dagnan NS, Tetchi EO, Aké O, Tiembré I, Zengbé P, et al. Description of sexual practices of women who have sex with other women to HIV/AIDS in Abidjan (Cote d'Ivoire). Bull Soc Pathol Extol. 2014;107(5):369–75.

Kong TS, Laidler KJ, Pang H. Relationship type, condom use and HIV/AIDS risks among men who have sex with men in six Chinese cities. AIDS Care. 2012;24(4):517–28.

Lane T, Mogale T, Struthers H, McIntyre J, Kegeles SM. "They see you as a different thing": the experiences of men who have sex with men with healthcare workers in South African township communities. Sex Transm Infect. 2008;84(6):430–3.

Lane T, Shade SB, McIntyre J, Morin SF. Alcohol and sexual risk behavior among men who have sex with men in South African township communities. AIDS Behav. 2008;12(4 suppl):S78–85.

Lau JT, Wang Z, Kim JH, Lau M, Lai CH, Mo PK. Acceptability of HPV vaccines and associations with perceptions related to HPV and HPV vaccines among men who have sex with men in Hong Kong. PLoS One. 2013;8(2):e57204.

Lau JT, Zhang J, Yan H, Lin C, Choi KC, Wang Z, et al. Acceptability of circumcision as a means of HIV prevention among men who have sex with men in China. AIDS Care. 2011;23(11):1472–82.

Liu J, Qu B, Guo HQ, Sun G. Factors that influence risky sexual behaviors among men who have sex with men in Liaoning province, China: a structural equation model. AIDS Patient Care STD. 2011;25(7):423–9.

Making love a crime: criminalization of same-sex conduct in Sub-Saharan Africa. London: Amnesty International; 2013.

Mayer KH, Wheeler DP, Bekker LG, Grinsztejn B, Remien RH, Sandfort TG, Beyrer C. Overcoming biological, behavioral, and structural vulnerabilities: new directions in research to decrease HIV transmission in men who have sex with men. J Acquir Immune Defic Syndr. 2013;63(suppl 2):S161–7.

Meyer IH. Minority stress and mental health in gay men. J Health Soc Behav. 1995;36:38–56.

Meyer IH. Prejudice, social stress, and mental health in lesbian, gay, and bisexual populations: conceptual issues and research evidence. Psychol Bull. 2003;129(5):674–97.

Millett GA, Jeffries WL 4th, Peterson JL, Malebranche DJ, Lane T, Flores SA, et al. Common roots: a contextual review of HIV epidemics in black men who have sex with men across the African diaspora. Lancet. 2012;380(9839):411–23.

Morineau G, Nugrahini N, Riono P, Nurhayati, Girault P, Mustikawati DE, Magnani R. Sexual risk taking, STI and HIV prevalence among men who have sex with men in six Indonesian cities. AIDS Behav. 2011;15(5):1033–44.

Mureithi MW, Poole D, Naranbhai V, Reddy S, Mkhwanazi NP, Sibeko S, et al. Preservation HIV-1-specific IFNγ+ CD4+ T-cell responses in breakthrough infections after exposure to tenofovir gel in the CAPRISA 004 microbicide trial. J Acquir Immune Defic Syndr. 2012;60(2):124–7.

Newcomb ME, Mustanski B. Internalized homophobia and internalizing mental health problems: a meta-analytic review. Clin Psychol Rev. 2010;30(8):1019–29.

Newman PA, Chakrapani V, Cook C, Shunmugam M, Kakinami L. Determinants of sexual risk behavior among men who have sex with men accessing public sex environments in Chennai, India. J LGBT Health Res. 2008;4(2–3):81–7.

Nyoni JE, Ross MW. Condom use and HIV-related behaviors in urban Tanzanian men who have sex with men: a study of beliefs, HIV knowledge sources, partner interactions and risk behaviors. AIDS Care. 2013;25(2):223–9.

Onyango-Ouma W, Birungi H, Geibel S. Engaging men who have sex with men in operations research in Kenya. Cult Health Sex. 2009;11(8):827–39.

Parry C, Petersen P, Carney T, Dewing S, Needle R. Rapid assessment of drug use and sexual HIV risk patterns among vulnerable drug-using populations in Cape Town, Durban and Pretoria, South Africa. SAHARA J. 2008;5(3):113–9.

Pawa D, Firestone R, Ratchasi S, Dowling O, Jittakoat Y, Duke A, Mundy G. Reducing HIV risk among transgender women in Thailand: a quasi-experimental evaluation of the sisters program. PLoS One. 2013;8(10):e77113.

Peacock E, Adndrinopoulos K, Hembling J. Binge drinking among men who have sex with men and transgener women in San Salvador: correlates and sexual health implications. J Urban Health. 2015;92(4):701–16.

Pham QD, Nguyen TV, Nguyen PD, Le SH, Tran AT, Nguyen LT, et al. Men who have sex with men in southern Vietnam report high levels of substance use and sexual risk behaviours but underutilise HIV testing services: a cross-sectional study. Sex Transm Dis. 2015;91(3):178–82.

Pisani E, Girault P, Gultom M, Sukartini N, Kumalawati J, Jazan S, Donegan E. HIV, syphilis infection, and sexual practices among transgenders, male sex workers, and other men who have sex with men in Jakarta, Indonesia. Sex Transm Infect. 2004;80(6):536–40.

Poteat T, Diouf D, Drame FM, Ndaw M, Traore C, Dhaliwal M, et al. HIV risk among MSM in Senegal: a qualitative rapid assessment of the impact of enforcing laws that criminalize same sex practices. PLoS One. 2011;6(12):e28760.

Poteat T, Wirtz AL, Radix A, Borquez A, Silva-Santisteban A, Deutsch MB, et al. HIV risk and preventive interventions in transgender women sex workers. Lancet. 2014;385(9964):274–86.

Prabawanti C, Dijkstra A, Riono P, Hartana TG. Preparatory behaviours and condom use during receptive and insertive anal sex among male-to-female transgenders (Waria) in Jakarta, Indonesia. J Int AIDS Soc. 2014;17(1):19343.

Pyun T, Santos GM, Arreola S, Do T, Hebert P, Beck J, et al. Internalized homophobia and reduced HIV testing among men who have sex with men in China. Asia-Pac J Public Health. 2014;26(2):118–25.

Risher K, Adams D, Sithole B, Ketende S, Kennedy C, Mnisi Z, et al. Sexual stigma and discrimination as barriers to seeking appropriate healthcare among men who have sex with men in Swaziland. J Int AIDS Soc. 2013;16(3 Suppl 2):18715.

Rispel LC, Metcalf CA, Cloete A, Moorman J, Reddy V. You become afraid to tell them that you are gay: health service utilization by men who have sex with men in South African cities. J Public Health Policy. 2011;32(suppl 1):S137–51.

Rosenberger JG, Reece M, Schick V, et al. Sexual behaviors and situational characteristics of most recent male-partnered sexual event among gay and bisexually identified men in the United States. J Sex Med. 2011;8(11):3040–50.

Ruan Y, Qian HZ, Li D, Shi W, Li Q, Liang H, et al. Willingness to be circumcised for preventing HIV among Chinese men who have sex with men. AIDS Patient Care STD. 2009;23(5):315–21.

Saavedra J, Izazola-Licea JA, Beyrer C. Sex between men in the context of HIV: The AIDS 2008 Jonathan Mann Memorial Lecture in Health and Human Rights. J Int AIDS Soc. 2008;11:9.

Safren SA, Thomas BE, Mimiaga MJ, Chandrasekaran V, Menon S, Swaminathan S, Mayer KH. Depressive symptoms and human immunodeficiency virus risk behavior among men who have sex with men in Chennai, India. Psychol Health Med. 2009;14(6):705–15.

Sanchez NF, Sanchez JP, Danoff A. Health care utilization, barriers to care, and hormone usage among male-to-female transgender persons in New York City. Am J Public Health. 2009;99(4):713–9.

Sohn AH, Srikantiah P, Sungkanuparph S, Zhang F. Transmitted HIV drug resistance in Asia. Curr Opin HIV AIDS. 2013;8(1):27–33.

Song D, Zhang H, Wang J, Han D, Dai L, Liu Q, et al. Sexual risk behaviours and their correlates among gay and non-gay identified men who have sex with men and women in Chengdu and Guangzhou, China. Int J STD AIDS. 2013;24(10):780–90.

Stromdahl S, Onigbanjo Williams A, Eziefule B, Emmanuel G, Iwuagwu S, Anene O, et al. Associations of consistent condom use among men who have sex with men in Abuja, Nigeria. AIDS Res Hum Retrovir. 2012;28(12):1756–62.

Taegtmeyer M, Davies A, Mwangome M, van der Elst EM, Graham SM, Price MA, Sanders EJ. Challenges in providing counselling to MSM in highly stigmatized contexts: results of a qualitative study from Kenya. PLoS One. 2013;8(6):e64527.

Ugarte Guevara WJ, Valladares Cardoza E, Essén B. Sexuality and risk behavior among men who have sex with men in León, Nicaragua: a mixed methods approach. J Sex Med. 2012;9(6):1634–48.

Wilson PA, Yoshikawa H. Experiences of and responses to social discrimination among Asian and Pacific Islander gay men: their relationship to HIV risk. AIDS Educ Prev. 2004;16(1):68–83.

Winter S. Lost in translation: transgender people, rights and HIV vulnerability in the Asia-Pacific region. Bangkok: United Nations Development Programme; 2012.

Wirtz AL, Kirey A, Peryskina A, Houdart F, Beyrer C. Uncovering the epidemic of HIV among men who have sex with men in Central Asia. Drug Alcohol Depend. 2013;132(suppl 1):S17–24.

Wirtz AL, Zelaya CE, Peryshkina A, Latkin C, Mogilnyi V, Galai N, et al. Social and structural risks for HIV among migrant and immigrant men who have sex with men in Moscow, Russia: implications for prevention. AIDS Care. 2014;26(3):387–95.

Wong FY, Huang ZJ, He N, Smith BD, Ding Y, Fu C, Young D. HIV risks among gay- and non-gay-identified migrant money boys in Shanghai, China. AIDS Care. 2008;20(2):170–80.

Xiao Z, Li X, Liu Y, Li S, Jiang S. Sexual communication and condom use among Chinese men who have sex with men in Beijing. Psychol Health Med. 2013;18(1):98–106.

Yoshikawa H, Wilson PA, Chae DH, Cheng JF. Do family and friendship networks protect against the influence of discrimination on mental health and HIV risk among Asian and Pacific Islander gay men? AIDS Educ Prev. 2004;16(1):84–100.

Yu L, Jiang C, Na J, Li N, Diao W, Gu Y, et al. Elevated 12-month and lifetime prevalence and comorbidity rates of mood, anxiety, and alcohol use disorders in Chinese men who have sex with men. PLoS One. 2013;8(4):e50762.

Appendix 1: Resources for LGBTQ Patients

Introduction

We have compiled information for you to pass on to your patients and have arranged them in the following sections:

1. Finding LGBT-friendly health care providers and community centers
2. Coming out to your health care provider
3. What to discuss with your health care provider
4. Trans health resources
5. Better sex, better relationships
6. Sexually transmitted infections
7. Alcohol and other drugs
8. Healthy minds and helplines
9. Exercise, nutrition, and body image
10. Family and parenting

Please feel free to photocopy and distribute this information, keeping in mind that some of the resources may not be appropriate for all audiences.

1. **Finding LGBT-friendly health care providers and community centers**
   - **Directory of LGBT-friendly providers – Gay and Lesbian Medical Association: Health Professionals Advancing LGBTQ Equality** (glma.org – navigate through Resources > For Patients > Find a Provider)

   - **Directory of LGBT Community Centers – Center Link: The Community of LGBT Centers** (https://www.lgbtcenters.org/)
   - **Directory of Transgender Specialists – World Professional Association for Transgender Health** (https://www.wpath.org/provider/search)

2. **Coming out to your health care provider**
   The Human Rights Campaign has created the following tips for coming out to your health care provider (hrc.org/resources/entry/coming-out-to-your-doctor):
   - **Tips for Finding and Being Open with Health Care Providers**
     - Ask for referrals. Ask friends or local LGBT centers for the names of LGBT-friendly health care providers. You can also check GLMA's Health Care Provider Directory.
     - Inquire by phone. When you call to make an appointment, ask if the practice has any LGBT patients. If you're nervous about asking, remember you don't have to give your name during that initial call.
     - Bring a friend. If you're uneasy about being open with your health care provider, consider asking a trusted friend to come with you.
     - Bring it up when you feel most comfortable. Ask your doctor for a few minutes to chat while you're still fully

J. R. Lehman et al. (eds.), *The Equal Curriculum*, https://doi.org/10.1007/978-3-030-24025-7

clothed – maybe even before you're in the exam room.

– Know what to ask. Learn about the specific health care issues facing LGBT people.

Also see the Fenway Health 'Do Ask, Do Tell': Guide to Talking to Your Health Care Provider About Being LGBT:

(lgbthealtheducation.org/wp-content/uploads/COM13-067_LGBTHAWbrochure_v4.pdf)

...as well as the Human Rights Campaign Guide to Coming Out:

(hrc.org/resources/entry/resource-guide-to-coming-out)

3. **What to discuss with your health care provider**

GLMA: Health Professionals Advancing LGBTQ Equality has put together a 'top 10 health issues' series to help guide LGBT primary care (Table A.1). See the GLMA website for more information on each topic (glma.org – navigate through Resources > For Patients > Top 10 Health Issues):

For further information on LGBT health care planning, check out the resources below:

- **Centers for Disease Control and Prevention - LGBT Health Information** (cdc.gov/lgbthealth)

  The CDC provides information on topics including STDs, substance abuse, mental health, suicide, and cancer.

- **National Women's Health Information Center, Lesbian and Bisexual Health Facts** (womenshealth.gov/publications/our-publications/fact-sheet/lesbian-bisexual-health.html)

  Information on lesbian and bisexual women's health.

- **Human Rights Campaign - Health and Aging Resources** (hrc.org/resources/category/health-and-aging)

  Information on health care proxies, advance directives, visitation, and other topics.

- **National Resource Center on LGBT Aging** (lgbtagingcenter.org/resources/index.cfm)

Table A.1 Summary of topics that LGBT patients should discuss with their health care providers

10 Things Gay Men Should Discuss	10 Things Lesbians Should Discuss
1. Come Out to your Health Care Provider	1. Breast Cancer
2. HIV/AIDS, Safe Sex	2. Depression/Anxiety
3. Hepatitis Immunization and Screening	3. Heart Health
4. Fitness (Diet and Exercise)	4. Gynecological Cancer
5. Substance Use/Alcohol	5. Fitness
6. Depression/Anxiety	6. Tobacco
7. STDs	7. Alcohol
8. Prostate, Testicular, and Colon Cancer	8. Substance Use
9. Tobacco	9. Intimate Partner Violence
10. HPV (virus that causes warts and can lead to anal cancer)	10. Sexual Health
10 Things Bisexual Persons Should Discuss	10 Things Transgender Persons Should Discuss
1. Come Out to your Health Care Provider	1. Access to Health Care
2. HIV/AIDS, Safe Sex	2. Health History
3. Hepatitis Immunization and Screening	3. Hormones
4. Fitness (Diet and Exercise)	4. Cardiovascular Health
5. Substance Use/Alcohol	5. Cancer
6. Depression/Anxiety	6. STDs and Safe Sex
7. STDs	7. Alcohol and tobacco
8. Prostate, Testicular, Breast, Cervical and Colon Cancer	8. Depression
9. Tobacco	9. Injectable Silicone
10. HPV (virus that causes warts and can lead to anal cancer)	10. Fitness (Diet & Exercise)

LGBT-specific health information related to aging.

- **Lambda Legal - Tools for Protecting Your Health Care Wishes** (lambdalegal.org/sites/default/files/ttp_your-health-care-wishes.pdf)

    LGBT-specific medicolegal considerations.

4. **Trans health resources**
- **Human Rights Campaign - Transgender Resources** (hrc.org/resources/category/transgender)

    Information on transgender visibility, inclusion, protection, and marriage.
- **Learning Trans** (learningtrans.org & vimeo.com/groups/learningtrans)

    Community-produced resources in transgender topics.
- **I Am: Trans People Speak** (transpeople-speak.org)

    This is a resource where people share transgender-related stories.
- **GLAAD - Transgender Resources** (glaad.org/transgender/resources)

    A comprehensive list of transgender resources, including tips for allies.
- **UCSF Center of Excellence for Transgender Health** (transhealth.ucsf.edu)

    Information on transgender health, primary care, STDs, cultural competency, and mental health.
- **American Medical Student Association - Transgender Health Resources** (amsa.org/AMSA/Homepage/About/Committees/GenderandSexuality/TransgenderHealthCare.aspx)

    Information on transgender language, health disparities, primary care, hormones, mental health, and surgery.
- **Canadian Professional Association for Transgender Health** (cpath.ca/resources/guidelines)

    Information on Canadian and international transgender care guidelines.

- **World Professional Association for Transgender Health** (wpath.org)

    Information on global transgender topics.

5. **Better sex, better relationships**
- **Go Ask Alice – Sexual Health and Relationships** (goaskalice.columbia.edu/sexual-and-reproductive-health & goaskalice.columbia.edu/relationships)

    This Columbia University Health Q&A provides information on relationships, erotica & pornography, fetishes & philias, kissing, masturbation, orgasms, toys, STIs, and other sexual topics.
- **ACON – Information on Lesbian Sex and Health/Information on Gay Sex and Health** (acon.org.au/womens-health/sex-and-sexual-wellbeing & acon.org.au/mens-health/sex-and-sexual-wellbeing)

    This Australian health promotion organization provides comprehensive information on gay men and women's sexual wellbeing, including relationships, sex, and STIs.
- **Autostraddle – Lesbian Safe Sex 101** (autostraddle.com/safe-sex-for-lesbians-45382)

    A guide to lesbian safe sex.
- **Gay Men's Health Services – Health & Wellness** (gaymenshealth.org/health-wellness)

    This resource provides information on anal health, kink, domestic violence, and more.
- **Gay Men's Health Charity – Better Sex/Sexual Problems and Solutions** (gmfa.org.uk/better-sex & gmfa.org.uk/sexual-problems-and-solutions)

    This UK organization gives up front information on sex techniques, premature ejaculation, erectile disfunction, hemorrhoids, messy sex & douching, and pain on intercourse.
- **The Healthy Bear – Guides to Douching & Butt Plugs** (thehealthybear.

com/a-guide-to-douching & thehealthy-bear.com/butt-plug-guide)

This Australian family physician provides information on douching, butt plug use, safe sex, drugs, and more.

Videos are also available at youtube.com/TheHealthyBear.

6. **Sexually transmitted infections**
   - **Centers for Disease Control and Prevention – LGBT Health, STDs & HIV Information** (cdc.gov/lgbthealth cdc.gov/hiv/risk/gender)

     Information about STDs and HIV/AIDS among gay and bisexual men, transgender people, and women.
   - **Gay Men's Health Services – STD Information & Positive Living** (gaymenshealth.org)

     Information on HIV/AIDS, chlamydia, warts, gonorrhea, viral hepatits, herpes, shigella, and syphilis.
   - **The Lesbian & Gay Foundation UK** (lgf.org.uk & lgf.org.uk/get-support/for-men/sexual-health-quickies)

     Information and videos on sexual health & safe sex, HIV/AIDS, cruising, saunas, and STDs.

     Sexual Health Quickies for men and women are available here: youtube.com/lgfonline
   - **The Healthy Bear – Gay Sexual Health Screening & HIV FAQ** (thehealthybear.com/gay-sexual-health-screening & thehealthybear.com/HIV-faq)

     This Australian family physician provides information on sexual health screening, HIV/AIDS, and more.

     Videos are available here: youtube.com/TheHealthyBear
   - **Gay Men's Health Charity – HIV & Sexual Health** (gmfa.org.uk/hiv-aids-and-sexual-health)

     Information on HIV/AIDS, STIs, and risky sex.
   - **The Body: The Complete HIV/AIDS Resource** (thebody.com)

     Comprehensive information about HIV testing, new diagnoses, medications, and more.

   - **AIDS.gov – the Basics of HIV/AIDS** (aids.gov/hiv-aids-basic)

     US Department of Health information about HIV/AIDS, prevention, diagnoses, and staying healthy.
   - **The Well Project** (thewellproject.org/hiv-information)

     Information about HIV for women.
   - **AIDS Map – Patient Resources** (aidsmap.com/resources)

     A UK-based organization that provides comprehensive information and tools for living with HIV.
   - **AVERT – HIV Prevention for Gay & Bisexual Men and Lesbian & Bisexual Women** (avert.org/sexuality-and-safer-sex.htm)

     A UK-based organization that provides information on HIV and safer sex for gay men and women.
   - **We All Test – STD Testing Reminders** (wealltest.com/test)

     Free online STD testing reminders.

7. **Alcohol and other drugs**
   - **Go Ask Alice – Drugs & Alcohol Information** (goaskalice.columbia.edu/alcohol-other-drugs)

     This Columbia University Health Q&A provides information on alcohol, caffeine & energy boosters, cigarettes & other nicotine, inhalants, LSD & other hallucinogens, marijuana & other cannabis, prescription & over-the-counter drugs, and sedatives & other depressants.
   - **Gay Men's Health Services – Drugs & Alcohol Information** (gaymenshealth.org/drug-alcohol-information)

     Information on alcohol, cocaine, ecstasy, GHB, methamphetamine, and ketamine.
   - **Gay Men's Health Charity – Drugs & Alcohol Information** (gmfa.org.uk/alcohol-and-drugs)

     This UK-based organization provides information on alcohol, crystal meth, GHB, mephedrone, ketamine, cocaine, MDMA/ecstasy, cannabis, poppers, heroin & opiates, crack, and tobacco.

- **Pride Institute Treatment Center** (pride-institute.com/about)

  Support and evidence-based treatment for LGBT people suffering from substance abuse and mental ill health.
- **SmokeFree.gov** (smokefree.gov)

  National resource to help quit smoking.
- **Substance Abuse & Mental Health Services Administration – Treatment Finder** (findtreatment.samhsa.gov)

  Find a local substance abuse treatment center.

8. **Healthy minds and helplines**
   - **Go Ask Alice – Emotional Health** (goaskalice.columbia.edu/emotional-health)

     This Columbia University Health Q&A provides information on depression, counseling, grief & loss, medications, obsessive & compulsive behavior, stress & anxiety, and suicide.
   - **GLBT National Help Center – GLBT National Hotline, Youth Talkline, and Peer Support Chat** (glnh.org)

     Free and confidential peer counseling, information, and resources to LGBT callers throughout the US. The GLBT national hotline is 1-888-843-4564. The youth talkline for callers under 26 can be reached at 1-800-246-7743. Online peer support instant messaging is also available.
   - **Fenway Health GLBT Helpline** (fenwayhealth.org/site/PageServer?pagename=FCHC_srv_services_tollfree)

     Free and confidential source of information, referrals, and support on coming out, HIV/AIDS, safer sex and relationships, and locating GLBT groups in the caller's local area. Call 1-888-340-4528, Monday through Friday, 6 pm–11 pm, Eastern Time. Webchat is also available.
   - **The Trevor Project – Youth Lifeline** (thetrevorproject.org)

     Crisis intervention and suicide prevention services for LGBT youth aged 13–24. Call 1-866-488-7386.

- **It Gets Better Project** (itgetsbetter.org)

  Testimonials from LGBT people around the world to support a better future.
- **Gay-Straight Alliance Network** (gsanetwork.org)

  National youth organization offering safe environments, peer support, leadership development, and training.
- **I'm From Driftwood** (imfromdriftwood.com)

  Inspiring first-person accounts of being LGBT in America.
- **American Psychological Association – Sexual Orientation Help Center** (apa.org/helpcenter/sexual-orientation.aspx)

  Information about sexual orientation, gender identity/expression, same-sex marriage, and more.
- **The Network/La Red – Partner Abuse Hotline & Safehome** (tnlr.org/get-support/hotline)

  This hotline provides emotional support, information, and safety planning for LGBT who are being abused or have been abused by a partner. Call 617-742-4911 (or call SafeLink toll-free at 1-877-785-2020 and asked to be transferred to the Network/La Red).
- **Anti-Violence Project – Violence Hotline** (avp.org/get-help/call-our-hotline)

  Free bilingual English/Spanish hotline that offers support to LGBT victims and survivors of violence. Call 212-714-1141.
- **National Coalition of Anti-Violence Programs** (ncavp.org/issues/default.aspx)

  Information for LGBT individuals who suffered hate-motivated/partner violence, rape, or sexual assault.
- **Substance Abuse & Mental Health Services Administration – Treatment Finder** (findtreatment.samhsa.gov)

  Find a local mental health treatment center.

9. **Exercise, nutrition, and body image**
   - **Go Ask Alice – Columbia University Health Q&A** (goaskalice.columbia.edu/nutrition-physical-activity)

Information on body image, eating disorders, fitness, food choices, nutrition, and weight gain/loss.

- **Fenway Institute – Take Charge! Series** (fenwayhealth.org/site/PageServer? pagename=FCHC_res_Information Documents)

  Guides to getting active, healthy eating, sleep habits, and more.

- **Gay Men's Health Services – Family Health Centers of San Diego** (gaymenshealth.org/health-wellness)

  Information on body image, fitness, and more.

- **US Department of Agriculture, Choose My Plate** (choosemyplate.gov)

  Information about nutrition, weight management, and physical activity.

10. **Family and parenting**

- **Human Rights Campaign – Parenting** (hrc.org/issues/parenting)

  Information on adoption, assisted reproduction, foster parenting, and schools for LGBT families.

- **PFLAG – Parents, Families, Friends, and Allies United with LGBT People** (pflag.org)

  The largest family and ally organization devoted to advancing equality and societal acceptance of LGBT people.

- **Family Acceptance Project** (familyproject.sfsu.edu/publications)

  Publications, tools, and peer-reviewed research aimed to promote LGBT health in the context of families.

Appendix 2: National Support Organizations

Introduction

This appendix is a resource to familiarize yourself as a health professional to some prominent LGBTQ support organizations. You may use this chapter as a springboard to better understand your LGBTQ patients and learn how you as a professional can encourage a network of social support. Some organizations have resources primarily for patients, others for providers, and some for both. The sections are as follows:

1. General
2. Transgender
3. People of Color
4. Youth and Young Adults

1. **General**
   - **Fenway Institute/National LGBT Education Center** (http://www.lgbthealtheducation.org/publications/lgbt-health-resources/)

     The Fenway Institute is an interdisciplinary center for research, training, education, and policy development, focusing on national and international health issues. For physicians, the National LGBT Education Center hosts live and recorded webinars on topics in LGBT health and counseling.
   - **GLMA: Health Professionals Advancing LGBTQ Equality** (http://glma.org/)

     GLMA's mission is to ensure equality in health care for lesbian, gay, bisexual and transgender individuals and health care providers. They host a comprehensive provider directory of LGBT-friendly and competent providers which can be found online. Online you can also find a cultural competency webinar series in four parts.
   - **GLAAD** (http://www.glaad.org/)

     The Gay & Lesbian Alliance Against Defamation (GLAAD) is dedicated to promoting and ensuring fair, accurate and inclusive representation of people and events in the media as a means of eliminating homophobia and discrimination based on gender identity and sexual orientation.
   - **GLSEN** (http://www.glsen.org/)

     The Gay, Lesbian & Straight Education Network strives to assure that each member of every school community is valued and respected regardless of sexual orientation or gender identity/expression.
   - **Human Rights Campaign** (http://www. hrc.org/)

     Founded in 1980, the Human Rights Campaign advocates on behalf of GLBT Americans, mobilizes grassroots actions in diverse communities, invests strategically to elect fair-minded individuals to office and educates the public about GLBT issues. Their Health Care Equality Index (HEI) ranks health care organizations on their policies and practices for both patients and employees.
   - **Immigration Equality** (http://www.immigrationequality.org/)

     Immigration Equality is a national organization that works to end discrimination

J. R. Lehman et al. (eds.), *The Equal Curriculum*, https://doi.org/10.1007/978-3-030-24025-7

in U.S. immigration law, to reduce the negative impact of that law on the lives of lesbian, gay, bisexual, transgender and HIV-positive people, and to help obtain asylum for those persecuted in their home country based on their sexual orientation, transgender identity or HIV-status.

- **Lambda Legal** (http://www.lambdalegal. org/)

  Lambda Legal is a national organization committed to achieving full recognition of the civil rights of lesbians, gay men, bisexuals, transgender individuals and those with HIV through impact litigation, education and public policy work.

- **Mautner Project** (https://whitman-walker. thankyou4caring.org/page.aspx?pid=625)

  The Mautner Project improves the health of lesbian, bisexual, and transgender women through advocacy, education, research, and direct service. They offer free e-mail and phone support for LBT women with practical support and information provided by trained volunteers.

- **National Center for Lesbian Rights** (http://www.nclrights.org/)

  The National Center for Lesbian Rights is a national legal organization committed to advancing the civil and human rights of lesbian, gay, bisexual, and transgender people and their families through litigation, public policy advocacy, and public education.

- **National LGBT Cancer Network** (http:// www.cancer-network.org/)

  The National LGBT Cancer Network works to improve the lives of LGBT cancer survivors and those at risk. You can find helpful resources for patients suffering or recovering from cancer including support groups nationwide.

- **National Resource Center on LGBT Aging** (http://lgbtagingcenter.org/)

  The National Resource Center on LGBT Aging is a technical assistance resource center aimed at improving the

quality of services and supports offere to lesbian, gay, bisexual and transgende (LGBT) older adults. The Center pro vides training, technical assistance an educational resources to aging providers LGBT organizations and LGBT olde adults.

- **Out & Equal Workplace Advocate** (http://www.outandequal.org/)

  Out & Equal Workplace Advocates edu cates and empowers organizations, huma resources professionals, employee resourc groups, and individual employees throug programs and services that result in equa policies, opportunities, practices, and ben efits in the workplace regardless of sexua orientation, gender identity, expression, c characteristics.

- **PFLAG** (http://www.pflag.org/)

  PFLAG promotes the health and wel being of gay, lesbian, bisexual and trans gender persons, their families and friend through support, education, and advocacy

- **Servicemembers Legal Defense Networ** (http://www.sldn.org/)

  SLDN is a national, non-profit legal se vices, watchdog and policy organizatio dedicated to ending discrimination an harassment of LGBTQ servicemembers.

- **Soulforce** (http://www.soulforce.org/)

  The purpose of Soulforce is freedom fc lesbian, gay, bisexual, and transgende people from religious and political oppre sion through the practice of nonviolen resistance. Their educational materials an programming highlight important way religion, politics and civil rights can have deep-seated impact on the health of patien and community.

2. **Transgender**

- **National Center for Transgende Equality** (http://www.transequality.org/)

  The National Center for Transgende Equality (NCTE) is a 501(c)3 social justic organization dedicated to advancing th equality of transgender people throug advocacy, collaboration and empowerment.

- **Center of Excellence for Transgender Health** (http://transhealth.ucsf.edu/)

    Based at the University of San Francisco, the Center provides services to health care providers, their patients, researchers and community organizers. An excellent resource for guidelines, reports, literature, and training materials. The organization is known for its Guidelines for the Primary and Gender-Affirming Care of Transgender and Gender Nonbinary People (http://transhealth.ucsf.edu/trans?page=protocol-00-00).

- **World Professional Association for Transgender Health** (http://www.wpath.org/)

    WPATH provides a wealth of information on global transgender topics in health. WPATH publishes the *International Journal on Transgenderism*, has an extensive directory of resources, and will connect patients with appropriate providers. They also publish the world's leading Standards of Care for gender-affirming treatment (https://www.wpath.org/publications/soc).

3. **People of Color**
    - **Black AIDS Institute** (http://www.black-aids.org/)

        The Black AIDS Institute is the first Black HIV/AIDS policy center dedicated to reducing HIV/AIDS health disparities by mobilizing Black institutions and individuals in efforts to confront the epidemic in their communities.

    - **The Center for Black Equity** (http://centerforblackequity.org/)

        The mission of The Center for Black Equity is to promote a multinational LGBT network dedicated to improving health and wellness opportunities, economic empowerment, and equal rights while promoting individual and collective work, responsibility, and self-determination.

- **National AIDS Education & Services for Minorities** (http://www.naesmonline.org/)

    National AIDS Education & Services for Minorities was created in an effort to counteract the increasing spread of HIV/AIDS in communities of color.

- **National Black Justice Coalition** (http://www.nbjcoalition.org/)

    The National Black Justice Coalition is a civil rights organization dedicated to empowering Black same-gender-loving, lesbian, gay, bisexual, and transgendered people. The Coalition works with our communities and our allies for social justice, equality, and an end to racism and homophobia.

- **National Minority AIDS Council** (http://www.nmac.org/)

    The National Minority AIDS Council has helped develop leadership in communities of color to address the challenges of HIV/AIDS since 1987.

- **NorthEast Two-Spirit Society** (http://www.ne2ss.org/)

    NE2SS works to increase the visibility of the two-spirit community and to provide social, traditional and recreational opportunities that are culturally appropriate to the two-spirit community. Based in New York City, the also provide national resources for Two-Spirit and LGBT American Indians.

4. **Youth and Young Adults**
    - **Campus Pride** (https://www.campuspride.org/)

        Campus Pride is the leading national nonprofit 501(c)(3) organization for student leaders and campus groups working to create a safer college environment for LGBT students.

    - **Children of Lesbians & Gays Everywhere** (http://www.colage.org/)

        COLAGE is a national movement of children, youth, and adults with one or more lesbian, gay, bisexual, transgender and/or queer (LGBTQ) parents. They work to bring together individuals with shared experiences to create a supportive community online. National retreats are also held around the country for LGBTQ families to attend.

- **Family Acceptance Project** (http://familyproject.sfsu.edu/)

  The Family Acceptance Project is a research, intervention, education and policy initiative that works to prevent health and mental health risks for lesbian, gay, bisexual and transgender (LGBT) children and youth, including suicide, homelessness and HIV in the context of their families. They have developed an assessment tool called the FAPrisk Screener for Assessing Family Rejection & Related Health Risks in LGBT Youth to screen for risk of depression, suicide, substance abuse, and STDs (http://familyproject.sfsu.edu/assessment). The organization will give providers training on using the screening instrument and recommendations on further counseling families.

- **Point Foundation** (http://www.pointfoundation.org/)

  The Point Foundation provides financial support, leadership training, mentoring and hope to meritorious students who are marginalized due to sexual orientation, gender identity and/or gender expression.

- **The Trevor Project (1-866-488-7386)** (http://www.thetrevorproject.org/)

  The Trevor Project operates the only nationwide, around-the-clock suicide prevention helpline for gay and questioning youth.

Appendix 3: Glossary

Active disclosure	Directly disclosing one's sexual orientation or gender identity
AIDS-related complex	A variety of clinical manifestations grouped under CDC category B conditions that occur in the months to years prior to the onset of major opportunistic infections in AIDS
Allies	Persons who are supportive of the struggles of sexual and gender minorities
Anatomic inventory	The current anatomy of the patient; the assessment of what organs the patient has or does not have
Anatomic sex	The sum of the structures that differentiate male from female
Asexual	Without sexual feelings or associations
Basic gender identity	A stage between the age of 2 to 3 years where most children begin to label themselves as boys or girls
Biopsychosocial model	A clinical paradigm incorporating biological, psychological, and social factors as highly interdependent determinants of mental health and illness
Bisexual	People who are attracted to people of the opposite sex or gender in addition to people of the same sex or gender
Bullying	The use of force, threat, or coercion to abuse, intimidate, or aggressively dominate others
Cisgender	Gender identity aligns with the sex assigned at birth; people who do not self-identify as transgender or gender-nonconforming
Clinical latency	A period of time during HIV infection when there are no clinical symptoms
Coming out	The process of disclosing one's sexual orientation and/or gender identity to others
Continuum of care	A system that guides and tracks patients over time through a comprehensive array of health services spanning all levels and intensity of care
Conversion therapy	Methods that attempt to cure individuals from same-sex attractions and/or behaviors, which in some historical cases involved electroshock therapy, genital mutilation, and even castration
Cross-dressers	People who dress as members of the opposite gender, occasionally or all the time
Cyber-bullying	The use of information technology to harm or harass other people in a deliberate, repeated, and hostile manner
Diathesis-stress model	A conceptualization that every person has an innate vulnerabilities (diatheses) to mental illness and that psychopathology emerges when these vulnerabilities encounter sufficient stress
Differences of sex development (DSD)	Variations in the typical path of anatomical sex development from conception to birth, ranging from minor to major
Disorders of sex development	See *differences of sex development*
Distal stressors	External stimuli (objective stimuli) that are characteristics of an individual's social environment
Elite controllers	Persons infected with HIV who maintain undetectable viral loads in the absence of treatment

© Springer Nature Switzerland AG 2020
J. R. Lehman et al. (eds.), *The Equal Curriculum*, https://doi.org/10.1007/978-3-030-24025-7

Family choice	One's desire to live in the company of partners, spouses, friends, biological family, and legal family that one has selected
Female-to-male (FtM)	Transgender person who has a sex assigned at birth of female and gender identity of male
Formication	A tactile hallucination of ants crawling one's skin
Founder virus	A single viral variant that accounts for the initial infection in the majority of incident HIV-1 infections
Gay	A sexual orientation of a man who identifies primary romantic feelings, sexual attractions, and/or intimate interactions toward people of the same sex or gender (may also be adopted by female or feminine-identifying persons)
Gay-related immunodeficiency (GRID)	(Defunct) syndromic early association of the AIDS illness with male-to-male sex
Gender affirmation surgery	Complex surgical procedures sometimes performed for the treatment of gender dysphoria; also called sex reassignment surgery, gender confirmation surgery, or gender reassignment surgery
Gender assigned at birth	A label assigned at birth based on the aggregate of sex characteristics, usually using a binary framework of male or female, assuming an infant's future gender identity
Gender discordance	A discrepancy between anatomical sex and gender identity
Gender dysphoria	Clinically significant distress or impairment in social, occupational, or other areas of function that occurs when the gender with which a person identifies does not match the sex that was assigned at birth
Gender expression	Outward manifestation of one's self-identified gender, including personal characteristics, mannerisms, choice of clothing, hairstyle, and specific behaviors
Gender identity	Self-defined and subjective internal experience of one's own gender
Gender identity disorder (GID)	An older term in the DSM that has been replaced by *gender dysphoria*
Gender incongruence	See *gender discordance*
Gender nonconformity	Gender identity, expression, or behavior that falls outside of culturally defined norms associated with a specific gender
Gender role	Role a person plays or is expected to play within a specific sociocultural framework based on gender
Gender variance	See *gender noncomformity*
Gender-affirming hormone therapy	Pharmacological alteration of the secondary sex characteristics of the patient's assigned or natal sex, replacing endogenous sex hormones matching the identified gender
Genderqueer	Neither male nor female but rather between, beyond, or some combination of genders
Hate crime	An illegal transgression in which the motivation is governed by intentional prejudice against the group
Health disparities	Differences in the overall rate of disease incidence, prevalence, morbidity, mortality or survival rates in a population as compared to another population; differences in health determinants between populations, such as income, smoking, and obesity or differences in access to health care and differences in quality of care received
Heteronormativity	A prevalent cultural and sociopolitical ideology that normalizes heterosexuality and male/female and masculine/feminine binaries
Heterosexism	A system of attitudes, bias, and discrimination favoring opposite-sex sexuality and relationships
Heterosexual	Literally, "different sex," referring opposite-sex or opposite-gender attraction; someone who experiences romantic feelings, sexual attractions, and/or intimate interactions toward people of the opposite sex or gender
Heterosexual assumption	The belief and practice that everyone is and should by default be treated as heterosexual until there is an indication otherwise